W0091151

Ecopoiesis

By the same author

Poiesis
The Language of Psychology
and the Speech of the Soul
Stephen K. Levine
ISBN 978 1 85302 488 7
eISBN 978 0 85700 074 3

Foundations of Expressive
Arts Therapy
Theoretical and Clinical Perspectives
Edited by Stephen K. Levine and Ellen G. Levine
ISBN 978 1 85302 463 4
eISBN 978 1 84642 185 3

Principles and Practice of
Expressive Arts Therapy
Toward a Therapeutic Aesthetics
Paolo Knill, Ellen G. Levine,
and Stephen K. Levine
ISBN 978 1 84310 039 3
eISBN 978 1 84642 032 0

Trauma, Tragedy, Therapy
The Arts and Human Suffering
Stephen K. Levine
ISBN 978 1 84310 512 1
eISBN 978 0 85700 193 1

Art in Action
Expressive Arts Therapy and Social Change
Ellen G. Levine and Stephen K. Levine
Foreword by Michelle LeBaron
ISBN 978 1 84905 820 9
eISBN 978 0 85700 270 9

New Developments in Expressive Arts
The Play of Poiesis
Edited by Ellen G. Levine and Stephen K. Levine
ISBN 978 1 78592 247 3
eISBN 978 1 78450 532 5

Philosophy of Expressive Arts Therapy
Poiesis and the Therapeutic Imagination
Stephen K. Levine
Foreword by Catherine Hyland Moon
ISBN 978 1 78775 005 0
eISBN 978 1 78775 006 7

Related titles

Nature-Based Expressive Arts Therapy
Integrating the Expressive
Arts and Ecotherapy
Sally Atkins and Melia Snyder
Forewords by Corrine Glesne
and Per Espen Stoknes
ISBN 978 1 78592 726 3
eISBN 978 1 78450 380 2

Emotional Resiliency in the
Era of Climate Change
A Clinician's Guide
Leslie Davenport
Foreword by Lise Van Susteren, M.D.
ISBN 978 1 78592 719 5
eISBN 978 1 78450 328 4

An Expressive Arts Approach
to Healing Loss and Grief
Working Across the Spectrum of Loss
with Individuals and Communities
Irene Renzenbrink
Foreword by Stephen K. Levine
ISBN 978 1 78775 278 8
eISBN 978 1 78775 279 5

ECOPOIESIS

A New Perspective for the Expressive and Creative Arts Therapies in the 21st Century

EDITED BY

Stephen K. Levine
and Alexander Kopytin

Foreword by Shaun McNiff

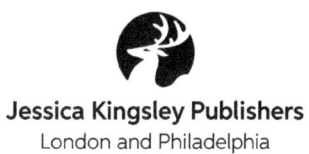

Jessica Kingsley Publishers
London and Philadelphia

First published in Great Britain in 2022 by Jessica Kingsley Publishers
An Hachette Company

1

Copyright © Stephen K. Levine and Alexander Kopytin 2022

All rights reserved. No part of this publication may be reproduced, stored
in a retrieval system, or transmitted, in any form or by any means without
the prior written permission of the publisher, nor be otherwise circulated
in any form of binding or cover other than that in which it is published and
without a similar condition being imposed on the subsequent purchaser.

A CIP catalogue record for this title is available from the
British Library and the Library of Congress

ISBN 978 1 78775 993 0
eISBN 978 1 78775 994 7

Printed and bound in Great Britain by CPI Group Ltd

Jessica Kingsley Publishers' policy is to use papers that are natural,
renewable and recyclable products and made from wood grown in sustainable forests. The logging and manufacturing processes are expected
to conform to the environmental regulations of the country of origin.

Jessica Kingsley Publishers
Carmelite House,
50 Victoria Embankment,
London, EC4Y 0DZ, UK

www.jkp.com

Contents

Part 2: Integrating Ecological and Sustainable Development Perspectives in Expressive/Creative Arts Therapies Practice with Individuals, Groups, and Communities

Part 3: Sustainable Development and Eco-Human Perspectives in the Contemporary Arts

Foreword: Artistic Expression as a Force of Nature

SHAUN MCNIFF

Alexander Kopytin and Stephen K. Levine have each greatly enhanced international understanding of the role that art can play in therapy as editors of many books and journals, and we now benefit from their new partnership to advance a deeper understanding of the integral relationship of art and nature. Their cooperation results in an ever-expanding international community of authors who offer a broad spectrum of timely ideas and methods to *Ecopoiesis: A New Perspective for the Expressive and Creative Arts Therapies in the 21st Century*.

I am privileged to have over 50 years of experience in engaging people from various regions of the world in studio communities where we explore how personal artistic expression can further well-being. This practical experience has reinforced my belief that the creative process can be best understood as an ecosystem of forces both inside and outside individual persons and inseparable from the whole of nature. The art that we make and bring forth from our distinct and individual interactions with life fulfills urges for expression that have always been fundamental to human presence on earth.

Throughout history there is consistent art evidence (McNiff, 2022) demonstrating how art heals by transmuting the most difficult circumstances into affirmations of life while also infusing persons and communities with creative energy. Nature offers what I consider to be the most convincing model, on both macro and micro levels, for understanding the creative process and how it heals in correspondence with the transformative dynamics of the physical world (McNiff, 2021).

The relationship between nature and well-being was fundamental to the first comprehensive public mental health programs in the United States during the mid-19th century. The large Massachusetts state hospital where I began my career was founded during this era, emphasizing humane and "moral treatment" based on compassion for all sectors of society, led by Dorothea Dix (1802–1887) and Thomas Story Kirkbride (1809–1883). The latter's "aesthetic" approach to care guided the ambitious creation of *asylum* structures in natural environments where contact with the earth was considered essential to well-being—therapeutic settings expressing a conviction that mental health afflictions were connected to alienation from life-sustaining natural elements. The perspective on asylums, originally suggesting sanctuary, haven, and regeneration, turned negative over the years to suggest institutions that enclose and separate unfit people from society.

Although this ambitious and nationally significant effort in America was not sustained as the country grew, and mental health practices progressively morphed into the scientized and technical methods of today, the fundamental principles survive, and they are being renewed as we once again appreciate how health is directly tied to mutual relations with all of life. The vision, like so many other universal human conditions, unfashionable to emphasize today, is intact. We study the past and worldwide traditions, such as Indigenous cosmologies and their reciprocal relationships with nature, East Asia's harmony with the Tao, and Hildegard of Bingen's (1098–1179) approach to health as *viriditas* (greening), not to "appropriate" but to understand processes and a common humanity that transcend ourselves and our ideologies, as nature does. Thus we are also able to further appreciate how what we do in our unique ways in a particular time, place, and community relates to continuous world experience and nature.

I was fortunate to work together with Maxwell Jones (1907–1990) whose leadership in social psychiatry and the development of the therapeutic community movement influenced my focus on therapeutic communities of art. His natural inclinations toward egalitarian and interdependent therapeutic environments ultimately led to conceiving these initiatives as manifestations of ecological principles consistent "with the biological systems found in nature" (Jones, 1982, p.155). I have similarly experienced all sectors of my practice as congruent with inherent processes of nature. Experience with art healing has returned me to formative college classes with Thomas Berry in the 1960s and affirmed the sacred and wondrous vision of the earth that he articulates through his studies of world cultures (1988, 1999).

It appears from the enduring transcultural definition of illness as a loss of soul, that it is the *nature* of soul to be lost in order to be restored, again in keeping with nature's cyclic patterns. And within the human community, artistic expression not only renews the lost soul but comes into existence and shapes itself across the millennia through participation in the process.

I ask why this proven art medicine is not more widely understood and universally accessible as a form of public health. Artistic expression is hindered by many human factors, many of which we inflict on ourselves in keeping with Shakespeare's Hamlet saying, "there is nothing either good or bad, but thinking makes it so" (Act 2, Scene 2). Our gift of thought has many shadows, especially in relation to spontaneous communication. Where we humans are prone to over-thinking, we can learn so much from animal life, as James Hillman did, about instinctive, attentive, and precise action. Yet the immobilizing features of self-judgment, doubt, and emotional vulnerability also reveal how we are often alienated from the intelligences of nature within us. Our wounds and afflictions are potential guides to renewal.

Society and its concepts of artistic value are another major restraining power. The most pervasive obstacles are stereotypic notions of so-called talent and the accompanying assumptions about who can and cannot participate in artistic expression. These restrictions in my experience are transcultural. In striving to help others access the universal and life-enhancing medicines of art, I have found it to be most helpful and convincing to base everything we do on the fundamental and empirical processes of the physical world. I introduce artistic expression as a force of nature, as accessible as breath (McNiff, 2015, 2021). To relax the mind and conceptual controls which reliably arrest fluidity, we approach all forms of artistic expression through the basis of bodily movement. I have described how the arbitrary separation of art forms and sensory intelligences is a construction of academic and professional institutions that goes against the grain of nature, where the constituent elements cooperate as necessary contributors to the creation, sustenance, and imagination of life (McNiff, 2020). The same applies to fixed methods of therapeutic practice and research which follow pre-ordained and often linear procedures, steps, or stages. In contrast, I have found that what might be described as radical simplicity and lightening the grip on the controls reliably opens us to the depths and infinite variations of creative expression—the simpler the deeper.

For example, with painting, I say if you can move, you can paint. Just make a gesture, repeat it, breathe with it and allow the successive movements to shape a composition. Let your actions lead with the mind relaxed and benefitting from what appears beyond its current sphere. In my studios, we might begin with simple black markers or Conte crayons and move with them on large pieces of paper. In my experience with people worldwide, I consistently see that the sustained making of these elemental gestures reliably results in significant and endlessly unique artistic expressions. Rather than the conventional concepts of talent and skill, we focus on authentic and natural gestures, energy and feeling, individuation within a common studio purpose that supports each person in doing new and different things, taking risks with the attendant vulnerability that accompanies acting outside our usual constraints and expectations. Conceptual ideologies and systems are discouraged in contrast to simply initiating and staying with the movement process, which, like nature, is always unique in relation to the individual person's presence and action. All the senses participate in this community of creation, and the mind too, which ideally takes on a supportive, reflective, and appreciative role rather than directing the process.

For those who might say that a nature focus is a sentimental and pastoral idealization, I would reply that although this is a potential concern that I share, that characterization does not represent a complete and all-encompassing perspective on nature, which includes disturbing, dark, and often chaotic forces as well as light and exultation. A *whole art* viewpoint engages difficult places together with comfortable ones. Artistic expression has proven throughout the millennia that this mix of toxins and anti-toxins, grief and joy, fear and daring, ultimately work together and often paradoxically need each other. The healing is based in doing something life-enhancing with disturbances in both our personal lives and the world at large. Rather than splitting perceptions of the natural world between positive and negative manifestations, a deeper and more realistic position embraces the whole.

My apprehension and caution for the future of art healing in relation to nature is to be wary of the tendency to focus therapeutic methods exclusively on bucolic qualities. If, like Jackson Pollock, we view ourselves "as nature," rather than approaching the natural world as distinct and separate from human existence, then every feature of our lives is a necessary participant in ecosystems of creation.

In *Earth Angels: Engaging the Sacred in Everyday Things* (McNiff, 1995), I emphasize how sanctity can be imagined as inherent to the most ordinary and sometimes debased places and things. It is the often unattractive, troublesome, and offensive expressions that present what we might need but cannot see or resist. Creative tension is a dependable contributor to creating new life and well-being; it moves us to do what we would not otherwise do, once again like the organic processes of nature. The healing happens when I dream with what I already have, and experience it in new ways, when I see that what may at first be unwanted presents an opportunity to understand how soulful experience is connected to the quality of attention that I can bring to it. Again, these principles are not new. They are arguably inherent to human experience. As Augustine of Hippo advised, try to extend the wonder experienced in response to the natural world to ourselves and the present moment, and maybe even the things that annoy us most.

We heal ourselves by aligning with the creative and life-sustaining processes of nature as a totality, realizing that our imperfections and struggles are integral to something much larger than ourselves which requires the participation of all life forms, no matter how small or seemingly insignificant. What might appear to be isolated actions make necessary contributions to the world at large. Just like people, nature and our human-made environments need our care. As we serve and cultivate them, we experience corresponding benefits, and they continue to care for us as they always have.

As an educator of those who work with the arts in therapy, I encourage truly *open access* to every person and community interested in participating in artistic expression as a form of public health. Experienced arts therapists are needed to lead, guide, and supervise but cannot exclusively appropriate and restrict forces of nature.

References

Berry, T. (1988). *The Dream of the Earth*. San Francisco, CA: Sierra Club Books.

Berry, T. (1999). *The Great Work: Our Way into the Future*. New York, NY: Three Rivers Press.

Jones, M. (1982). *The Process of Change*. Boston, MA: Routledge & Kegan Paul.

McNiff, S. (1995). *Earth Angels: Engaging the Sacred in Everyday Things*. London and Boston, MA: Shambhala Publications.

McNiff, S. (2015). *Imagination in Action: Secrets for Unleashing Creative Expression*. London and Boston, MA: Shambhala Publications.

McNiff, S. (2020). Whole art expression: Going with the grain of nature. *POIESIS: A Journal of the Arts and Communication*, 17, 28–35.

McNiff, S. (2021). Revisioning art and nature: Toward a depth psychology of creation. *Ecopoiesis: Eco-Human Theory and Practice*. (2)1. https://en.ecopoiesis.ru/articles/article_post/ mcniff-shaun-revisioning-art-and-nature-toward-a-depth-psychology-of-creation.

McNiff, S. (2022). Art is the Evidence: Convincing Public Communication of Art-Based Research and its Outcomes. In R.W. Prior, M. Kossak, & T. Fisher (eds), *Applied Arts and Health, Education and Community: Building Bridges*, pp.16–30. Bristol/Chicago, IL: Intellect and University of Chicago Press.

Preface

STEPHEN K. LEVINE

When Alexander Kopytin first contacted me, asking me to become co-editor-in-chief of a new Russian-English journal, *Ecopoesis: Journal of High Eco-Humanitarian Technologies*, I was a bit sceptical. I had used the term "ecopoiesis" (with an "i") before to designate what I called a "poietic" approach to the environment, one that understood our relationship to the world around us as based on the concept of *poiesis*, the human ability to transform the world with a view to beauty. However, I was not sure what "eco-humanitarian" meant. If anything, the term was an indication to me of the difficulty of collaboration with someone from another culture with a different language. Alexander assured me that he did not mean humanitarian in the ordinary English sense of a process designed to help people in need. Instead, he said he was using it to indicate our essential relationship to the world around us. After an exchange of emails, Alexander suggested "eco-human." Similarly, "technologies" did not necessarily mean technical ways of being in the world. This was an important clarification, since I saw our ecological crisis as brought about primarily through the mis-application of technology.

Finally, it became clear to me. Alexander was an experienced and knowledgeable art therapist, and he wanted to use what he had gathered from his field as a way of relating to the environmental crisis that we were in. "Eco-human" to him indicated that our existence was not capable of being understood without taking into account the fact that we were worldly beings, that indeed human existence was ecological itself. "Technologies" meant the extension of the arts therapies, their basic concepts and methods, to ecological thought. "High" in the original name was a way of distinguishing an aesthetic approach from a merely technical one.

This exchange of views not only showed me that cross-cultural communication was possible, but that in our correspondence we could each deepen our own individual understanding. In the end, we agreed that the new journal would be called *Ecopoiesis: Eco-Human Theory and Practice*, a name which clarified our mutual perception of the need for a change in our relation to the world around us that was necessary in this time of environmental crisis.

Why ecopoiesis? *Poiesis* was a word that I had brought into expressive arts therapy to ground the foundations of the field in a philosophy of human existence, rather than in a psychological framework. I took it from the work of Martin Heidegger, who formulated an understanding of human existence in terms of a poietic or artistic relationship to the world, as I explain in my chapter in this book. Human beings are fundamentally eco-human, that is, we cannot separate our existence from the world around us. This has become clear in our own time, the Anthropocene, in which human activity has transformed the world. However, to exist *as* human is not to take an instrumental attitude towards the world, one in which we can impose our will on what is around us. Rather, our essential capacity is to shape the world in a way that respects its otherness. The poietic disclosure of the world shows us its inherent possibilities. Through an attitude of respect, we can shape our world to let things shine as they are, in other words, to let their beauty be seen.

What does this perspective have to do with the arts therapies? It seems to me that this is the fundamental attitude of therapeutic work, and especially the work of the arts therapies. In therapy, we do not impose our will on the other person and try to make them be who we think they should be. Rather, we take a receptive attitude to help them see their own possibilities for development. This attitude is usually called "holding," a term originally used by D.W. Winnicott to indicate the relationship of the mother to the child but also the relationship of the therapist to the client. If the child is held according to their own needs rather than those of the mother, she can have a secure basis on which to act in the world. For Winnicott, the child finds herself through play. Similarly, the holding of the therapist makes a frame within which clients can find themselves through a playful letting-be.

Moreover, Winnicott understands play as the basis of creativity. In the creative process, the artist plays with materials and helps them find a new form. Art-making may be a "shaping," but a shaping that takes place through a letting-be similar to the practice of the therapist. This letting-be is what Heidegger calls "poiesis." In the arts therapies, the fundamental attitude is a poietic one. Thus, the arts therapies seem to me to be particularly suitable as examples of an ecopoietic relationship to the world, as the chapters in this book demonstrate.

Introduction

ALEXANDER KOPYTIN

We are proud to present this book pioneering the eco-human perspective on the arts and arts therapies. During this critical period of human existence, the book is designed to be a forum for innovative ideas and practices based on the values of the environmental movement, ecopsychology and deep ecology; it aims to support human health in close connection to environmental well-being. As populations all over the world—as well as the global web of life itself—are being threatened with environmental crisis, and its wide-ranging social, psychological, and economic impact, we are challenged to search for a new platform for our professional mission incorporating the humanities, the arts and ecology. Global civilization appears to be fragile when destructive consumerist human activity brings greater entropy to the world. Yet at the same time, both humans and the global web of life are revealing their resilience and their capacity for life-affirming creative responses.

The book highlights the position of ecological, earth-based, nature-assisted arts therapies as one of such creative responses in the face of demands for sustainable development. It establishes the eco-human understanding of the arts and arts therapies and outlines their role in the process of paradigm change, the development of environmental awareness and values, and the movement towards the goal of sustainable development. It also presents "eco-human technologies" that embrace a wide spectrum of nature-assisted, ecological creative endeavors and their application in various segments of life.

The book aims to promote innovative ideas and practices based on recognizing the *ecopoietic* nature of human beings, their ability to shape the world in order to fulfill their needs and to take care of the environment with the aim of being able to experience and create beauty.

The objectives for this book are as follows:

- To present ideas and practices based on the union and co-creation of human beings and nature, in order to make a sustainable world realizable.
- To promote eco-human values, supporting human health and well-being in close connection with caring for the environment.
- To demonstrate the important role of the arts in their alliance with ecology and the human sciences for the restoration and development of constructive human relations with nature, and the promotion of environmental consciousness and sustainable lifestyles.
- To support cross-disciplinary dialogue and cooperation between the expressive and creative arts (the visual arts, creative writing, dance/movement, drama, and music) and the new eco-human approaches and sciences, such as ecology, ecopsychology, eco-therapy, environmental education, eco-aesthetics, ecological management and other related fields.

Though a growing number of publications on nature-assisted arts therapies have appeared in the last few years (Atkins & Snyder, 2018; Berger & Lahad, 2013; Kopytin & Rugh, 2016, 2018), this book hopes to be a decisive step further in building a new perspective for the expressive and creative arts therapies in the 21st century.

The idea for this book arose from the spirit of natural and cultural ecology, on the basis of a renewed understanding of the role of the arts and arts therapies in human and planetary life. The words that sum up this vision are "ecological," "earth-based," and "nature-assisted": arts therapies that promote the capacity of human beings to respond to and transform difficulty and suffering through their creative ability to bring health, well-being, and beauty into their existence and the world around them.

The concept of *ecopoiesis* is introduced in the book, based on the idea of the poietic nature of humans, supporting the idea of humans as "environmental subjects." This concept is intended to provide the foundations necessary to consider human beings in their relations with the more-than-human realm, the web of life, as willing and able to take care of their "earthly home," guided not only by their needs, but also by the desire to maintain biodiversity and ecological well-being. We believe that the book is the first one to present the ecopoietic perspective. We understand that the human creative function—poiesis, our capacity to shape the world around us—is fundamentally ambiguous, in the sense that we as humans can either support or destroy the environment. However, we believe that humanity can use its ecopoietic capacity to move the world of more sustainable living for humans and the more-than-human world from the realm of possibility to that of reality. Such a transition requires our creative imagination and action congruent with an ecospheric perspective that serves the interests of human and planetary life. We invite the reader to consider the perspectives presented here and to go further in helping to develop the emerging field of ecopoiesis.

References

Atkins, S. & Snyder, M. (2018). *Nature-Based Expressive Arts Therapy: Integrating the Expressive Arts and Ecotherapy*. London and Philadelphia, PA: Jessica Kingsley Publishers.

Berger, R. & Lahad, M. (2013). *The Healing Forest in Post-Crisis Work with Children*. London and Philadelphia, PA: Jessica Kingsley Publishers.

Kopytin, A. & Rugh, M. (eds). (2016). *Green Studio: Nature and the Arts in Therapy*. Hauppauge, NY: Nova Science Publishers.

Kopytin, A. & Rugh, M. (eds). (2018). *Environmental Expressive Therapies: Nature-Assisted Theory and Practice*. New York, NY & London: Routledge/Taylor & Francis.

PART 1

In Search of the Eco-Human Paradigm in Expressive Arts, Therapy, and Education

Theory, Methodology, Concepts

Chapter 1

The Awakening Roar of Beauty

SALLY ATKINS

Our experience of intimacy with the natural world is shaped by our personal sensual encounter with nature and by the stories we tell ourselves about who we are and our place within the world. Throughout history, humans have turned to story, myth, and metaphor to understand the mysteries of the world. In her novel, *Ceremony*, Leslie Marmon Silko tells us this about stories, "I will tell you something about stories... They aren't just entertainment... They are all we have... You don't have anything if you don't have the stories" (Silko, 1977, p.2).

On a warm day in early autumn, I was returning home from my customary walk in the forest near my home. Suddenly ahead and slightly to the left of my way, I noticed a dark shape moving slowly. Several thoughts immediately came to mind. First, the dark shape was a black bear, a very large one. Second, she had several cubs with her. Third, the distance to my door, while not very far, was greater than that between the bear and me. Fourth, bears can run much faster than humans.

Bear sightings are not unusual in my area of the Appalachian Mountains. In fact, we had recently experienced a visit. A large male bear sat in our driveway for a long time, contentedly eating berries from a tree. I know several things about black bears. I know that they are rarely aggressive, with the notable exception of a mother bear with cubs. I know that you should not run away, nor look directly at a bear. However, when this bear stood up on her hind legs looking directly at me, although I knew that this stance was more a sign of curiosity than aggression, I stood for a moment transfixed, fascinated, and afraid, with my heart racing wildly, before I walked quickly to my doorway. Safely at the door, I turned to look once more as the bear returned to all fours and, with her three cubs, slowly moved away. Experiences like this one leave no doubt that I have been met by a being with consciousness and agency. This was an experience of fear, aliveness, and respect, a strong reminder of the beauty and terror that we encounter in our intimacy with the natural world.

The lion's roar

James Hillman (2007) tells a story that comes from the folk traditions of animal psychology about the lion's roar. Among early cultures, the story was told that because newborn lion cubs are immobile, blind, and seemingly without breath, they must be awakened into life by the roar of the lioness. That awakening roar, according to the story, can be heard from as far away as eight kilometers. We live in a time of exploitation of cultures and natural resources, mass extinction of species, and pollution of our lands, water, and air, fed by consumer capitalism, obsession with technology, and the destruction of many aspects of the social, political, and natural fabric of life. In this time of environmental urgency, we need this story, this image of a mother caring for new life by roaring, to awaken to the roar of the earth, the call to awaken and care for the beautiful and fragile life we are given.

Most meetings with the consciousness and agency of the beings in our world are not so dramatic as hearing the roar of a lion or my story of the bear. Yet, if we are present, aware, and noticing, we are surrounded by a myriad of wonders. Today, tiny shoots of spring flowers are pushing their way up through the winter snow. A fallen leaf is floating beside the ice in the pond. The wind is creating a dance of bare branches against the grey sky. Not everything here is beautiful. Not far away, bulldozers are plowing through trees and earth to widen the traffic-snarled highway. North of here, more than 500 mountaintops of this ancient range have been destroyed by strip mining. The nearby river must be checked regularly for trash and pollution.

Some years ago, a personal experience of accidental environmental destruction led me to rage and then to question, as I have again and again, how we are to live, how I am to live in this time.

MADWOMAN
I remember
That afternoon
I heard
The chainsaws.

In the woods
Behind my house
I saw bodies of trees
Locusts stacked high,

The other trees ravaged
By their downing.
They took only locusts,
The toughest wood.

Especially good
For fence posts.
They took
All of them.

I heard a voice,
Ferocious, screaming rape
I scared myself
The loggers stopped.

Pure rage too late,
The mistake already made,
Only doing their job,
They said, and left quickly.

The old man with four fingers
Offered to replant some trees
For the misunderstanding.
Hemlocks, I said,

Not because I really wanted them,
But because they grow fast
And he needed to make
Some gesture of atonement.

The locusts will come back
On their own, but not
In my lifetime
Or my children's

I live in a house of wood,
I keep a fire in winter.
What reparation do I make?
And tell me, how am I to live?

(Atkins, 2005)

Poiesis, ecopoiesis, sympoiesis

The question of how we are to live in this time leads me to consider the concepts of *poiesis*, *ecopoiesis*, and *sympoiesis*.

Poiesis

In the literature of expressive arts therapy, Stephen Levine (2019) writes extensively about the concept of *poiesis*. Levine defines *poiesis* as the creative capacity to respond to the world and to shape what is given. He emphasizes that this capacity of knowing by creating is basic to human existence. Levine has deepened and elaborated on this concept and its central importance for the field and for our lives over many years. *Poiesis* remains for me a fundamental idea for my understanding of the creative process inherent in expressive arts and in life. Levine (2020) says that to address the environmental challenges of this time what is needed now is an ecopoietic perspective, one in which aesthetic responsibility, the capacity to respond to the world in order to bring about beauty, is central.

Ecopoiesis

Ecopoiesis is the theme of the 2009 volume of *Poiesis: Journal of the Arts and Communication* edited by Stephen Levine. With this theme, Levine offers an invitation to think broadly about the earth, nature, the body, ecology, and our ways of thinking. He inspires us to reconceive ourselves as part of the ongoing *ecopoietic* system of the world and to imagine how we might walk more gracefully on the earth.

Alexander Kopytin (2020), a founder of the *Ecopoiesis: Eco-Human Theory and Practice* journal, likewise uses the concept of ecopoiesis to emphasize the interaction and interpenetration of different living systems in an ecological intimacy, an aspect of the co-creation and co-evolution of the human being and nature. Kopytin emphasizes that the eco-human process is not just individual self-expression or shaping the world only to fulfill human needs. The creative eco-human process is one of creating in support and in service of nature and life, to contribute to the well-being of the environment, with the aim of beauty.

Ecopoiesis is human participation with what Mary Richards (1973), noted poet, philosopher, and teacher at the famous Black Mountain College, calls the formative forces of continual creativity in the world. Richards also points out that human creativity is a capacity larger than formal art-making. As human beings, we are creative in all aspects of our lives. We create with food, with space, with our children, and with our lives. Richards (1989, p.41) says that, "All the arts we practice are apprenticeship. The big art is our life."

Sympoiesis

Philosopher and scientist Donna Haraway (2016) proposes the concept of *sympoiesis*, meaning making-with, creating-with the complex and interpenetrating systems of the world. She underscores the need to understand that in order to survive the spiraling ecological devastation of our times, we must see our relationship with nature as becoming one with the earth and all its inhabitants. In ecological literature, the current epoch in which we live is generally referred to as the Anthropocene. Built on the prefix *anthro* (man), the name emphasizes the understanding that human actions have overtaken our ability to reverse the effects of human consumption and capitalism on the earth. Haraway presents the image of the spider as a generative concept for imagining and living in our current epoch. She suggests calling our current epoch the Chthulhucene, emphasizing the necessity of becoming-with in order to live together on a damaged planet. The image of the *cthulhu*, the spider, is intended to evoke thinking with and relating with other beings, not in a linear hierarchy of dominance, but in an entanglement that includes nature, humans, and other-than-human relationships. This entanglement is like the strands of a web and the legs of the spider with which she feels and senses her environment.

Stories of separation and belonging

Since the beginning of human history, image and story have shaped the way we understand who we are and our place in the world. Narratives exert strong control over how we live. Stories that shape our understanding come from many sources, from history, science, religion, philosophy, popular culture, and now from the internet and social media. Today we have many examples of conflicting narratives, narratives of separation from the natural world, as well as narratives of interconnection and belonging.

Stories of separation

Many of the stories we are living today are stories of separation from nature, of objectification of and dominion over the earth. Such stories have supported a world of massive destruction. Many environmental writers believe that the current state of our personal and planetary dis-ease is less a matter of ignorance and apathy but rather due to the western industrialized world's stories of separation from and objectification of the earth. Physicist and novelist Alan Lightman (2005) warns of the particular hazards of the stories of our wired world of today. These are stories in which we experience a constant overload of information and stimulation and an obsession with speed, consumption, and material wealth.

We must change the way we live on and within this earth, and to do so we must listen to the different stories that are emerging today from environmental scientists, philosophers, artists, and poets—stories that also echo the wisdom of Indigenous and earth-based cultures.

Stories of belonging

In contemporary ecological sciences, significant changes are occurring in our scientific understanding of human life embedded in the systems and cycles of the living earth. Likewise, stories told by environmental philosophers and writers reflect in literal and metaphorical ways ideas of the interrelationship of all of life. Stories of ecological writers also reflect in many ways the relational ontology of Indigenous wisdom.

Stories of environmental science

General system theory, outlined first by biologist Ludwig von Bertan-lanffy (1968), tells a story of the complexity and relational reality of living systems beyond the reductionist perspectives of classical science. Since the time of von Bertanlanffy, insights from systems theories have been applied widely in many fields of the physical and social sciences, including theories of self-organization, cybernetics, and complexity studies. These approaches examine the structure of systems as well as how systems interact and communicate.

The British anthropologist Gregory Bateson (1972), considered the father of contemporary family therapy, helped to found the science of cybernetics, extending the concept of systems theories to the social and behavioral sciences. Bateson emphasizes the importance of context, understanding that things cannot be understood in isolation from the ecology of relationships in which they participate and communicate. He says that the most important task of our time is to think in new ways, to move from seeing the world as things, as our noun-oriented language encourages, to seeing the world as creative, interdependent, and interrelated. Bateson emphasizes that the most important task of our time is to embrace the epistemological shift from objectification of the world to understanding the world as a system of interdependent, creative, and multi-layered relationships, "the pattern that connects" (p.462) within the wholeness of the universe.

In the field of psychology, German psychologist Jurgen Kriz (2006) emphasizes systems thinking and a process-oriented perspective of reality. This view embraces the awareness that the world consists of continually changing complex systems of processes, ongoing processes of becoming in which humans are intimately involved.

Norwegian psychologist, economist, and expressive arts therapist Per Espen Stoknes (2015) calls for a turn from an anthropocentric worldview to an ecocentric one in which it is understood that each being has inherent value. As a striking example of ecopoiesis, he discusses the poiesis of the air. He sees the air as a living being actively involved in being and becoming, continuously creating the worlds in which our bodies exist. Stoknes says that what we think of as the self is actually a web of interrelationship. Our very breathing is interconnected with the trees and forest, with the phytoplankton in the oceans, and with each other.

Stories of eco-philosophers

Poets, writers, and philosophers share in telling stories of belonging. Eco-philosopher, eco-theologian, and cultural historian Thomas Berry (1988, 1999, 2009) is one of the leading scholars exploring the fundamental story of our human relationship with the earth. Berry describes our current anthropomorphic stories of the earth by pointing out our human "autism" toward the world, suggesting that we have lost our conversation with trees, rivers, mountains, and animals, and our understanding of ourselves as participatory in this conversation. He reminds us that plants and stones, lakes, rivers, and mountains all have something to teach us, and that our loss of capacity to participate in this great conversation is what allows us to pollute and degrade our environment. He calls also for awakening to a consciousness of the sacred dimensions of the earth to see the universe as a communion of subjects rather than a collection of objects.

Ecologist and philosopher David Abram (1996) agrees that our current commodification of nature is related to the stories we tell about reality and also to our linguistic structure that privileges materialism, rationality, and objectivity. He highlights the fact that our very act of perception is actually a reciprocal interaction of our living body and the living world that we inhabit. Each of us is both subject and object. He calls us to remember the wisdom older than our thinking minds, our "age old reciprocity with the many-voiced landscape" (p.ix). He reminds us that when we enter a forest we see and are seen by all of the animals and plants around us.

Stories of Indigenous wisdom

Contemporary stories of belonging from environmental writers echo the stories of belonging told by writers of Indigenous wisdom. Thomas Berry (1988) points out that some of the most integral understanding of our human intimate relationship with the earth is reflected in the stories of native peoples. He says that even a small amount of contact with native peoples can enhance our capacity to experience the immediacy of the living world. This has been true of my own personal experiences of many years with teachers and artists from Hopi, Zuni, Acoma, Chochiti, the Navaho Nation and the Qualla Boundary of the Eastern Band of the Cherokee People (Atkins & Snyder, 2017).

Indigenous philosophies emphasize the vital materiality of nature and the relational reality of the world. Professor of environmental biology and member of the Potawatomi Nations Robin Wall Kimmerer (2013) says that to be Indigenous means to live as if our material and spiritual lives and those of our children depend on how we live in relationship to the land we inhabit. She asks us to recognize that we are walking among beings worthy of respect: the rock people, the standing people, the beaver people, the bear people:

> Imagine the access we would have to different perspectives, the things we might see through other eyes, the wisdom that surrounds us. We don't have to figure out everything by ourselves: there are intelligences

other than our own, teachers all around us. Imagine how much less lonely the world would be. (p.58)

Beauty and aesthetic responding

In expressive arts therapy, an *aesthetic response* is the feeling of being emotionally moved or touched, enlivened in a strong way by a work of art and the experience of art-making (Levine, 2019) or by experiences in nature (Atkins & Snyder, 2017). The capacity for aesthetic responding is strongly related to love, wonder, and beauty. The writer Herman Melville (1852) speaks of it as an interior responding wonder. Alexander Kopytin emphasizes that ecopoiesis requires love for the earth and all of its beings, including ourselves.

Beauty, says Hillman (2007), is the roar that awakens the heart. Beauty is the lioness roar that awakens our sleeping sense of being alive. This beauty is more than a pleasing appearance or a source of objectified pleasure. It is not a characteristic to be possessed. Hillman (2007) writes that beauty is the manifestation of the *anima mundi*, the soul of the world, reflecting a deep and exquisite appreciation of the world. For Hillman, seeing the world as ensouled honors the inherent value, sovereignty, and mystery of each being. The absence of soul leaves us with a dead, empty, barren place, a world with no inherent dignity and nothing that is sacred.

Philosopher Sandra Lubarsky (2018) says that beauty brings us alive and thus is necessary for the sustainability of our species. She maintains that our current environmental crises are intimately related to our culture's *anaesthesis*, our numbness to beauty. It is this numbness to beauty that enables us to poison our air and pollute our lands, rivers, and oceans. Beauty as a powerful force that affects our ecological practice as well as our emotions and aesthetic values is often under-emphasized in the discursive landscape of ecology. Lubarsky says that the decline of beauty and the decline of the natural world are directly related. Both are victims of mechanism and materialism and disregard the importance of our sensuous connection with the natural world. She urges us to remember that in the arts and in nature we must honor ways to be more fully alive.

Irish poet and philosopher John O'Donohue (2005) also believes that in some ways the many crises of the world today are about the nature of beauty. O'Donohue says that when we awaken our hearts and minds to the call of beauty, we both awaken and surrender, and we become aware of the mysteries of the world: "At its deepest heart, creativity is intended to serve and evoke beauty" (p.7).

The aesthetic encounter in the arts and in nature is one that involves the senses and the imagination. The capacity for aesthetic responding carries with it the *aesthetic responsibility* to respond to the life that is given to us. In her instructions for living a life, the poet Mary Oliver (2008) tells us just that: to pay attention, be astonished, and tell about it. Telling stories of astonishment and wonder in response to beauty often goes beyond the capacity of ordinary language. Here the arts have much to offer, pointing to what cannot be said in ordinary language. For me, poetic words are often my way of aesthetic responding. My aesthetic response to the forest is reflected in the following poem.

RITUAL
When you enter
The spell of the forest
Come with curiosity
And questions.

Come after the rain
To the protection of pines
Lick the droplets
Left on needle tips,
Taste slowly
These holy sacraments.

Breathe in the generosity
Of the living air
Where the smell of sap
Rises fierce and pungent.

Come at night
To the dark mystery
Of a moonlit mountain path,
Look up at the sky
Through the calligraphy
Of branches.

Touch with both hands
The muscled integrity
Of the great black oak
Where time is written
In slow circles, languages
Older than words.

Listen to the songs of trees
Listen with your secret ear
Listen to the sounds
You cannot hear.

(Atkins, 2020)

Personal ecopoiesis

The concept of ecopoiesis offers us a perspective with which we can find ourselves within a story of belonging, of finding our place, as the poet Mary Oliver (1986) says, within the family of things. For me, ecopoiesis begins with my own place and story, the place I inhabit and the stories that inform my understanding of who I am and my place in the world. I am a mountain woman. I pay attention to the direction of the wind, the phases of the moon, and the annual cycle of seasons. I live among remnants of the earth's oldest forests and mountains and the two oldest rivers on the North American continent. My Celtic ancestors have lived and survived in this land since the 1700s. While I have traveled and taught in many places around the world, this is my landscape of belonging, and this landscape inhabits my psyche.

In the early morning darkness, I arise quietly in order not to disturb my husband sleeping beside me. I make my way to the bathroom and begin my day, as I always do, with cold water. Four times I splash my face, once for each of the four cardinal directions, east, south, west, north, reminding myself that this is what I am, what I am made of: air, fire, water, earth. These elements also represent the cycles of life in which I am always imbedded: morning, noon, evening, night; spring, summer, autumn, winter. I recall the Cherokee animal teachers of each direction, the far vision of eagle in the east, the playfulness of raccoon in the south, the introspection of black bear in the west, and the gentle wisdom of deer in the north. I drink the cold water from my hands, grateful for clean water, recalling drinking this way from mountain streams. This is how I find where I am in relation to everything bigger than myself. Indigenous wisdom, the Celtic imagination of my ancestors, and my own sensuous experience tell me that the earth is alive and creating and that I am a part of this.

The great American civil rights leader Dr. Martin Luther King held a vision of community in which justice prevailed and all people were treated with respect. He called it the beloved community. In the spirit of ecopoiesis, could we envision a beloved community to include the earth and all of her beings, marked by respect and care for the human and the more-than-human world? In this urgent time, in a beloved community, everything becomes dear.

NOW EVERYTHING BECOMES DEAR
The sound of rain on the tin roof
And the stream rushing its way
Over stones toward the quiet of the lake
The moment the pale, still present sun
Casts shadows across the mountains

Tiny sparrows who keep on
Building their nest under the eaves
In the corner of the porch
Three wild turkeys
Marching bravely toward the forest

The creaking rhythm of a rocking chair
The crackling comfort of fire
On the broad stone hearth
The voice of a loved one on the phone
The look of wonder on a child's face

Now everything becomes dear
Clean water, simple food
Time
This slow day
This deep breath.

Sally Atkins, previously unpublished

References

Abram, D. (1996). *The Spell of the Sensuous*. New York, NY: Pantheon Books.

Atkins, S. (2005). *Picking Clean the Bones*. Blowing Rock, NC: Parkway Publishers.

Atkins, S. (2020). "Ritual." *Hermit Feathers Review*. Clemmons, NC: Hermit Feathers Press.

Atkins, S. & Snyder, M. (2017). *Nature-Based Expressive Arts Therapy: Integrating the Expressive Arts and Ecotherapy*. Philadelphia, PA: Jessica Kingsley Publishers.

Bateson, G. (1972). *Steps to an Ecology of Mind*. San Francisco, CA: Chandler Publishing Co.

Berry, T. (1988). *The Dream of the Earth*. San Francisco, CA: Sierra Club Books.

Berry, T. (1999). *The Great Work: Our Way into the Future*. New York, NY: Bell Tower.

Berry, T. (2009). *The Sacred Universe: Earth, Spirituality and Religion in the Twenty-First Century*. New York, NY: Columbia University Press.

Haraway D.J. (2016). *Staying with the Trouble: Making Kin in the Cthulhucene*. Durham, NC: Duke University Press.

Hillman, J. (2007). *Mythical Figures* (Uniform Edition Vol. 6). Putnam, CT: Spring Publications.

Kimmerer, R.W. (2013). *Braiding Sweetgrass: Indigenous Wisdom, Scientific Knowledge, and the Teachings of Plants*. Minneapolis, MN: Milkweed Editions.

Kopytin, A. (2020). Archetypal psychology in the context of the eco-human approach. *Ecopoiesis: Eco-Human Theory and Practice*, 1(2), 6–16.

Kriz, J. (2006). *Self-Acrualization*. Norderstedt: Herstellung und Verlag.

Levine, S.K. (2019). *Philosophy of Expressive Arts Therapy: Poiesis and the Therapeutic Imagination*. London & Philadelphia, PA: Jessica Kingsley Publishers.

Levine S.K. (2020). Ecopoiesis: Towards a poietic ecology. *Ecopoiesis: Eco-Human Theory and Practice*, 1(1), 17–24. [open access internet journal].

Lightman, A. (2005). *A Sense of the Mysterious: Science and the Human Spirit*. New York, NY: Pantheon Books.

Lubarsky, S. (2018). Personal communication.

Melville, H. (1852). *Pierre; or, The Ambiguities* (book III, chapter I). New York, NY: Harper & Brothers.

O'Donohue, J. (2005). *Beauty: The Invisible Embrace*. New York, NY: Harper Perennial. (Original edition published 2003 under the title *Divine Beauty*.)

Oliver, M. (1986). *Dream Work*. New York, NY: The Atlantic Monthly Press.

Oliver, M. (2008). *Red Bird*. Boston, MA: Beacon Press.

Richards, M.C. (1973). *The Crossing Point: Selected Talks and Writings*. Middletown, CN: Wesleyan University Press. (Original work published 1966.)

Richards, M.C. (1989). *Centering in Pottery, Poetry and the Person* (second edition). Hanover, NH: University Press of New England. (Original work published 1962.)

Silko, L.M. (1977). *Ceremony*. New York, NY: Penguin Books.

Stoknes, P.E. (2015). *What We Think About When We Try Not To Think About Global Warming: Toward a New Psychology of Global Warming*. White River Junction, VT: Chelsea Green Publishing.

von Bertanlanffy, L. (1968). *General System Theory: Foundations, Development, Applications*. New York, NY: George Braziller.

Chapter 2

Nature-Assisted Creative Arts Therapies and the Paradigm Change: What Arts Therapists Can Do in the Face of New Global Challenges

ALEXANDER KOPYTIN

Introduction: The crisis of ecology and the humanities

The global environmental crisis has become a reality. Its transition into an ecological catastrophe is a matter of time during which humankind can either take certain steps to prevent it, or remain on the same track of uncontrolled exploitation of the planet's natural resources. Attempts are being made to solve the global environmental crisis in various ways, in particular by implementing a sustainable development model, which, among other things, assumes the need for technological reorganization, as well as introducing environmental education to support the development of environmental awareness.

The environmental crisis is taking place against the backdrop of many complex social issues, demonstrating the fragility of the existing order in which, due to globalization, everything is dependent on everything else. From the perspective of ecological theory, this is a relatively stable system but a system without resilience. The crisis in the humanities appears to be at the core of the current global situation. According to Arran Gare (2019), the most promising avenue for defending the humanities and their values is to claim intrinsic value for all life. The crisis in the humanities coming at a time of accelerating ecological destruction threatening not only most terrestrial species but the future of humanity supports radical ideas in ecology. "These held out the last hope for upholding the humanities and humanistic human sciences, and avoiding the political consequences of denying value to living beings except as instruments" (Gare, 2019, p.637).

Nature and culture work as autonomous but synergetic systems: both are parts of the whole system of life on this planet. Both of them need to be engaged in order to empower human beings and the global life web to cope with our various challenges and to restore themselves. I refer here to both human and environmental resilience, with their capacity for creation, which can enable us and the earth to recover. Realizing our creative, *poietic*, capacity, together with the more-than-human world, we support both an inner and outer ecology.

Nature-assisted creative arts therapies arose from the spirit of these ideas, to bring the arts therapies and the ecological perspective into their original interconnection on the basis of a renewed understanding of the role of the arts, nature, and the human sciences in the life of the planet.

Defining nature-assisted, ecological, creative arts therapies

Ecological or nature-assisted creative/expressive arts therapies represent an emerging therapeutic cluster, based on the new understanding of the role of the arts in providing public and environmental health and establishing more harmonious and mutually supporting relations of humans with nature. These forms of therapy belong to an established group of mental health professions or specialized therapeutic approaches, such as art therapy, music therapy, dramatherapy, dance-movement therapy, and expressive arts therapy. These disciplines focus on the therapeutic use of creative/expressive processes of clients and their relationship with the therapist. Ecological arts therapies are characterized by a new perspective on health issues and the role of the arts in providing public and planetary health and well-being. They are supported by scientific approaches such as ecopsychology and ecophilosophy and demonstrate a new perspective on our understanding of the therapeutic role of human bonds with nature.

The spectrum of expressive forms, used as environmental creative responses embraced in these therapies, is broad and includes visual art, drama and ritual, music, dance and movement, and creative writing, as well as practices that integrate the expressive arts in terms of interacting with animals and plants, wilderness journeys, contemplative presence in nature, and so on. Ecological/nature-assisted arts therapies, together with ecotherapy, environmental philosophy, environmental education, and the contemporary environmental arts, support the emerging eco-human approach and the growing field of constructive innovations and eco-human technologies. These can be applied in education, medicine, and the wider social context in order to counteract the environmental crisis and enable a more harmonious co-evolution of human beings and the more-than-human world: the eco-sphere.

The emergence of nature-assisted or ecological arts therapies marks a decisive moment in the development of these therapies, because they mean something more than just a set of innovations that can be implemented in already established therapeutic approaches. Rather, they strive to form a new and even revolutionary platform for empirical forms of therapeutic and health-promoting work, supported by a constellation of distinct theoretical ideas and values.

Environmental psychology, ecopsychology, environmental education, deep ecology, the environmental arts/eco-arts, ecological arts therapies, as well as some forms of environmental activism belong to the environmental movement. This movement challenges the basic foundations of our current civilization and can even be considered to be related to a paradigm shift, since paradigms, according to Kuhn (1962), are not simply theories, but the entire worldview in which theories exist, and all of the implications that come with it. A significant part of the environmental movement is concerned with the need for radical change in personal beliefs, and the need for ideas about complex systems and organizations to replace former ways of thinking about human beings and organizing social and economic life in its relationships to the global life web. Ecological arts and arts therapies, together with environmental psychology/ecopsychology, environmental humanities, environmental education and deep ecology, become a major source of ideas in the tradition of anti-reductionist thinking in science and in the humanities and bring forth the new environmental paradigm which reverses modernist, Cartesian thinking and perception of the human being and the world as machines.

Nature-assisted arts therapies and other branches of the ecological movement aligned to the need for a paradigm shift bring a new perspective to our understanding of health and pathology and new ways to address personal and collective mental distress, since at their most ambitious they seek to redefine mental health within an environmental context and invite us to re-examine the human psyche as an integral part of the global web of life.

Nature-assisted arts therapies can involve experiences of becoming embedded in the ecosystem and empathic attuning to the living environment and forms of life. This process has the potential to allow us to actualize and bring to the conscious mind certain aspects of the human experience, in particular those related to our biological history and our "ecological unconscious," according to Theodore Roszak (2001). The results of this include improved health and well-being, and support for our perception of ourselves as "ecological subjects": our eco-identity (Næss, 1989, 2003). Nature-assisted arts therapies can bring changes to humans' perception of themselves in their interconnectedness with the life web and by doing so, they provide a modest but compelling act of regeneration, an adaptive response to healing not only of human beings, but of the multitude of places on the planet that experience distress and "illness." They strive to achieve multiple therapeutic goals, embracing both the micro and macro levels, since they not only deal with individual needs and health issues, but with environmental issues as well.

One of the characteristics of nature-assisted or ecological arts therapies can be summarized as follows. These practices usually include either outdoor or indoor activities that involve direct interaction with the natural world or natural materials and often lead to the perception of the environment and its inhabitants as other forms of life, which are then engaged with ethically. The activities can include series of exercises that awaken sensory awareness through relaxation, breathing, exploratory mindful walks, body scanning, journaling and other tasks which help to develop receptivity, focus attention and increase a sense of embodiment in the living environment.

How can we address these issues that are usually ignored in most conventional therapies?

As arts therapists, we can address these issues in different ways. We can offer our clients the possibility to engage in creative non-instrumental environmental activities, to learn how to see and create beauty around themselves and how to develop effective self-regulatory skills and coping strategies that can be used both in therapy and in everyday life to improve and promote their health and well-being.

We can also help our clients to enrich their ecological knowledge, develop their ecological consciousness and thus decrease their possible destructive impact on the natural environment and prevent the risk of various physical and mental issues as a result of unsustainable ways of living and pathogenic environmental factors. We can do this, in particular, through waste reduction and an environmentally conscious attitude to our use of materials.

Nature-assisted arts therapies recognize that people have the fundamental need and right to live in a "healthy," beautiful and unthreatened environment, and that such a need and a right must be fulfilled. According to the tenets of sustainable development, the balance between economic growth, care for the environment and social well-being are interconnected and must be guaranteed.

Unfortunately, arts therapists are not trained in the environmental paradigm and do not learn how to address these issues on both theoretical and practical levels. Therefore, special modules for arts therapists during their training and professional work, and even a specialization in the field of nature-assisted or ecological arts therapies, should be developed, so that our professional field can contribute to human and environmental health and well-being to a greater degree.

Defining human relationships to the environment

While considering the postulates and basic theoretical ideas that could be relevant for the emerging field of nature-assisted or ecological arts therapies, the eco-human multi-professional approach, which is formed out of growing environmental crisis as well as crisis in the humanities, appears to be a central option.

The eco-human approach recognizes that the key problem of the humanities—the problem of understanding ourselves as "environmental subjects"—cannot be solved within the framework of Cartesian science that separates a person (the subject) from the external world of objects. Rather, the eco-human approach posits that the subject be considered in relation to the living environment, the natural, more-than-human world. We believe that ecology in the broad sense of the term, as a worldview, needs a new conception of the human as much as the modern humanities need ecology and the environmental perspective.

According to the current definition of the eco-human approach (Kopytin, 2020; Levine, 2020), individuals should be considered as living in relationship to the living environment—the web of life—and seeking to reveal their own selves as well as their environmental subjectivity, through their reciprocal intersubjective communication. In doing so, they shape both the world and themselves. The eco-human approach is aimed at overcoming the environmental crisis and the crisis in the humanities by strengthening the links of the humanities with environmental knowledge and ecology. This implies the task of developing the ecological consciousness and sustainable lifestyle that characterize "environmental subjects," individuals with an "ecological identity" (Næss, 1989, 2003).

According to Arne Næss, the underlying cause of the ecological crisis is the psychological organization of a personality which has been formed by industrialization and scientism. Accordingly, in order to overcome the environmental crisis, it is necessary to form a different psychological organization of the personality, based on the concept of environmental identity: eco-identity. This concept of eco-identity allows us to recognize and further develop theories that help a) to exemplify a more ecological, or systems, view of the person, b) offer an understanding of how an expanded self-concept might affect the functioning of individuals and their surrounding environment, and c) suggest how self-constructs might be changed.

This approach postulates the "poietic" or creative nature of human beings, that is, their ability to shape the surrounding world and themselves. Humans exist in the mode of possibility; they can choose to shape the world and themselves in a way that is not yet actual but that is contained to bring forth beauty by propagating with the other. From the perspective of the eco-human approach, a person's ability to love and support life can be considered to be a property of the human being in its acts of co-creation with nature.

According to Levine (1992, 2020), poiesis indicates our basic capacity to shape the world:

> The human being is distinct from other creatures in that it is not pre-adapted to a particular environment. Instead it has the ability to build radically different worlds suitable (or not) to life in a wide diversity of surroundings. In building its world, the human shapes the environment, and as it does so, it shapes itself. World building is self-building. (Levine, 1992, pp.23–24)

Based on the idea of poiesis, the concept of ecopoiesis (from the Greek *Οἶκος* meaning home, housing, and *ποίησι*, meaning making, creating) is an important part of the eco-human approach, supporting the idea of humans as "environmental subjects" (Kopytin, 2020; Levine, 2020). This concept is designed to provide the foundation necessary to consider humans in their relations with the living environment as willing and able to take care of their "earthly home." It recognizes the need for humans and their habitat to become a niche in the life web and for humans to live non-destructively with other species.

Ecopoiesis designates a quality and mechanism of the co-evolution of humans and nature, a conscious and responsible co-creation of humankind with nature, based on our physical, emotional, and spiritual connection with it. Through ecopoiesis, human beings, together with nature and as part of it, continue and support themselves, as well as various forms of earthly life and the eco-sphere. Creative acts perceived from the ecopoietic perspective are rooted not so much in the need for individual creative "self-expression" in the traditional sense of this word, but in the motivation to support and serve nature and life and to achieve non-duality, a balance between natural and cultural milieu. Ecopoiesis cannot be achieved without love for the earth and for the beings that inhabit it, including ourselves.

> Ecopoiesis shifts the focus from the ego, the "I" that sees the world and writes about the world, to the world itself and how the world poietically writes itself, or poietically expresses itself. Ecopoiesis is the expression of the eco-sphere and we are always already part and parcel of that eco-sphere. (Morris, 2021)

Ecopoiesis as a creative human function is expressed through humans' initiatives to care for and respect the environment, and to see ecosystems as a source of health and well-being for themselves and others who belong to both the human and more-than-human worlds. It implies a fundamental human need and ability to connect to the web of life, to arrange the life space and do something meaningful, beautiful, and healing, both for themselves and the ecosphere, and with nature. This can mean various things, in particular gardening, animal encounters, simply spending more time in ecologically healthy settings, or more actively working on maintaining and restoring eco-health, and being involved in environmental action. The ecopoietic function can make one socio-politically active, able to engage further in eco-health promotion and become an agent of change in the educational, public health and environmental spheres.

As a constructive component of the eco-human approach, eco-human technologies can be defined as methods of transforming the human being in its attitude to the environment and itself. Eco-human technologies can be used in the field of pedagogy, psychology, medicine, and other fields, in a wide cultural domain, forming environmental awareness and values, contributing to preserving and developing the human and natural resources of the planet (Kopytin, 2020).

The role of the arts in providing meaningful human connection to nature

The visual and performing arts, as well as other forms of organized and meaningful human-environmental interaction, existed in human history long before the civilized mind came to an understanding of creative acts as primarily the result of individual activity. The wider environmental perception of the arts can be found in many world traditions, especially in those characterized "by ideas about the interconnectedness of all things, perpetual movement, impermanence, and how small and humble acts generate larger changes in the world" (McNiff, 2015, p.12). Such perception of the arts is also implied in the contemporary environmental movement and represents the perennial need of human beings to keep their intrinsic connection with nature around and in themselves.

Considerable similarity can be found between modern environmental and ecopsychological understanding of the arts and world traditions, and their environmental practices that support mind-body-spirit integration. Both contemporary ecotherapy and Indigenous cultural traditions can be characterized in their perception of the arts as implying the vital function of supporting healthy bonds with nature, the web of life, and in doing so giving voice and articulate meaning for earthly life. According to such a conception of the role of the arts, natural environments and various life forms can be highly attractive to humans, not only due to their pragmatic value, but also to their aesthetic, emotional, and spiritual significance.

In the context of creative/expressive arts therapies, the role of the arts in providing meaningful human connection to nature should be emphasized. The arts possess their own means of solving the environmental and human issues that face us. The spectrum of ways to engage with nature through the arts is wide and involves the participant taking different roles, from objective observer to active interventionist. The functions of the arts that can be relevant for the goals of ecological/nature-assisted arts therapies are outlined below:

The arts support meaningful action leading to changed perception of the natural environment. Study of the cultural history of humankind helps us to recognize that making art brings new meaning to human relations with nature; raises consciousness of our place in the natural world and our interdependence; encourages people to transcend their own personal problems and develop a sense of being part of a bigger whole, thus allowing the spiritual awareness of a relationship with the natural world, to develop the self-directed need to be caring and to preserve and respect the natural world and develop lifestyles that will aid this (Clinebell, 1996). Making art with and in nature also helps to reach such goals of ecotherapy as facilitating healing and experiencing well-being as an inner state of wellness, including a physical, mental and emotional state of consonance which exists in a healthy environment and is based on a harmonious connection with its ecology.

According to environmental psychology, meaningful action is the opportunity to make a useful contribution to a genuine problem. It may involve being effective at a large scale (e.g., the choice of livelihood, a life-long struggle for environmental justice or food security), but perhaps more often it involves actions at a modest level (e.g., participating in a stewardship activity, community involvement, voting). The meaningfulness experienced is less a consequence of the scale of the effort involved and more about deriving a sense of making a difference, being respected and listened to, and feeling that we have a secure place within our social group.

Reasonable behavior is more likely when people feel that they are needed and that their participation matters. A number of studies indicate that doing something judged worthwhile or making a difference in the long run are primary motives underlying voluntary environmental stewardship behavior (Greese et al., 2000; Maller et al., 2006). In these studies, the notion of meaningful action emerges as one of the most significant sources of satisfaction.

One of the main effects of making art with and in nature is that the arts give natural landscapes and objects some kind of "distinctive meaning, relevance and status" (Sontag, 1990, p.28). Making art as a form of environmental activity can help people to recognize the meaningfulness and beauty of nature, even if they initially didn't recognize such qualities. If a person is focused even on the most depressed, sad, and colorless environment and starts looking beneath the superficial exterior of things or places using the arts, they will often see some spark of life, unique, individual aspects that characterize those objects or places.

However, this necessarily requires "turning ourselves inside out, with the heart as the site of reconnection" (Chalquist, 2007), in order to be able to dissolve through "the art of biophilia" (Kopytin, 2016) the psychological barriers that characterize the history of our progressive alienation from the land and fuel the environmental crisis.

The arts help people to feel in control of the environment and participate in its management and restoration. Art-making can be used to promote individuals' and communities' active position in their relationship with the environment and develop their perception of themselves as people who are able to exert a certain amount of influence on it.

In being involved in environmental expressive/creative activities, people can "personalize" and appropriate the environment. This can also be a significant factor in their feeling safe and in control of the space they occupy. This controlling function of the arts can be especially important in ecotherapy activities, when the client perceives the environment as lacking control (which is natural for most outdoor activities) and evoking anxiety. The arts mediate one's interaction with the space involved and help to provide equilibrium between the dynamic quality of the natural environment and the more static nature of certain artworks.

The active stance in the human relationship to nature is the main characteristic of "contemporary ecotherapy" (Burls, 2007); a significant factor of mutuality can also support collective behavioral change. According to Halpern and colleagues (2004), behavioral interventions tend to be more successful where there is an equal relationship between the influencer and the influenced and where both parties stand to gain from the outcome (p.25). In public mental health, such mutuality can be seen in the relationships between practitioners and service users, where the latter assume greater responsibility. For Burls (2007):

> In ecotherapeutic approaches, there seems to be a further level of mutuality: the role of the influencer is adopted by people who would normally be classed as the influenced. In benefiting from personal lifestyle changes and associated recovery, the service users help to develop a framework

for reciprocity towards the environment and the community. In doing so, the community is influenced to care for and respect the environment and, in addition, to see their local green spaces as a source of health and well-being. (p.35)

The arts can be considered as a form of ecological personalization and subjectification. Our perception of the constructive human interaction with nature through the arts can be enriched by concepts such as personalization of the environment (Heimets, 1994; Laurence, Fried, & Slowik, 2013). This concept is related to psychosocial aspects of a person's experience, for example their territoriality and need to maintain a sense of belonging, ownership and control over their space. Personalization can also be understood as a human behavior that aims to express certain distinctive features of the individual in their surrounding environment. Environmental art can be understood as an ecological form of personalization based on the empathic and supportive human interaction with the natural world.

The expressive arts and acts of creative personalization of the environment can promote an environmental ethic, and a more active and participatory position in people's relationship with the world around them, as well as supporting their self-esteem and empowerment.

Personalization of the environment and natural objects through the ecopoietic stance in the world can also imply subjectification of natural objects, their being perceived as having their own subjectivity, able or being in some form of reciprocity, having a dialogue and communication with human beings. Subjectification implies both empathy and identification with natural objects and environments and plays a crucial role in the process of developing the human relationship to the more-than-human world; it also enables an ethical perception of nature to be established.

Engaging in environmental art supports mindfulness and a sense of physical presence in the environment, connecting the symbolic forms of the arts and language to the immediate physical experience of the natural world (the life process). Some environmental arts-based activities can be considered as a way of developing somatic awareness and an embodied sense of self in one's relation to the environment. This effect is most obvious as a result of environmental arts-based activities which balance time between mindfulness and creative expression, when emphasis is placed on meditative journeys or path-working (walkabouts) as a form of mini-pilgrimages in the "green area," accompanied with or followed by participants' involvement in making art (drawing, taking photographs, making environmental constructions, botanical arrangements, etc.). Other expressive forms, such as dance and movement, ritual, music improvisation, narrative-construction in order to express and integrate complex experiences, can expand the scope of expressive/creative arts therapeutic techniques.

Embodiment effects can be easily facilitated through various environmental creative activities, or mindful journeys that help us to feel more embedded in the web of life. Often, the projective nature of the arts enables one's identification with natural objects and environments on a physical level, projecting one's perception of the body or its parts onto natural processes and environments. Through this process, the symbolization of somatic phenomena and processes is possible.

Mindful creative activities can be integrated into ecotherapy practices and support the goals of ecotherapy by fostering reconnection and returning to experiencing ourselves in the here and now as embodied beings. This requires attention to physical sensations in their relation to mental states evoked by one's presence and interaction with the environment. It should be emphasized that the curative powers of nature are enhanced by the degree of mindfulness and mental focus one brings to these interactions. People can immerse themselves in "quiet fascination" (De Young, 2013, p.24) and a state of presence in the environment, as well as be encouraged to use different arts and instrumental media like photography to explore experiential awareness and practice mindful attention by documenting responses to sensory stimuli. For instance, they can be asked to take pictures of what they move toward as pleasant and also to photograph what they experience as unpleasant, as was done in one new mindfulness-based art therapy intervention (Peterson, 2013), a good example of a palliative environmental program.

Whichever particular expressive arts are used, participants can be encouraged to immerse themselves in a kind of meditation with their absorption in physical and emotional processes, on the one hand, and attentiveness to the environmental stimuli, on the other. They can walk or act mindfully, keeping a sense of their presence in the environment with immediate experience here and now, appreciating their physical contact with the natural objects and sensory qualities of the "green space" with its "field effects."

Mindfulness-based environmental expressive arts therapy programs can include an introduction with mindfulness instruction and emphasis on the role of attention in health. Warming-up activities involving breathing and relaxation, and exploratory walkabouts in certain environments, can be introduced to provide deeper effects (DeYoung, 2013; Linden & Grut, 2002).

Ecological, eco-human perspective on health and illness

The eco-human approach recognizes a synergy between human health and well-being and environmental integrity. It emphasizes a new perspective on our understanding of health and pathology and ways in which personal and collective insanity could be cured, since this approach seeks to redefine sanity within an environmental context. It contends that seeking to heal the soul and the body without reference to the ecological system of which we are an integral part is a form of self-destructive blindness. The eco-human approach draws on the ecological sciences to re-examine human health and well-being as an integral part of the web of life. If we are embedded in the wide web of life we somehow feel what happens "out there," as we are a mindful part of this web, and we respond to the deteriorating global situation deeply in our body, mind, and psyche. Ecopsychology recognizes and seeks to address how the pain of the ecological world shows up as pain within and between human beings.

Ecopsychology, together with environmental philosophy, has come to understand that ecosystems can be healthy or unhealthy, and that their condition is in synergy with their constituent parts of the person. From the eco-human point of view, "health" is characterized by mutual augmenting of the whole community and the component communities of each other at multiple levels, facilitating their continued successful functioning, their resilience in response to new situations and stresses, and motivating ongoing change and development to maximize developmental options.

Climate change is currently the great issue of planetary health, together with other complex issues which we respond to deeply in our body, mind, and psyche. However, we suffer even more, both individually and collectively, when we find ourselves unable to respond to the situation around us, when our creative response to reality is restricted and we experience ourselves as being in a helpless situation. The work of the change agent in the ecological arts therapeutic mission, then, is to restore and develop our capacity for ecopoietic creative action that we as individuals or communities are often lacking.

One of the characteristics of the increasing global environmental and human "'pathology'" is the human relationship to beauty. Beauty has become a cultural fetish, a triviality, something relative and subjective, that is used to sell; it is today primarily an object and instrument of commodification. However, beauty is actually a core quality of life, bringing health and resilience, and is one of the key concepts associated with ecopoiesis; the ecopoietic attitude of human beings to the web of life and nature around and in themselves. The ecological idea of beauty with its connection to health is not limited to the sphere of human experience. It is not tied to the notion that beauty is inherent only in human beings with their capacity for artistic and aesthetic activity, but is a manifestation of natural life and part of our cultural experience: the cultural activity of human beings with their ability to aesthetically respond to the world and organize it in accordance with their ideas and experience.

Beauty in its environmental meaning is strongly connected to human and environmental health in their reciprocal relations with each other and their ability to support and cherish each other. Beauty is also an expression of the human and ecosystems' capacity to continue to exist, adapt, cope with various challenges, flourish, and multiply. However, beauty as a property of "healthy" nature and culture is not limited to any one state of childhood, youth, and maturity, but rather characterizes the whole lifespan of any organism. The ecological idea of beauty is connected to the concept of the limitations that are inherent in any living organism. Our sense of beauty also implies our ability to meet with the limitations of our existence and our capabilities, to respond to them and to experience a mixture of trepidation, delight, and humility. This vision of beauty with its connection to human and environmental health and sustainability provided in the arts can serve as a guideline for all our acts in our relationships with both culture and nature.

The environmental and ecopsychological perspective on personality formation

Whereas in most conventional therapies, the categories of nature and the living environment/web of life are simply ignored, or considered to be secondary with regard to one's relation to the human world, for our primary caregivers (parental figures) and other people with whom significant relations can be established throughout the lifespan—from our perspective, one's relations with the more-than-human world—the web of life implies an equal significance in the eco-human approach.

According to environmentally or ecologically grounded personality theory, one's relationship with nature occupies a special role, being considered as a vital factor of healthy personality formation; establishing an eco-identity has the same significance as one's relations with people. Emotional bonds with nature and the attachment of human beings to nature, together with their bonds with other people, serve as a vital factor of healthy personality formation, beginning with the early developmental phase and ending with the final stage of the human lifespan.

Barrows (1995) points out that Piaget, Stern, Fordham and others whose theories inform our work now may serve as a bridge to a more ecologically based understanding of child development:

> The place where transitional phenomena occur, then (to use Winnicott as a sort of bridge to a new formulation), might be understood, in this new paradigm of the self, to be the permeable membrane that suggests or delineates but does not divide us from the medium in which we exist. It is in this realm that distinctions between subjective and objective begin to blur and intersubjectivity is possible. (Barrows, 1995, pp.106–107)

From an eco-human perspective, personality development takes place within a wider matrix of being and relationships that enables the formation of eco-identity. The notion of an eco-identity can be pre-eminent for the fields of ecopsychology and ecotherapy; it challenges most "conventional" personality theories. It can be defined as the interiorized dynamical structure of our relationship with nature that embraces both the human and more-than-human worlds and serves as one of the significant foundations for self-perception and self-concept. This is a kind of self-perception and self-understanding that is linked to one's mutually sustaining relationship with nature and implies one's responsibility and care for nature. Ethical and aesthetic perception of the natural environment and some practical action aimed at its preservation and cultivation serve as important factors of one's own health and well-being.

Eco-identity is considered to be opposed to a "consumer false self" (Kanner & Gomes, 1995), "an ideal that is taken to heart as part of a person's identity… The consumer false self is false because it arises from a merciless distortion of authentic human needs and desires" (p.83).

Nature as the third part in therapeutic relationships

Ecotherapy is sometimes believed to be "radical" in regard to most modern therapies due to its different perception of the conditions, goals and therapeutic relationship involved. Ecotherapy, like most other therapies now, is based on relational theories of therapeutic action, with their focus "on the larger relational system established by the client and the therapists, within which psychological phenomena crystallize and in which experience is continually and mutually shaped in a dialogue of the client and the therapist" (Bridges, 1999, p.292). However, while the main parties in this relational system in most therapies are client and therapist, nature assumes the role of the third party in ecotherapy and ecological arts therapies. Within this relational system, the crucial role is given to affective attachment both to the therapist and nature in the process of therapeutic change.

Nature is perceived here as a subject of a certain kind and requires environmental ethics that include emotional and subjective elements built on a relationship of care between human beings and the more-than-human world—the different subjects of the living environment, the ecosystem. Ecotherapy invites clients to get involved in the relationship with nature, to develop a sense of reciprocity and empathy in human relationships to nature and to identify with various forms of natural life as a significant factor of therapeutic action. Clinebell (1996) postulated that ecotherapy is characterized by the three-way relationship of person, therapist, and nature, in which nature is considered to be a kind of a co-therapist or educator.

Understanding nature as the third party in therapeutic relationships implies specific psychological, ethical and existential attitudes towards it. Perceiving nature as a subject with which some affective bond can be established is also possible as a result of intensified human-nature relationships typical within ecotherapy. Our experience of interaction with various life forms as a source of protection and nurture enables this effect. Corbett and Milton (2011) even emphasize that, therapeutically, the natural world could bring another dimension into the transferential relationship. Further exploration would be required to develop this, for example drawing on the work of various attachment, personality and object relations theorists. If we recognize that nature has provided human beings with care for millions of years, then our affective bond and attachment to the natural environment is possible, though its quality can vary depending on the developmental circumstances of the particular individual.

It should be recognized, however, that ecotherapy and ecological/ nature-assisted arts therapies, like any other therapy, require an appropriately structured and accompanied therapeutic process. The presence of the therapist throughout a whole course of therapeutic work provides the client with the sense of safety, containment, order, and comprehensibility and helps them to shape and crystallize their experience.

Environmental and ecopsychological perception of the therapeutic setting

According to the traditional clinical model of the arts therapy setting, it is in both "an environment conducive to creativity" (Malchiodi, 2007, p.80) and a container for powerful and unregulated experiences (Killick, 2000) that "the space in which the relationship between therapist and client develops" (Case & Dalley, 1992, p.19). The need for a client to reach a certain state of mind to provide symbol formation in the atmosphere of the arts therapy setting has been emphasized. Symbol formation as a means of effective therapeutic communication and the main focus for therapeutic discourse is given a central importance in clinical arts psychotherapy. It is postulated that "visual imagery—the quintessential stuff of symbolism—is the raw material of art therapy" (Wilson, 2001, p.40) which then can materialize through art-making. Since the symbol is defined as a representational object that can be evoked in the absence of an immediate stimulus, the therapeutic environment is arranged to evoke symbol formation based on the client's immersion in their inner realm rather than in the outer reality and to help the client to begin using images as a reflection of their inner world based on the concept of "drawing from within" (ibid., p.56). Such perception of the symbol formation and the art as a reflection of our inner world is more typical for the clinical, psychoanalytic model, which is different from the perception of the art in the framework of poiesis/ecopoiesis, in which the art that is made brings something new into the world.

In the arts therapies, clients' relations to the outer environment is sometimes discussed to offer them additional opportunities for connecting to their inner worlds. As Case and Dalley (1992) explain:

> The outer environment in which the institution is set will also directly and indirectly impinge upon and influence the sessions as clients make use of the content of the rooms and whatever is offered by the external

environment (for instance, offering clients views of the outside world can evoke memories, feelings and fantasies). (p.32)

However, it is unusual for most arts therapists, especially those following a psychodynamic orientation, to consider environmental factors implied in socio-cultural and natural surroundings as having much significance in the therapeutic process or action. The emphasis is rather placed on interpersonal therapeutic interaction and the psychological exploration of the arts product as a reflection of the client's symptoms and their inner dynamics connected to therapeutic relations, with minimum or no attention given to immediate environmental stimuli. A client's connection to the wider environment and expanding therapeutic boundaries is usually considered to be less significant and even counterproductive.

The eco-human approach, in particular environmental ecopsychology together with socially sensitive approaches in arts therapies and in contemporary therapies in general, however, has expanded our understanding of the therapeutic setting and therapeutic environment. Contemporary understanding of the therapeutic action also includes the healthcare facilities and "therapeutic team" as well as the community. The therapeutic environment is designed and applied not only to support and facilitate state-of-the-art medicine and technology, patient safety, and quality patient care, but also to embrace the patients' family and caregivers in a psychosocially supportive therapeutic space. It is believed that the characteristics of the physical, social, and psychological environment in which a patient receives care affect patient outcomes, patient satisfaction and safety, staff efficiency and satisfaction as well as organizational outcomes. Ecopsychology and ecotherapy seem to be congruent with this idea of the therapeutic environment, but give even more importance to natural environmental factors.

Since both ecopsychology and ecotherapy recognize the synergy between human health and well-being and the health and ecological integrity of the natural environment, eco-therapeutic practices usually take place within natural environments or in other ways are somehow related to nature. Though some ecotherapy practices, at least during certain parts of the session, can take place indoors, special significance is given to participants' involvement in certain activities outdoors. Outdoor spaces used throughout these activities can vary considerably.

The wide continuum of environments used in nature-based or eco-arts therapies can embrace spaces with prevailing natural objects and characterized by greater biodiversity, on the one hand, and those with mostly built objects, on the other. The answer to the question "How much nature is needed in order to practice eco-arts therapies?" would include a wide variety of environments in which nature is present in one or another form. It could be the garden in a mental hospital or a public school, or more distant wilderness areas, "as long as the setting is maintained as a central reference to the process and its conduction" (Berger, 2009, p.240).

The Green Studio model was introduced (Kopytin, 2016) to define a special place where eco-arts therapeutic sessions can take place. The Green Studio/Eco-Studio can be characterized as a therapeutic indoor or outdoor space with a certain abundance of natural living forms and materials, possibly some natural landscape, a part of the natural environment that can be chosen, maintained, and personalized by the client or community. Sometimes it cannot be as permanent as the traditional therapeutic setting and is characterized by a unique equilibrium of static and dynamic qualities. Its dynamic qualities are dependent on greater transparency of its boundaries and the natural processes involved.

As we have defined it (Kopytin, 2016, p.20), the Green Studio can be created as an accessible green area, a part of the institution (hospital, rehabilitation center, shelter, residential home), or aligned with a private practitioner's office. It can also be a kind of "portable studio" (Kalmanowitz & Lloyd, 2005, 2011) arranged in the municipality (park, garden, beach, etc.) or in the "wild" environment. But even in this latter case, a sense of order, permanence, and comprehensibility for the client is possible as a result of their relationship with the therapist and the various activities which give them a possibility to personalize a natural space.

The Green Studio can be perceived as the space in which the human function of ecopoiesis can materialize. It is possible and even necessary to perceive the Green Studio as providing a two-pronged system to achieve both individual health (at the micro level) and public and environmental health outcomes (at the macro level) (Burls, 2007).

Conclusion

The field of community and social action therapies, including creative/ expressive arts therapists' interest in exploring new ways of therapeutic work with environments, has been growing in the last decades. Ecological or nature-assisted creative and expressive arts therapies tend to constitute an increasingly significant part of the spectrum of contemporary ecotherapeutic methods characterized by an active stance in professionals' and clients' relationship to the environment.

The key presuppositions and theoretical foundation of ecological/nature-assisted arts therapies, a branch of contemporary ecotherapy and the ecological movement at large, have been presented. Though these forms of therapy belong to an established group of mental health professions or specialized therapeutic approaches, they are characterized by a new perspective on health issues and the role of the arts in providing public and planetary health and well-being. Ecological arts therapies have been seen to be supported by such scientific approaches as ecopsychology and ecophilosophy, and they demonstrate a new perspective on our understanding of the therapeutic role of human bonds and forms of environmental activity with nature.

Together with ecotherapy, environmental philosophy, environmental education, as well as the contemporary environmental arts, ecological arts therapies are aligned with the emerging eco-human multidisciplinary approach and the growing field of constructive innovations that can be applied in education, medicine, and the wider social context in order to counteract the environmental crisis. These therapies can also be used to enable a more harmonious co-evolution of human beings and the more-than-human world. The eco-human multidisciplinary approach should be seen as a worldview and a system of eco-human constructive innovations that recognize a synergy between human well-being and the health and ecological integrity of the natural environment. This is a perennial idea that has gained new currency and a sense of urgency in the modern environmental movement, particularly in its "deep ecology" wing.

Such key concepts of ecological expressive therapies as human health and illness, eco-identity formation, nature as the third part in therapeutic relations, the therapeutic setting, and the role of the arts in providing meaningful human connection to nature have been considered from the eco-human perspective, inviting mental health professionals to explore a new vision of the sustainable future and their role in bringing it to fruition. The eco-human approach maintains a rich network of researchers and practitioners who share the goals of creating durable behavior change at multiple levels, promoting an environmental ethic and maintaining harmonious human-nature relationships. Today, this approach as well as the fields of environmental psychology, conservation psychology, and ecopsychology are helping society to form an affirmative response to emerging environmental and natural resource constraints. This is a great challenge, since the response must plan for, motivate, and maintain environmental stewardship behavior through a period of significant energy and resource depletion.

We as humans exist both in the mode of reality and in the mode of possibility; we can choose to shape the world and ourselves in a way that is not yet actual but that is contained potentially in what is already given. This ability is our creative, ecopoietic function, which means shaping the world around us, producing different phenomena and "products," which either support or destroy the environment. We can use our poietic function to move the world of more sustainable living for humans and the more-than-human world, the web of life, from the realm of possibility to the realm of reality, but this transition requires our creative imagination, intention, and activity, together with the living environment.

While our multicultural community is striving to go through this transition, nature-assisted or ecological arts therapies can play a greater role in helping our clients and societies to survive, be healthy, and form an affirmative response to the constraints in the environmental and natural resources that are emerging now and that we will continue to face in the future.

References

Barrows, A. (1995). The Ecopsychology of Child Development. In T. Roszak, M.E. Gomes, & A.D. Kanner (eds), *Ecopsychology: Restoring the Earth, Healing the Mind* (pp.101–110). San Francisco, CA: Sierra Club Books.

Berger, R. (2009). Nature Therapy: Developing a Framework for Practice. A PhD thesis. School of Health and Social Sciences, University of Abertay, Dundee.

Bridges, N.A. (1999). Psychodynamic perspective on therapeutic boundaries. *The Journal of Psychotherapy Practice and Research*, 8(4), 292–300.

Burls, A. (2007). People and green spaces: Promoting public health and mental well-being through eco-therapy. *Journal of Public Mental Health*, 6(3), 24–39.

Case, C. & Dalley, T. (1992). *The Handbook of Art Therapy*. New York, NY: Routledge.

Chalquist, C. (2007). The environmental crisis is a crisis of consciousness: Bringing the psychological dimension into the discussion. Speech delivered at Voices for Change, organized by students at Sonoma State University.

Clinebell, H. (1996). *Ecotherapy: Healing Ourselves, Healing the Earth: A Guide to Ecologically Grounded Personality Theory, Spirituality, Therapy and Education*. Minneapolis, MN: Fortress.

Corbett, L. & Milton, M. (2011). Ecopsychology: A perspective on trauma. *European Journal of Ecopsychology*, 2, 28–47.

De Young, R. (2013). Environmental Psychology Overview. In S.R. Klein & A.H. Huffman (eds), *Green Organizations: Driving Change with IO Psychology* (pp.17–33). New York, NY: Routledge.

Gare, A. (2019). Report on the 19th Annual Gathering on Biosemiotics in Moscow. *Sign Systems Studies*, 47(3/4), 627–640.

Greese, R.E., Kaplan, R., Ryan, R.L., & Buxton, J. (2000). Psychological Benefits of Volunteering in Stewardship Programs. In P.H. Gobster & R.B. Hull (eds), *Restoring Nature: Perspectives from the Social Sciences and Humanities* (pp.265–280). Washington, DC: Island Press.

Halpern, D., Bates, C. Mulgan, G., & Aldridge, S. (2004). *Personal Responsibility and Changing Behavior: The State of Knowledge and its Implications for Public Policy.* London: Cabinet Office.

Heimets, M. (1994). The phenomenon of personalization of the environment. *Journal of Russian and East European Psychology*, 32(3), 24–32.

Kalmanowitz, D. & Lloyd, B. (2005). Inside the Portable Studio: Art Therapy in the Former Yugoslavia 1994–2002. In D. Kalmanowitz & B. Lloyd (eds), *Art Therapy and Political Violence: With Art Without Illusion* (pp.106–125). New York, NY: Routledge.

Kalmanowitz, D. & Lloyd, B. (2011). Inside-Out Outside-In: Found Objects and Portable Studio. In E.G. Levine & S.K. Levine (eds), *Art in Action. Expressive Arts Therapy and Social Change* (pp.104–127). London and Philadelphia, PA: Jessica Kingsley Publishers.

Kanner, A.D. & Gomes, M.E. (1995). The All-Consuming Self. In T. Roszak, M.E. Gomes, & A.D. Kanner (eds), *Ecopsychology: Restoring the Earth, Healing the Mind* (pp.77–91). San Francisco, CA: Sierra Club Books.

Killick, K. (2000). The Art Room as Container in Analytic Art Psychotherapy with Patients in Psychotic States. In A. Gilroy & G. McNeilly (eds), *The Changing Shape of Art Therapy* (pp.99–114). London and Philadelphia, PA: Jessica Kingsley Publishers.

Kopytin, A. (2016). Green Studio: Eco-Perspective on the Therapeutic Setting in Art Therapy. In A. Kopytin & M. Rugh (eds), *Green Studio: Nature and the Arts in Therapy* (pp.3–26). Hauppauge, NY: Nova Science Publishers.

Kopytin, A. (2020). The eco-humanities as a way of coordinating the natural and human being. *Ecopoiesis: Eco-Human Theory and Practice*, 1(1), 6–16.

Kuhn, T. (1962). *The Structure of Scientific Revolutions*. Chicago, IL: The University of Chicago Press.

Laurence, G.A., Fried, Y., & Slowik, L.H. (2013). My space: A moderated mediation model of the effect of architectural and experienced privacy and workspace personalization on emotional exhaustion at work. *Journal of Environmental Psychology*, 36, 144–152.

Levine, S.K. (1992). *Poiesis: The Language of Psychology and the Speech of the Soul.* Toronto: Palmerston Press/Jessica Kingsley Publishers.

Levine, S.K. (2020). Ecopoiesis: Towards a poietic ecology. *Ecopoiesis: Eco-Human Theory and Practice*, 1(1), 17–24.

Linden, S. & Grut, J. (2002). *The Healing Fields: Working with Psychotherapy and Nature to Rebuild Shattered Lives.* Published in Association with the Medical Foundation for the Care of Victims of Torture. London: Frances Lincoln.

Malchiodi, C.A. (2007). *The Art Therapy Sourcebook* (second edition). New York, NY: McGraw-Hill.

Maller, C., Townsend, M., Pryor, A., Brown, P., & St. Leger, L. (2006). Healthy nature healthy people: "Contact with nature" as an upstream health promotion intervention for populations. *Health Promotion International*, 21, 45–54.

McNiff, S. (2015). *Imagination in Action: Secrets for Unleashing Creative Expression.* London and Boston, MA: Shambhala Publications.

Morris, M. (2021). An eco-theology of (post)human animal grace. *Ecopoiesis: Eco-Human Theory and Practice*, 2(1), 12–24. [open access internet journal].

Næss, A. (1989). *Ecology, Community and Lifestyle: Outline of an Ecosophy*. Cambridge: Cambridge University Press.

Næss, A. (2003). The Deep Ecology Movement: Some Philosophical Aspects. In: H. Rolston (ed.), *Environmental Ethics* (pp.112–127). Oxford: Blackwell.

Peterson, C. (2013). Mindfulness-Based Art Therapy: Applications for Healing with Cancer. In L. Rappaport (ed.), *Mindfulness and the Arts Therapies: Theory and Practice* (pp.64–80). London: Jessica Kingsley Publishers.

Roszak, T. (2001). *The Voice of the Earth*. Grand Rapids. MI: Phanes Press.

Sontag, S. (1990). *On Photography*. New York, NY: Straus and Giroux.

Wilson, L. (2001). Symbolism and Art Therapy. In J. Rubin (ed.), *Approaches to Art Therapy: Theory and Technique* (second edition) (pp.40–53). New York, NY: Brunner-Routledge.

Chapter 3

Ecopoiesis: Towards a Poietic Ecology

STEPHEN K. LEVINE

In the age of the Anthropocene, ecological thinking needs to go beyond the opposition between humanity and nature and instead be based on *poiesis*, the human capacity to shape what has been given to us. *Poiesis* is traditionally thought of as referring solely to art-making, but it has the wider significance of shaping the world in response to our needs and, in so doing, shaping ourselves. The western philosophical tradition, based on the search for eternal principles behind changing appearances, is unable to recognize the importance of *poiesis*, which validates the historical nature of sensory experience and the changing forms to which it gives rise. When *poiesis* is restored to its rightful role as a basic human mode of existence, we can formulate an *ecopoietic* approach to ecology, one in which the concept of aesthetic responsibility—the capacity to respond to the world in order to bring about beauty—is central. This perspective has important implications for ecological theory and practice.

Introduction: Philosophy and ecology

Can a philosophy based on *poiesis* contribute to ecological thinking? Does it even make sense to talk of nature as being like a work of art? In order to begin thinking about these questions, we first have to deconstruct the concept of nature itself. Too often, "nature" is understood as a transcendental signifier, something that in its pristine essence underlies all our making and doing. The goal of ecological practice is envisioned as a "return to nature," a doing away with all the depredations which humans have wrought on it. The concept of "wilderness" is a corollary to this way of thinking. From this point of view, wilderness is pure and good, but civilization has ruined it.

In fact, "nature" is always a product of "culture." The two concepts belong together. Moreover, human beings are poietic "by nature"—we are shaping animals. Our instincts are not pre-adapted to our environment, as they are with other creatures. Rather, we must shape the world around us in accordance with our needs. Thus even "wilderness" is what we make by declaring an area to be territory that is off-limits to human use. It is "marked" as such and delimited; often it continues to be affected in accordance with our designs—trails are laid down, controlled burns are set, and so on. "Nature" is something we make, not something we find. We cannot "get back" to nature, but we can shape it in a way that makes sense to us.

Often, however, our shaping does not "make sense," that is, it is not pleasing to the senses. If the need according to which we shape the surrounding world is one of maximizing profit, then we run the risk of making the world "senselessly." Good illustrations of this form of shaping can be seen in the work of Edward Burtnysky, photography that vividly shows the ugliness of our designs.[1]

As we shape the world, moreover, we also shape ourselves. We form our way of life by affecting the world around us. Thus, we draw petroleum from the earth to fuel the cars that we use as transportation. We then become "drivers," beings who move by means of machines that have required fossil fuels to work. It is impossible to overestimate how deeply the automobile has affected our existence. Our whole way of life, our economy as well as our ecology, is based on it. If we ever were to shift to other forms of transportation, we ourselves would become different beings.

What can *poiesis* contribute to ecological thinking? First of all, we must understand what we mean by this term. In Greek, the word *poiesis* means making in general. All forms of production are comprehended by it. At the same time, *poiesis* can also refer to the particular mode of making in which something is made so that it can appear *as* made. The poietic work, what we call "the work of art," shows itself, and in showing itself it shines forth as what it is. This showing manifests itself to the senses. Thus, the statue is meant to be seen, the music to be heard, and

---

1   www.edwardburtynsky.com

so on. The work is sensible; it can only be apprehended by the senses. Beauty, then, can be understood to be the sensible manifestation of appearance.

The traditional philosophical antipathy to the arts is easy to comprehend from this perspective. If philosophy aims to go beyond appearance toward essence, not to the way a thing *seems* to be but to the way it *is*, then *poiesis*, which aims at appearances, can only be an inferior mode of existence. For Plato, the arts deal with the changing world of the senses, whereas philosophy seeks the unchanging object of the intellect. For him, the chaos of sensible appearance is a hindrance to true understanding, based on the unitary essence of unchanging truth. *Poiesis*, then, is seen as the enemy of truth (Plato, 1987, 607e)

From this point onward, what Plato called "the ancient quarrel between poetry and philosophy" is weighted on the side of philosophy (Plato, 1987, 607b). Even in Aristotle's thinking, in which *poiesis* is understood as a kind of knowing (i.e., knowing by making), it is seen to be inferior to *theoria*, the kind of knowing that does not depend on the senses and which can grasp pure form by the intellect alone. In general, the tradition of philosophy either denies *poiesis* any insight into truth or considers it to be subordinate to intellectual understanding.

It is not until Nietzsche that *poiesis* is restored to its central place as our fundamental mode of being and knowing. For Nietzsche, even philosophy is something *made*, and as such can be considered art, in spite of its own self-understanding. Nietzsche's rehabilitation of *poiesis* implies a greater valuation of the sensible world as well. He even accuses the philosophers of a "hatred of the earth" in their attempts to reach a realm of existence beyond the world of the senses. Philosophy's "Being," for Nietzsche, is only another name for what religions call "God"—the eternal principle beyond the ever-changing world of sensible appearance (Nietzsche, 1962).

It is possible to see Heidegger's phenomenological ontology as a continuation of Nietzsche's fundamental project of restoring *poiesis* to the center of human existence. Heidegger's task is to think what is as it appears to us; the opposition between essence and appearance, intellect and sense, being and becoming, is overcome once we give up the idea of an eternal unchanging world behind the world of appearance. Rather, Being *shows* itself; the task of philosophy is to grasp its mode of disclosure (Heidegger, 1962, p.263).

However, the temporal manifestation of truth means that it appears in different ways in different epochs of history. We are historical beings, we live in worlds that are illuminated in different ways at different times. The philosophical understanding of truth as unchanging essence is a mode of disclosure that reveals the world to us in a particular way; but this understanding itself is historical and subject to revision.

In *Being and Time*, Heidegger tries to think the way in which our own existence manifests itself within the perspective of time. At this point in his thinking, Heidegger sees our temporal mode of being revealing itself as what it is not in our everyday ongoing life, in which one moment seems to follow another, and shows itself as what it is only when we are shaken out of our complacency by an experience of dread (angst), an experience in which everyday concerns fade away and we suddenly realize that we will die. If we do not try to escape from this moment of insight but instead grasp our mortality resolutely, then we can choose to exist "authentically," that is, to grasp our possibilities in a way that is proper to our own existence as finite beings (Heidegger, 1962, p.311).

From the beginning, Heidegger's thinking was oriented primarily toward Being; his analytic of existence (*Dasein*) was a way to grasp our own being as a pathway toward the understanding of Being itself. As his thinking developed, however, it underwent a "turning" (*Kehre*) in which he attempted to look directly at the way in which Being is disclosed. In his essay "The origin of the work of art" (1971), Heidegger considered the primary manifestation of Being to take place in the work of art, through *poiesis*. For Heidegger, *poiesis* is understood to be a mode of disclosure proper to finite beings, who live their temporality within a historical horizon. Art does not reveal eternal essences; rather, a work is of its time; indeed, it shapes its time by disclosing possibilities that were previously hidden.

Since art is itself a mode of showing, it is particularly suited to the disclosure of Being, a disclosure that is always historical. The work reveals the world in a new way; it shows the possibilities of our historical existence. At the same time, however, this setting-forth of the world is only accomplished by what Heidegger calls a setting-back into the Earth. There is something in the work that resists manifestation. The work itself is a struggle between World and Earth, between manifestation and hiddenness, a struggle that is put into place in the figure (*Gestalt*) (Heidegger, 1971, pp.63ff.).

Heidegger's concept of "Earth" is difficult to understand, primarily because "Earth" refers to that which resists understanding. In one sense, it refers to the "material" of the work, that out of which the work is made.

However, Heidegger does not intend the opposition between World and Earth to be understood as one between "form" and "matter." Thinking in terms of form and matter implies a violent imposition of a structure on an inchoate material; this kind of thinking is still within the framework of the Will to Power, which, as Nietzsche saw, was the fundamental project of philosophy—to master the world by understanding it.

"Earth," therefore, is not to be understood or mastered, it is that out of which knowing and willing emerge. There will always be something that is unknown in the artwork; this is what makes interpretation both possible and necessary. Nevertheless, an interpretation proper to the work does not seek to go beyond its appearance to an underlying essence; rather, it tries to let what shows itself show itself from itself—to let the work manifest itself more fully. "Earth" is what prevents the work from being subject to a totalizing knowledge; it is also what enables us always to go further in our understanding of the meaning of the work.

Heidegger's thinking of *poiesis* remains to some extent within the tradition of philosophy, even though he aims to deconstruct aesthetics as that tradition has configured it. The works to which Heidegger refers still possess the "aura" which, as philosopher Walter Benjamin tells us, is in decline; they are the "great works" of high culture that the discipline of aesthetics has always prioritized. For the most part, Heidegger is only interested in the works that can change the world, the founding works of a historical epoch that compel us to understand our existence in a fundamentally different way.

Poiesis and aesthetic responsibility

In the field of the expressive arts, as it has been developed at The European Graduate School and elsewhere, the Heideggerean notion of *poiesis* has been extended to apply to other modes of change, both individual and communal. Expressive arts in all their forms (therapy, coaching, education, conflict-transformation and peace-building) rely on an essentially poietic mode of understanding: we shape ourselves by shaping the world. The arts have the special capacity to take us into an imaginal world that enables us to see new possibilities in our daily lives. The role of the change agent, then, is to help others shape this world of the imagination in a way that affects them, that touches, we say, their "effective reality," a notion analogous to H.G. Gadamer's notion of "effective historical reality," the history which affects our understanding of our own existence (Gadamer, 1975, p.267). The sign of this effectiveness lies in what we call the person's "aesthetic response," that sensory-emotional experience which is literally "breath-taking," which makes us stop and compels our attention to what is happening in the moment. It is akin to what Aristotle tells us is the beginning of philosophy: the sense of wonder. It is also, we might say, an experience of beauty.

The responsibility of the change agent is to help the other person find their aesthetic response, that which feels "just right," the "felt sense" of what is needed at the moment. "Aesthetic responsibility," then, is an essential component in all actions that aim to bring about change (Knill, Levine, & Levine, 2005, pp.136–145). Change agents cannot "produce" or "make" change; what they can do is to help others find the possibilities for change and the resources that are needed to accomplish it. Art-making then becomes an analogue for everyday life; we shape our world as we shape our works—and our works are one way we shape our world.

This shaping, again, is not a willful imposition of form on the materials of a life. Rather, it is a letting-be analogous to the ways in which images appear in art-making. Heidegger calls this *Gelassenheit*, letting something show itself as what it is (Heidegger, 1966, p.55ff.). How can the individual or community take what has been given and allow it to find the possibilities proper to it? We cannot escape the historical context in which we exist, but we can act in such a way that we can discover new possibilities for meaning and beauty to emerge.

What would this perspective mean in ecological thought and practice? Can we speak of an "aesthetic responsibility" toward the earth? This would imply that it is our responsibility to shape the world in a way that "makes sense," that is pleasing to the senses, that, we can even say, is beautiful. We have to overcome the traditional opposition in aesthetics between "interest" and "beauty," between what we need and what we value for its intrinsic form. "Beauty," as Stendhal said, "is the promise of happiness" (Stendhal, 1975, p.66). Ecology thus takes place within what Marcuse called the "aesthetic dimension," the world that is manifested to the senses (Marcuse, 1978, p.xxiiff.). It "makes no sense" to think of an "an-aesthetic ecology," a world in which sensible appearance is secondary to instrumental goals. We suffer in such a world, and we make others suffer as well.

A poietic approach to ecology would not begin with an abstract blueprint; "planning" is too often the imposition of an idea on an environment unsuited to it. Rather, we must ask, what does the earth need? What possibilities are contained within our surroundings that can be developed in a way that touches our effective reality? This approach presupposes that there is a fit between the human and the environment, an a priori between what used to be called "man" and "world." Despite all evidence to the contrary, it rejects the notion that a human being is essentially destructive and that the only way to "heal" the environment is to remove it from human concerns, to, in effect, de-humanize it.

Certainly, much of what we have done to the planet has been destructive; we cannot ignore the depredations that we have wrought on the world around us and on the creatures within it, including ourselves. But can we not see this violence as a consequence of our unwillingness to accept our limited place within the world, an attempt to become "masters of the universe," to go beyond our finitude and ascribe unlimited powers to ourselves? The earth then becomes, as Heidegger tells us in his writings on technology, a "standing-reserve" (*Ge-stell*) for human purposes (Heidegger, 1993, p.331ff.). Nature becomes "natural resource," something at our disposal without inherent existence of its own.

We need to deconstruct the opposition between the "natural" and the "human," an opposition which leads to the alternatives of a dream of unlimited control over the earth, on the one hand, and the vision of a nature "pure" from human contact on the other. As finite historical beings, we are "thrown" into a world we have not ourselves made; yet it is within our power to choose those possibilities which exist within this world in order to develop it in a "suitable" way, a way that is fitting for the habitation of finite beings.

This would mean, however, that we would have to acknowledge our own poietic nature, our existence as creatures who shape ourselves by shaping the world around us. It would also mean acknowledging our aesthetic responsibility for the ways in which we shape this world. How can we affect the world in a way that makes sense, a way that is pleasing to the senses, a way, indeed, that brings forth beauty? A poietic ecology would have to take these questions seriously without falling into the trap of a romantic conception of the natural.

The romantic perspective implies a world without the human or, at best, with a humanity that lives in "harmony" with the world without disturbing it. The pastoral image of the shepherd is sometimes used to evoke this: the human who dwells in pastoral simplicity by "tending" what is given to him. The metaphor of "shepherding," however, does not begin to grasp the human situation. We are not shepherds living harmoniously in pastoral simplicity, we are builders and shapers who form both urban and rural communities in which to dwell. We *work* the materials that are given to us; we do not simply receive them. But this does not mean that we can disregard them, that we can simply bend them to our purposes. We are not creator gods; rather we take what is given and *respond* to it. In doing so, we give it a new form—we transform it in accordance with its own possibilities.

There is a truth to the romantic view, however, that we need to pay attention to. The image of nature "in itself," not distorted by human needs to master it, points to the hidden character of "Earth" of which Heidegger speaks. Beyond all our projects, there is something that fundamentally resists our capacity for mastery. "Earth" is what remains beyond our power; at the same time, it reveals itself as capable of transformation in specific ways, depending on the historical period in which we live. This quality of "Earth" shows itself in all our projects; in whatever we do, we encounter the limits of our power. We have to take account of the consequences of our shaping activities; in this sense, there is no "free lunch" in a poietic ecology. No technology, no matter how "sustainable," will be without consequences with which we have to deal—and then the process of shaping will begin again. Of course, this does not mean that we cannot choose between technologies, taking into account both their effectiveness and their destructive potential; but it does imply that there is no technological fix for our environmental concerns, nothing that will provide a "final solution" to our relation to the environment.

Principles of a poietic ecology

What, then, might be the principles of a poietic ecology? The following are some of the perspectives that it could embody:

1. The human being is a shaping animal. We exist by shaping the world around ourselves.
2. In this process, our shaping is a response to what has come before us. We always exist in a particular historical world, and we take the form appropriate to this world.
3. Nevertheless, we are not determined by the world in which we live, nor by the form in which we find ourself at any given time. Rather, we exist in the mode of possibility; we can choose to shape the world and ourselves in a way that is not yet actual but that is contained potentially in what is already given.

4. Human existence is finite. Not only do we come to an end, as all beings do, but we can grasp ourselves *as* finite. This implies that we can respect our limits and recognize that we are not the masters of the world around us, nor even of ourselves.

5. To shape the world in a way that is appropriate to human finitude would mean developing an attitude of *respect for otherness*. "Earth" will always be beyond our power. In this sense, our proper attitude toward it is *awe*.

6. As finite beings, we are in the world in an embodied way. We live in a sensible world, and we experience the world primarily through our senses. This is a receptive capacity, but at the same time it has a shaping aspect to it. We see what we look at, and we look at what engages our attention. Sensing is not passive, but neither is it pure activity – it is a responding to what is there.

7. Sensing has a cognitive capacity; our senses "make sense" of the world. It is not the case, as Kant thought, that the senses are "blind" and that it requires the logical intellect to impose categories on sense data for meaning to emerge. Rather, there is a "pre-formation" of meaning in sensible experience; this provides the material on which the intellect works by developing its potential significance. In English, as in the Romance languages, "sense" means both sensory capacity and significance; the two are not divorced.

8. If we are to live in a world that makes sense, then this world must be appropriate to our senses. It follows that we have a responsibility to shape the world "aesthetically." *Aisthesis*, in its original sense, means pertaining to the senses. Aesthetics, then, refers to the way we sense the world; *poiesis* to the way we shape it according to our senses (i.e., aesthetically). Thus we can say that we have an *aesthetic responsibility* to the world.

9. Beauty is what pleases us aesthetically. It is what touches us through the senses and takes our breath away. The beautiful need not be harmonious and perfect in its form, as traditional aesthetics would have it. Rather beauty, within the framework of a poietic ecology, is understood to emerge from the awe with which we regard the world and the beings within it. A poietic conception of beauty has some of the quality traditionally ascribed to the sublime—that which surpasses our finite capacity to grasp it. Beauty could thus be said to be the apprehension of "Earth" in the world.

10. The arts have a special role to play in this framework. As modes of showing, they can reveal the ways in which we have made the world ugly; they can confront us with our an-aesthetic and destructive acts. At the same time, they can point towards what is possible. In their imaginative explorations, the arts show us what *can be*, not only what *has been*. The vision of beauty provided in art can serve as a guideline for all our shaping acts.

11. To speak of a poietic ecology is to imply that nature can be considered as a work of art. This might be seen to be a romantic attitude, were it not that within this framework, art itself is not understood in terms of the imposition of form on matter, as it is in the traditional ontology that underlies Romanticism without its knowing it. If the work of art is itself a struggle between "World" and "Earth," between revealing and concealing, and if "Earth" is essential to the work as its bearing ground, then to consider nature as a work of art is not to imply mastery over the environment. Rather, this perspective points to a different attitude toward the world around us, one in which we accept our responsibility for shaping the environment in a way that respects its otherness as well as our own capacity for affecting it.

Conclusion: Poietic ecology and environmental practice

The implications of a poietic ecology for environmental practice remain to be worked out. Nevertheless, we can point to many examples where this framework has implicitly been employed. Any time when we see, for example, the development of a landscape that takes into account its natural contours and the particular materials which make it up, we can see a poietic ecology at work. Similarly, when urban redevelopment is designed in terms of the culture of the people involved and their way of life, there is an element of *poiesis* involved.

I am particularly fond, in this context, of Rousseau's image of the contrast between the French and the English garden. The French garden, as he describes it, is developed according to an abstract plan. It has a formal quality which is appropriate to the social position of those for whom it is designed. The English garden, on the other hand, looks wild, as if it has developed "naturally." In fact, it has been carefully tended to, but its shaping has taken into account the "natural" capacities of the land and the plants that can grow there. In Rousseau's eyes, this "natural" chaos is much more beautiful than any "artificial" order. "Nature" here, of course, means not that which is wild and untouched, but that which has been shaped in a way that respects its otherness (Rousseau, 1968, Part IV, Letter XII). Perhaps we should understand Rousseau's concept of "natural man" in the same way: "natural" human beings are the ones who shape themselves in accordance with their own capacity for beauty—in the words of Hölderlin, as quoted by Heidegger, we can "dwell poetically upon the earth" (Heidegger, 1949, p.270).

Human existence is poietic by nature, and nature is what we shape through *poiesis*. If we can accept our responsibility as shaping beings, our aesthetic responsibility, while at the same time respecting the limits of our powers as finite, then perhaps it will make sense to see "nature" as the work of art that it always has been. And then, perhaps, we can honor the earth, for in our relation to it, to paraphrase St. Paul, "...we live and move and have our being" (Acts 17:28).

References

Gadamer, H.G. (1975). *Truth and Method*. New York, NY: The Seabury Press.

Heidegger, M. (1949). *Hölderlin and the Essence of Poetry: Existence and Being*. Chicago, IL: Henry Regnary Company.

Heidegger, M. (1962). *Being and Time*. New York, NY: Harper & Brothers.

Heidegger, M. (1966). *Discourse on Thinking*. New York, NY: Harper & Row.

Heidegger, M. (1971). The origin of the work of art. *Poetry, Language, Thought*. New York, NY: Harper & Row.

Heidegger, M. (1993). *The Question Concerning Technology: Basic Writings*. New York, NY: HarperCollins.

Knill, P.J., Levine, E.G., & Levine, S.K. (2005). *Principles and Practice of Expressive Arts Therapy: Toward a Therapeutic Aesthetics*. London and Philadelphia, PA: Jessica Kingsley Publishers.

Marcuse, H. (1978). *The Aesthetic Dimension: Toward a Critique of Marxist Aesthetics*. Boston, MA: Beacon Press.

Nietzsche, F. (1962). *Thus Spoke Zarathustra*. Baltimore, MD: Penguin Books.

Plato (1987). *The Republic*. London: Penguin.

Rousseau, J.J. (1968). *Julie, or the New Eloise*. University Park, PA: Pennsylvania State University Press.

Stendhal (1975). *Love*. London: Penguin.

Chapter 4

The Role of Attention in Expressive Art and Nature-Based Healing

MADELINE M. RUGH

Introduction

Therapists of any persuasion, including expressive arts therapists, need to first experience and understand how our attentional patterns are affecting our experience of the world. If we seek to incorporate "nature" into our therapeutic practices without this critical awareness, our work may devolve into use-based "techniques" without touching deeper levels of cultural healing that our western mind requires.

> Attention...is not just another "cognitive function"—it is actually nothing less than the way in which we relate to the world. And it doesn't just dictate the kind of relationship we have...it dictates what it is that we come to have a relationship with, changes what kind of thing comes into being for us: in that way it changes the world. (McGilchrist, 2019, pp.13, 28)

The "world-changing" type of attention described by Iain McGilchrist (2019) is what is required of us now for true healing to take place with people and planet. Nothing less will provide the health and wholeness we so crave. The Earth (people and the planet) needs us to *heal our minds* in order to restore our health, which is also her (the Earth's) health. Therapy, in this context, could be understood from the Greek origin of the word, meaning to "attend": attending in a new way, specifically for the western Eurocentric mind. What I am calling a "new way" is actually an old way which has remained intact for most Indigenous cultures of this planet, whose wisdom and understanding of our coherence with the living world is a healing salve, providing a template for recognizing when we are in relationship and harmony.

Expressive therapists have an advantage and an especially close affinity to nature-based therapy due to their understanding and application of non-verbal modalities. The expressive arts provide learning and healing in ways which are mirrored in the beauty and forms of nature: colors, sounds, shapes, textures, and movements, the language of a living world. The characteristics and qualities of the expressive arts, then, are already in alignment with the voice of the myriad and marvelous beings of this world. However, our training in traditional concepts (and thus perceptions) of western psychology may subtly derail our knowing and trust in the processes of creation, connection, and imagination called for when attending to both our inner and outer nature. For those of us bringing nature into our practice in a heartfelt way, we will need to look for the incongruities in traditional therapeutic behaviors and expectations when attempting to connect with the more-than-human world. How we "language" our work with nature and therapy is one incongruity I wish to call attention to (no pun intended!) in this chapter. For example, current and very important research on the therapeutic qualities of the natural world is couched in an unspoken word: *use*. Seeking to "use" nature for our therapy without reciprocity or recognition of our interconnection and coherence with all that lives will not bring us or the planet to the place of integration and wholeness that is the hallmark of therapy and health. However, it needs to be noted that most expressive therapists who are currently working with nature, as well as eco-therapists in general, orient to the living world with the intention to connect, to recognize our belonging, and to establish a reciprocal relationship.

Another incongruity from my perspective is, paradoxically, the over-reliance on "seeing" or vision as our primary attentional modality. When engaging and listening in a heart-centered way with the life of other beings of the world we access the felt level or heart-based perception. This kind of seeing with the "eye of the heart" will be addressed later in this chapter, but for the moment let me say the felt capacity of the heart contains emotion but is much more than emotional. So, it is not "seeing" that is the problem; rather, it is the *way* we see that limits or reinforces our preconceived ideas about nature. Our seeing has been sequestered by a deeply ingrained cultural attitude of use, of nature as a backdrop to our dramas, of nature not being sentient and subjective, which means we do not see at all...or superficially at best.

> ...our relation to the earthly world is that of spectators looking at a kind of spectacle, it ensures that there is no real reciprocity between the perceiver and the perceived, no real affinity between humankind and the rest of the earth. (Abram in Sewall, 1999, p.xv)

The third incongruity, briefly addressed earlier, is embedded in the use of the word "therapy" and nature. For many people, the word therapy signals a way of relating that is often a code word for those suffering from mental or emotional illness. It implies you must have something "wrong" with you to participate. The word "therapy" somehow boxes in the mystery of relating to the sacred dimensions of life and the multidimensional complexities of the more-than-human world. It is a "safe" and familiar word, letting us feel productive and purposeful. It potentially participates in *use* as we are using nature for our therapy. It also has the quality of *doing* something in nature rather than *being* with nature. One way in which I have tempered this dilemma is to hold it within its original Greek meaning, to attend, and thus giving or offering our attention to a person or place. Perceptual psychologist Laura Sewall (1999) recommends employing the word "offering" our attention rather than the more common "paying" attention. For me, this small shift creates a spaciousness, an open, heartful way for being present to a person or a plant with fewer preconceived expectations.

As has been noted, the "incongruities" that might compromise our healing efforts are almost all language based, which is to say these seemingly small words—use, see, therapy—embody and sustain our perceptual worldview of the isolated, "rugged" individual rather than a human who is aware of our interdependence.

In this chapter, I am indebted to the many wonderful ecotherapy clinicians, educators, artists, and arts therapists who already understand the issue with the western mind and the worldview healing that is required. Simply stated by psychotherapist Sarah Conn, "Our task is to open ourselves to the presence of the more-than-human world" (Buzzell & Chalquist, 2009, p.112). My hope is that the ideas presented here will alert therapists, helpers, and guides to the need to refine our own nature-connected work and to recognize the subtlety and pervasiveness with which our western sense of separation operates.

The sources of my thinking for this chapter are based on direct personal experience with an animate living world from early childhood, and on the integration of ideas offered by many thoughtful writers and researchers in the areas of ecology, art, and healing. In the remainder of this chapter, I will elaborate on some of the ideas and "incongruities" presented in this introduction to serve as a rudimentary guide into a "world-changing" and "word-changing" shift in the quality of our attention and presence.

Attention and western psychology

According to Laura Sewall (1999) western theories of attention are concerned with what it is and how it works. The phenomenology of attention is a different matter (p.98). In modern psychology, attention is defined as *the ability to choose and concentrate on relevant stimuli*. Attention is the cognitive process that makes it possible to position ourselves toward a *relevant* stimulus and consequently respond to it. This very important cognitive ability is an essential function in our daily lives. Luckily, attention can be trained and improved with the appropriate cognitive training. Psychology recognizes four major types of attention beyond the initial state of arousal. Arousal refers to level of alertness, whether we are tired or energized.

1. Focused attention: the ability to focus attention on a stimulus.
2. Sustained attention: the ability to attend to a stimulus or activity over a long period of time.
3. Selective attention: the ability to attend to a specific stimulus or activity in the presence of other distracting stimuli.
4. Alternating attention: the ability to change focus (attention) between two or more stimuli, also referred to as divided attention or multitasking.

We use attention in our daily lives in a countless number of tasks. From the time we wake up to when we go to bed, we are constantly using these different types of attention (Kendra, 2021). I would like to remind the reader of Iain McGilchrist's statement in the introduction of this chapter (2019, p.5). Working from a phenomenological orientation to attention, he states that attention is no mere cognitive function: it is a worldview, it is how we view and create the world we experience. It is important to juxtapose this awareness with the usual ways in which the "cognitive faculty" of attention is treated in a western science context, as evidenced in the description above.

Many years ago, I was listening to an audio recording by professor of religion and Asian studies Rick Jarrow on a subject matter not related to attention. I have never forgotten his statement, however, which I am paraphrasing here as: "Attention is our most valuable asset—everybody and everything wants it: television commercials, online ads, politicians, students, children, bosses, partners and pets." I felt the deep truth of this statement and wondered frequently about the effects of the demand for my attention on me. I wondered, what exactly is my ability to attend? Who or what is attending? What happens when my attention is constantly sequestered by others? What does it mean to "attend" in the first place? What is the effect of "my" attention on others, including the other-than-humans of the living world? Recent research amplifies the significance of Jarrow's statement in the following quote:

> The unique role of attention has also been recognized in the new digital technologies of the modern "attention economy", in which the human gaze is increasingly being monetized and mined as a resource, again pointing to its central position in the landscape of the twenty-first century. (Tweedy in McGilchrist, 2019, p.x)

Not only is the human gaze (attention) being "mined" and "monetized" but the imagistic content of our inner world and imagination have been sequestered and colonized. We no longer have genuine access to, nor do we honor, our naturally arising inner images. I believe our inner images (dreams, art, imaginings) are intimately connected to nature, so the lack of access and honor is highly problematic. Expressive arts therapists represent a force for the protection and preservation of this wilderness of inner images and imaginings, usually called the unconscious. According to depth psychologist Robert Romanyshyn (1997):

> What we call the unconscious is the many faceted consciousness of creation. The unconscious needs to be re-imagined as the consciousness of animals and plants, minerals and stars, of angels and atoms. The unconscious needs to be freed from the notion that it describes

our ignorance about ourselves and re-imagined as the epiphany of other kinds of consciousness. (pp.168–169)

This is a radical thought, one worth adding to our reflections as expressive therapists for whom the image is almost always the domain of individual psychology rather than a potential threshold for communion and communication with the living world.

Many of the studies documenting the healing and healthful attributes of nature have noted the effectiveness of the natural world to restore our capacity to "attend," both in adults under the duress and stress of overly focused attention and in children diagnosed with attention deficit disorder or attention deficit hyperactivity disorder (Louv, 2005).

In the following section I will briefly explore two exemplary kinds of research that highlight nature-based healing.

Nature-based health and healing research

According to research that began in earnest in the 1980s and gained momentum through to the present moment, natural environments have the capacity to restore our attention, improve our performance on tasks, and build our resistance to and recovery from stressful life events (please note that these are all instrumental "use"-based outcomes). There are long lists of benefits, including faster recovery from illness, reduced pain and anxiety, reduced stress, and fewer stress-related emotional and physical conditions. Individuals who want to know more can find a wealth of studies online. There is no question about the efficacy of nature in human health and well-being. For the purposes of this chapter, I will limit my writing to a closer look at two contrasting models that have been in the popular media recently: Kaplan & Kaplan's (ART) (see Ackerman, 2020) attention restoration theory and forest therapy or forest bathing from Japan.

With the notable exception of forest therapy, the implications of these investigations in nature-assisted therapy do not involve connecting or communicating with nature: rather the focus is on "using" nature to help us feel better. Which is good! Not bad, just not enough given the deeper need in our culture to change our worldview and the attentional patterns that sustain it.

ART has as its central observation the negative consequences of continued engagement of "focused or directed" attention and fatigue affecting our ability to solve problems with the possibility of making critical life-threatening errors in work such as that of first responders or emergency medical personnel.

Kaplan and Kaplan suggest that the natural environment can help resolve health problems of modern people's daily lives caused by focused attentional stress and subsequent fatigue. Kaplan and Kaplan also emphasize stress relief and restoration of "directed" attention in healthy adults. But what does this mean? To what are we restoring attention, for what use? More business (or busyness) as usual? Directed or focused attention is certainly an important skill for noticing and thus responding to the natural world; however, its use here may be more related to being able to get back to our grueling stress-filled jobs and still focus. I am suggesting that this is both important and not enough. For example, challenging the way in which we work-to-live following an industrial model might be more therapeutic than helping us stay "adjusted" to it.

Kaplan and Kaplan propose that there are four states of attention that adults experience as they move toward restoration of "focused" or directed attention (Ackerman, 2020):

1. *Clearer head:* thoughts, concerns, worries from whatever was demanding one's attention are allowed to pass through the mind and fade away.

2. *Mental fatigue recovery:* focused or directed attention makes it easy to feel depleted and drained. This stage allows directed attention to recover and be restored to normal levels.

3. *Soft fascination:* nature allows the individual to be gently distracted and engaged in a low-stimulation activity (viewing or being in nature), which reduces the internal noise and provides a quiet internal space to relax.

4. *Reflection and restoration:* evoked by spending a long period of time in an environment that meets all four of the requirements of a restorative environment; being away, soft fascination, extent, and compatibility. The individual is then able to relax, restore their attention, and reflect on their life.

Two of these areas are of special consideration in this chapter: extent and compatibility both indicate that the environment must not have unexpected features, it must be familiar. Total familiarity with a living, moving, changing environment is a desire and function of the left hemisphere of the brain, which I will describe shortly. But suffice it to say, one would need to establish this "familiarity and friendship" *first* through right hemisphere orientation. The demands that the environment be a particular way highlights for me the emphasis on the primacy of human need, not on relating to nature. This is evidenced when Kaplan and Kaplan note six other dimensions of compatibility:

1. *Distraction:* the environment should not be distracting or stimulating.
2. *Deficit of information:* the individual should already have all the information needed to understand and enjoy the environment.
3. *Danger:* the environment cannot be dangerous in any sense of the word.
4. *Duty:* the individual should not feel drawn to the environment out of a sense of duty or responsibility.
5. *Deception:* the individual should not be experiencing a discrepancy between the task they are doing and their true feelings about it.
6. *Difficulty:* the environment must not be one in which individuals need to prepare for or anticipate difficult situations to navigate.

I would like to contrast this model with the perspective of forest therapy originating in Japan. Forest therapy is a research-based framework for supporting healing and wellness through immersion in forests and other natural environments. Forest therapy is inspired by the Japanese practice of shinrin-yoku, which translates to "forest bathing." Studies have demonstrated a wide array of health benefits, especially in the cardiovascular and immune systems, and for stabilizing and improving mood and cognition (Park *et al.*, 2010). Forest therapy builds on those benefits and looks beyond, to what happens when people remember that we are a part of nature, not separate from it, and are related to all other beings in fundamental ways.[1]

Researchers Kyung Hee Oh, Won So Shin, Tae Gyu Khil, and Dong Jun Kim identified a six-step process model for nature-based therapy (2020). Their study involved 180 self-reported essays on "forest therapy experiences" submitted to the Korea Forest Service. Results revealed that the healing attributes of a nature-based therapy process contained six steps: stimulation, acceptance, purification, insight, recharging, and

---

[1]   www.natureandforesttherapy.earth

change. When in the natural environment, participants first experienced positive emotional change, followed by cognitive and behavioral changes. This study revealed that the nature-based therapy process did not consist of just a single element or step but involved an integrated way of healing with emotional and cognitive changes.

The six steps were defined as follows. Please note, I have italicized statements that stand in profound contrast to western studies such as ART:

1. *Stimulation:* on visiting the forest, participants felt better and refreshed by five sensory effects of the forest. They also experienced emotions such as happiness, fascination, curiosity, and joy. *Their senses and sensibilities were recovered.* Participants who had experienced such positive stimulation tended to visit natural environments more actively and frequently. Therefore, the *experience of positive stimulation* in the natural environment is an important starting point for healing and change.

2. *Acceptance:* in this stage, participants experienced receptive feelings in the forest, including the sense of consolation and comportment. The forest was a place where participants could rest and relax at any time. *Participants felt that the forest accepted everything about them. They felt consolation and comfort in the forest as if they were in their mother's arms. Their tiring and exhausting lives were relieved when they communicated emotionally with the nature.* Their minds were opened.

3. *Purification:* in this stage, participants overcame and dissolved their negative feelings. They vented and released their negative energy in a quiet forest. Their minds and emotions were then lightened and cleansed. This led them to experience relief from stress. Their pain and anger then disappeared. They also forgot worries while they walked through the forest. They could honestly recognize their own feelings of avoidance in the tranquil forest alone. *They confided stories from their heart that they usually could not tell others. They communicated with nature, emptying and washing away their mind and emotions. They became relaxed and generous so they could afford to look back and reflect on themselves.*

4. *Insight:* this is the most important and meaningful stage in the nature-based therapy process. Participants experienced awakening through self-reflection and meditation in nature. They then communicated with themselves and talked with their inner self.

They knew what they really wanted. They found a new way of life. They regained their identity. They also discovered the meaning and purpose of their life and reinterpreted the meaning of their pain. The most important phenomenon at this stage was "change of thought". Participants could make a choice for new life through "change of thought." Factors that can promote insight in nature are survival methods of animals and plants, strong vitality, and the order of nature.

5. *Recharging:* the forest filled participants with positive energy, such as hope, courage, and confidence. Recharging involved both psychological and physiological aspects. *In the natural environment, participants developed the will and desire for life.* Hope, courage, confidence, and positive thoughts became energy that could overcome difficulty and create a new life. Recharged with positive energy, participants could go back into the world they were once afraid of and avoided.

6. *Change:* participants could now live a life with changes such as relationship restoration, re-employment, advancement, new challenges, and accomplishments. In addition, the value of life could be changed. They described having a more positive attitude, leading to a satisfying life. These changes ultimately led to self-realization.

There are some similarities with ART, highlighting the power of nature in stress relief and fatigue recovery. However, the role and nature of attention is considerably expanded in forest therapy, and there is a strong element of relationality and reciprocity. One reason for these important differences in results may be related to the research method but also to the history of Shinto as a spiritual practice in Japan. Shinto recognizes that all life is ensouled, every life form is alive and aware: it is an animistic orientation. Having a cultural history in Shinto may have prepared the participants for an attentional worldview pattern that was open to experiencing nature in a deeper more spiritual way rather than an instrumental way evident in western studies. The statements that I italicized are significant in addressing the healing of our western fragmented and alienated attentional patterns. For example, the emphasis in stimulation of the senses and restoration of sensory sensitivity rather than restoration of directed attention as a cognitive function. The indication that people returned to nature on their own with more frequency suggests a sense of attachment and caring. Probably the most striking element for me was the feeling of being accepted by the forest—this is transformational territory. Statements were made such as: "The forest accepted everything about them and it felt as if they were in their mother's arms." In the area of "purification," "they confided stories from their heart that they usually could not tell others," they "communicated with nature," all of this leading to deeper inner-self-reflection and finally to a transformed life. Now that's healing and health! But it is clear that the way in which these participants spontaneously attended to and participated with the living world made all the difference.

Comparing these two studies helps to demonstrate how our attentional models are guided by our culture and the need for western people to expand attention and be open to these deeper relational and reciprocal potentials of the living world. Do we know how to do this? Certainly, applying the expressive therapies to nature-guided work is a powerful mechanism for attentional change that incorporates seeing and the senses in abundance, with excellent examples from publications on ecotherapy (Burns, 1998; Buzzell & Chalquist, 2009) and on expressive arts and nature-based healing (Atkins & Snyder, 2017; Kopytin & Rugh, 2017). Perhaps our therapeutic training in learning how to attend to our clients contains an overlooked and highly relevant element, which will be examined next.

Attention and therapeutic training

Attention of the finest quality is the fundamental instrument of the therapist. Given its basic importance, it is thus quite astonishing that so little explicit discussion of attention is to be found in the clinical literature (Speeth, 2003, p.83). Gurdjieff scholar Kathleen Speeth, practiced in many esoteric traditions, and a licensed psychotherapist, describes the training of counselors and therapists as focusing on all manner of "attentional maneuvers." This includes maintaining unconditional positive regard; monitoring countertransference; being authentic; establishing and maintaining rapport; and sustaining sensitive contact regardless of subject matter, emotional tone, or context. Without further training, such requirements are about as easy to follow as the esoteric "Love thy neighbor as thyself" (Speeth, 2003, pp.83–84). Dr. Speeth goes on to say that most sacred traditions have very clear and systematic practices in "taming and mastering" human attention through meditation and prayer. Psychotherapy training does not, as evidenced in the earlier description of the four types of attention.

In therapeutic encounters, the attentional pattern can be understood best as a two-way process in which we move from outer focused awareness of the client (body postures, eye contact, words, breathing) to inner focused "proprioceptive" awareness and responses of our own sensations, feelings, thoughts, and so on. In addition to the focused attentional domain, there can be a shift to panoramic attention (called "splatter vision" by professional trackers). This kind of attention takes in the whole sensory realm and experience of the therapeutic encounter equally. Attention then shifts from inner/outer focused to panoramic.

There is also a third kind of attention, a form of "meta" awareness which has strong spiritual roots. Speeth refers to this as witness consciousness— our ability to be aware that we are aware. Speeth imagines these three attentional capacities as an equilateral triangle with the witness at the top and a continuum of narrow (focused or directed) attention to panoramic (unspecified broad and contextual) forming the base. These two major types of attention (focused and panoramic) also form the matrix for the research by Iain McGilchrist on the attentional worldview patterns of the hemispheres in the brain, which I will discuss shortly.

Another form of attentional training described by Speeth is the ability to deeply identify with a client in order to more fully comprehend their inner world and experience. This is an empathic attentional function that requires letting go of our own identity temporarily though not completely. It is also a shamanic practice within which there are specific requirements for not abandoning one's sense of self totally. These kinds of merger technologies are ancient. Recent utilization of them comes in relation to work with animals, especially horses, and is referred to as "joining up." Identification with other animals, plants, trees, land, water, and mountains is a powerful way of coming into relation but holds the discernment issue of anthropomorphic projection versus direct reception of the Other. This way of non-anthropomorphic receiving is guided by the perception of the heart.

Attention of the heart: Himma

Himma is an Islamic word popularized by the work of Islamic scholar Henry Corbin: it means "spiritual perception of the heart". In most Indigenous and world spiritual traditions, the heart is the center of being (not the head) and is a source of communion with the real but invisible sacred realms of spirit. Recent research especially from the HeartMath Institute and the new field of neuro-cardiology has recognized that the heart is an *organ of perception*: a brain with neurons, neurotransmitters, and hormones. The heart has a memory separate from the brain—it feels, thinks, and knows; it is an attentional organ. The heart's electromagnetic field is five thousand times stronger than that of the brain. With each pulse, especially the space between each pulse referred to as heart rate variability (HRV), information is gathered and shared from the living world and from within the person.

When the fluctuating electromagnetic field of our heart touches another field—whether from a person, rock, or plant—we feel a range of impressions from our experience of the information encoded within those organisms: electromagnetic fields. This is, in fact, the source of the deep feelings that come from our immersion in wild landscapes. This kind of information exchange is embedded deeply within our cellular memories. We are made for the nature of each thing to pass into us through our hearts, which thinks about it, stores memories about it, and engages in dialogue with it (Buhner, 2004, p.94).

Buhner further suggests that asking the beings of the more-than-human realm how they feel draws your attention into the heart as the locus of awareness and communion. The awareness of the heart plays a crucial role in opening to the living world. It is the organ designed to do just that. When we speak of the heart as an organ of perception, of seeing and sensing, of knowing and remembering we are clearly not talking just about emotion. Feeling is another word we need to be mindful of as it is often confused with emotion. They are not the same. I can "feel" hungry but that is not an emotion, or I can "feel" angry, and that is an emotion. The use of the word "feel," then, should be understood to encompass emotion but is much more than emotion. The felt experience is the language of the heart and the "gregarious" body as David Abram (1996) poetically describes our bodies' enthusiastic participation in nature through the senses and the heart.

Our western attention has been sequestered by an obsession with the cranial brain with very little awareness of the heart as a brain and a perceptual organ. I will briefly highlight the research of Iain McGilchrist, a psychiatrist whose work, *The Master and His Emissary* (2009), explores the nature of the hemispheres of the brain beyond the usual descriptions, coming to a profound conclusion very relevant to our exploration of attention.

Attention and the brain

Tweedy in McGilchrist (2019, p.x) states, "I am my attention," indicating the depth of meaning this word implies. According to McGilchrist, the kind of attention we give to nature and life in general is directly related to the orientation of the two hemispheres of our brain. This is not about the former ideas of hemispheric functions (left—language, right—emotion), which is inaccurate as both hemispheres are involved in emotion and language (for example). Rather, his research has highlighted a surprising and profound understanding of hemispheric differences; that each hemisphere specializes in a particular "worldview." The hemispheres embody two "discrete" and "distinct" modes of attention that can be understood at their most basic level as "focused" and "panoramic," similar to Speeth's description of therapeutic attention. Our western industrialized culture has developed a significant over-emphasis on the worldview of the left hemisphere, while actively thwarting the presence and expression of the right. The hemispheres are both important but not equal. The left should depend on the wholistic contextualized empathic worldview of the right, but as in the story of the Master (right hemisphere) and his Emissary (the left hemisphere), the left has usurped the role of master.

Albert Einstein encapsulated this truth when he called *the intuitive or metaphoric mind a sacred gift and the rational mind a faithful servant* (Samples, 1976). We have created a society that honors the servant and has forgotten the gift.

McGilchrist provides a simple explanation about how the two modes of attention function effectively in the split brain of a bird. Birds pay narrow focused attention to the seeds in gravel with the right eye (left hemisphere) while keeping their left eye (right hemisphere) open with panoramic attention for predators. They use their left eye (right hemisphere) when seeking relationships for mating and nesting. A summarized and greatly oversimplified list of the attentional qualities of each hemisphere will further our understanding of this vital piece of information.

The left hemisphere is overly optimistic in its self-appraisal, unaware of its limits and thinks it knows it all, can "go it alone," is in denial of its shortcomings, and disinclined to change its mind. It is the source of the "inner voice" that harangues us. It doesn't trust, so emphasis is on self-protection, paranoia, and isolation. It operates in a closed loop, rehashing and replaying out old but familiar patterns. It sees the human body and the natural world as discrete pieces and parts. It favors fixed perspectives and directed, focused attention and needs to be in control.

It is abstract and mechanical and generalizes things into categories. It is better attuned to tools, especially tools and things it has made. It sees things as flat (like a computer screen) and detached from us. Living presences are no longer accessible to this form of attention, and meaning is mainly related to how something can be used.

The right hemisphere enables us to see ourselves connected to and, in the human case, to empathize with, whatever is other than ourselves. The right hemisphere has no voice; rather, it operates through the felt level and images. It is wholistic, sees the big picture, is contextual, compassionate, and empathic. All experiences come through the right hemisphere first, received in their fullness without bias and are only dealt with by the left after they have become familiar. It is better at making connections between things, sees things as wholes, and works from whole-body awareness. The right hemisphere experiences and expresses self-doubt, wonders, and sees the world of humans and nature as a net of interdependencies (McGilchrist, 2019, pp.24–25).

McGilchrist believes that we have built a world in western culture that is an extension of the left hemisphere and its worldview in which nature is something we use for our benefit, not something we exist within or relate to. The study by Kaplan & Kaplan, for example, suggested that the environment has to be familiar in order to help restore focused attention...AND...focused attention belongs primarily to the left hemisphere so it is very clear that these studies will not support or encourage a relationship with nature.

The essential difference between right and left hemisphere is that the right pays attention to the Other: to whatever it is that exists apart from ourselves with which it sees itself in profound relation. It is deeply attracted to and given life by relationships, the betweenness that exists with the Other. By contrast, the left pays attention to the virtual world that it has created which is self-consistent and self-contained, ultimately disconnected from the Other, making it powerful and also impotent as a closed loop, only able to operate on and to know itself through the things it has made (McGilchrist, 2019, p.23).

Attention: Seeing, sensing, and the expressive arts

John Berger (in Sewall, 1999, p.135), author of *Ways of Seeing*, stated that "visually everything is interdependence." In the world of visual art education there are three main drawing (seeing) practices that are commonly taught with forms of hand-eye listening: contour drawing, gesture drawing, and negative space drawing. I learned each of these methods in my early training as a visual artist and remember their effect on me. I recognized them as forms of sacred practice, of visual mindfulness and meditation. As Berger states (in Sewall, 1999), it prepared me (or reinforced in me the already existing tendency) to see connections, to see in a relational way as opposed to the current cultural malaise of seeing nature as discrete objects for our use and exploitation—a left-hemisphere dominance effect.

As expressive arts-based healers and helpers we are neither surprised by nor resistant to perceiving interconnections between people and the myriad expressions of life. This chapter is an attempt to bring our full attention to what our discipline may take for granted or may have lost in our educational training, which relies heavily on western psychology and gives little or no attention to the rest of the world in descriptions of human health and development.

Though most expressive therapists may be very familiar with contour drawing, gesture drawing and negative space drawing, I would like to briefly explain for the non-visual arts readers what each of these ways of seeing entails so that music, dance, and drama practitioners may see their own connections.

Contour drawing, often referred to as blind contour, involves slow and tender attention to the "outlines" and "in-lines" or contours in and around a form. Blind contour means you rarely look at your paper but keep your eye and hand holding a pencil or pen in slow motion, not unlike a seismograph needle recording subtle vibrational shifts in the Earth's crust. Gesture drawing is a specialty of the sumi-e tradition of Japanese ink and brush artists: it involves hours of open-hearted present-centered observation similar to contour drawing but seeking to take into your heart the essence or spirit of the land, a bird, or a tree. Then, in a sudden quick explosion of brush and ink, you depict your relationship and the inner sense of spirit expressed in its outward form in nature. Negative space drawing involves noticing the shape of the space between objects and drawing that space as shape. For me, this method has always been the most exciting. What we think of in our culture as nothing—empty space—actually forms the so-called solid objects which are usually the sole focus of our attention.

These three methods of seeing/drawing, especially negative space, hark back to Berger's statement that "visually everything is interdependence." I would like to push this recognition that we as visual artists are trained for perceiving relationships a little further, with one more critical recognition if we are to engage the living world in healing and helpful ways.

Attention and the senses

*Those of us conditioned by western values tend to bring little aware-
ness to the exchange between ourselves and our surroundings. We
seldom consider the degree to which belief and consciousness shift
and determine our particular way of seeing, or the way in which
perception is a shared flux of fire, emanating from both sunlight and
soul...to envision the act of seeing as the marriage between viewer
and viewed to be woven into the fabric of a shifting field of light, of
energy, beauty and all that one may lay eyes upon.*

Sewall, 1999, pp.58–59

When we gaze at another being or form with an open heart and welcoming eye, seeing is not just me looking at you or "it" (never an "it"!), but is
actually reciprocal! "Vision is a deeply reciprocal event, a participatory
activity in which both the seer and the seen are dynamic players. To
see is to interact with the visible, *to act and be acted upon*" (Abram in
Sewall, 1999, p.xv). It is to shake up this *very* entrenched notion that we
are the sole actors in perception of the Others which are "out there,"
separate from us, static objects that we then perceive by turning our
attention to "it". Seeing it, naming it, then moving on to "see" something
else is erroneous at best and one primary source for maintaining our
pathological sense of alienation and disconnect from the living world
(clearly left hemisphere in outlook). "Nature is something we look *at*,
not something we are *in* and *of*" (Abram in Sewall, 1999, p.xvi).

As expressive therapists interested in joining the natural world as
a therapeutic act, we must understand the reciprocal nature of seeing
and attention, and practice ways of experiencing the truth of it. David
Abram, in his book *The Spell of the Sensuous* (1996), states:

My senses connect up with each other in the things I perceive, rather
each perceived thing gathers my senses together in a coherent way, and it
is this that enables me to experience the thing itself as a center of forces,
as another nexus of experience, as an Other. (p.62)

Our senses and acts of perception belong not to us alone but exist
between ourselves and the Others. If a stone catches my attention, I
need to realize that it called and I respond with my gregarious body and
heart. To experience this is a profound revelation that once embraced,

alerts you to your permeability and allows you to take your place in the family of all beings.

Looking at the example of Barbara McClintock, a famous cytogeneticist who won the Nobel prize for her work with corn chromosomes, we see all our attentional possibilities for restoring our connection with a living world in action: perception of the heart, right-hemisphere attention, identification or joining up, the role of the senses, and seeing, and the left hemisphere taking its proper role in support of these other capacities of engaging and knowing.

The scientific community is still very much attached to linear, reductionistic, hyper-rational ideas of the world, for a study to be valid then, it must be "objective". McClintock, on the other hand, employed a deeply personal method of cognition thoughtfully relating to the "other" (in this case corn genome) with friendly curiosity and heart-felt imagination. Her method of conducting research actually involved relating to the corn genome which allowed her the ability to listen and learn at a remarkably "subjective" level. Though her results remain dynamic and valid to this day, her "method" of study rendered her and her results suspect and she was actively shunned. The rejection and censorship of McClintock may reflect the consequences of left-hemisphere dominance and what Buhner calls "perceptual sensory gating": "You must not extend awareness further than your culture wants it to go...you must not experience the metaphysical background of the world..." (Buhner, 2014, p.44).

In describing her process, McClintock stated:

> First, you must learn to see and have the time to look, the patience to hear what the material has to say to you, the openness to let it come to you and above all, one must have a feeling for the organism... The more I worked with the chromosomes the bigger and bigger they got, and when I was really working with them I wasn't outside, I was down there, part of the system, right down there with them and these were my friends. Seeing without the feeling of caring, without an empathic feeling sense of the thing observed, is merely looking. (Buhner, 2014, pp.324–327)

Concluding thoughts

What might happen if we, as counselors and expressive therapists, set an intention to approach the natural world with the same kind of attention we give to a client, as described by Speeth? What might be the response from the natural world if given unconditional attention of the heart? Do we already, as trained therapists, possess the right-hemispheric attentional skills to recognize and experience our belonging? If we do, then do we need to consciously acknowledge our training in relational sensitivity, supporting the more active expression of the right-hemisphere worldview?

In a world that has become increasingly dominated by one particular mode of attention, one rooted in and promoted by the left hemisphere of the brain, if we consciously alter our habitual mode of attention to one based on a more integrated, empathic, relational, and embodied sense of relationship, it could have dramatic, perhaps even revolutionary, consequences (McGilchrist, 2019, p.xi).

References

Abram, D. (1996). *The Spell of the Sensuous*. New York, NY: Vintage Books.

Ackerman, C.E. (November 9, 2020). *What is Kaplan's Attention Restoration Theory (ART)?* https://positivepsychology.com/attention-restoration-theory.

Atkins, S. & Snyder, M. (2017). *Nature-Based Expressive Arts Therapy: Integrating the Expressive Arts and Eco-Therapy*. London and Philadelphia, PA: Jessica Kingsley Publishers.

Buhner, S.H. (2004). *The Secret Teachings of Plants: The Intelligence of the Heart in the Direct Perception of Nature*. Rochester, VT: Bear & Co.

Buhner, S.H. (2014). *Plant Intelligence and the Imaginal Realm*. Rochester, VT: Bear & Co.

Burns, G.W. (1998). *Nature-Guided Therapy: Brief Integrative Strategies for Health and Well-Being*. Philadelphia, PA: Brunner/Mazel.

Buzzell, L. & Chalquist, C. (eds.) (2009). *Ecotherapy: Healing with Nature in Mind*. San Francisco, CA: Sierra Club Books.

Kendra, C. (February 10, 2021). *How Psychologists Define Attention*. www.verywellmind.com/what-is-attention-2795009.

Kopytin, A. & Rugh, M. (eds) (2017). *Environmental Expressive Therapies*. London and New York, NY: Routledge/Brunner & Mazel.

Louv, R. (2005). *Last Child in the Woods: Saving Our Children from Nature-Deficit Disorder*. Chapel Hill, NC: Algonquin Books.

McGilchrist, I. (2009). *The Master and His Emissary: The Divided Brain and the Making of the Western World*. New Haven, CT: Yale University Press.

McGilchrist, I. (2019). *Ways of Attending: How Our Divided Brain Constructs the World*. New York, NY: Routledge.

Oh, K.H., Shin, W.S., Khil, T.G., & Kim, D.J. (2020). Six-step model of nature-based therapy model. *International Journal of Environmental Research and Public Health*, 17(3), 685. https://doi.org/10.3390/ijerph17030685.

Park, B.J., Tsunetsugu, Y., Kasetani, T., Kagawa, T., & Miyazaki, Y. (2010). The physiological effects of Shinrin-yoku (taking in the forest atmosphere or forest bathing) evidence from field experiments in 24 forests across Japan. *Environmental Health and Preventative Medicine*, 15, 18–26. https://doi.org/10.1007/s12199-009-0086-9.

Romanyshyn, R.D. (1997). Egos, Angels, and the Colors of Nature. In D. Fideler (ed.), *Alexandria: The Order and Beauty of Nature* (pp.165–180). Grand Rapids, MI: Phanes Press.

Samples, B. (1976). *The Metaphoric Mind: A Celebration of Creative Consciousness*. Reading, MA: Addison-Wesley.

Sewall, L. (1999). *Sight and Sensibility: The Ecopsychology of Perception*. New York, NY: Jeremy Tarcher Putnam.

Speeth, K.R. (2003). On Therapeutic Attention. In M. Brady (ed.), *The Wisdom of Listening* (pp. 83–107). Boston, MA: Wisdom Publications.

Chapter 5

Culture and Nature: The Play of Ecopoiesis

VARVARA SIDOROVA

Culture is guiding and limiting,
Being born and being destroyed,
The human world of meanings,
The other, the others, the strangers, and oneself.
A polyphony of meanings going out
to the invisible dome of the temple,
woven from the meanings and sounds of words.
Bodies and Body, permeated with threads of belonging.
Sandcastles of civilizations.
The taste of different continents,
originating where there were no words,
dances, songs, rhythm, and lines drawn on the body.
Each day we draw patterns on the body of the earth,
illuminated by the one Sun and one Moon that we share
And by our starry sky, visible through the eyes of our ancestors
And through the eyes of each of us.
The sense of family and belonging
The voice that calls us in old age and is not appreciated in childhood.
That invisible landscape of human meanings
that continues to shape us every second
and which we too shape,
weaving a carpet of such familiar and different human ways of being,
without which we would not be human.

Varvara Sidorova

Let me begin with the basic principles that I hold:

- Culture and nature are inseparable. They exist in mutual poietic interaction.
- The natural and geographical location, combined with the characteristics of a particular culture, affect how each culture manifests itself both externally and internally: they affect the culture of perception, thinking, and corporeality as a whole—the culture of the work of consciousness (Sidorova, 2005; Sidorova & Vasilyuk, 2009).
- There is a connection between the larger body of nature and human bodies, conditioned by culture at different stages of development.
- In the modern world, as a result of urbanization, globalization, and technocratization, there is a disruption in the connection with one's own body, with the natural world, with traditional cultures and natural creativity.
- The pandemic has launched a process of change in our relationship to nature, between the body of nature and one's own body, weakening the process of attunement to nature.
- The practice of intermodal expressive arts therapy can help to establish connections at these breakpoints. It can enhance body awareness and promote an understanding of the body as a thinking and feeling body. The body then becomes a space for the birth of meanings that are lived through the creation of art forms.
- The art forms of both traditional and modern cultures can be mediators and channels for the psychic energy of consciousness, a bridge and a meeting place; they can be used in the context of expressive arts therapy, in the context of both nature-oriented and culture-oriented expressive arts therapy (Sidorova, 2020).

Human beings have two parents: nature and culture. Just as a person cannot exist without nature, with which we are in constant exchange, inhaling and exhaling, consuming food and sunlight, dependent on weather and slight fluctuations in temperature, neither can that person exist without culture, that invisible space of human meanings and ways of being and perceiving the world that makes someone human. It is not enough to be born in a human body to become a human, you need to grow up in the field of people.

We can imagine nature without a person and without cultural influence, but we can't imagine a person without nature and culture—our body is a part of nature. Were it not for the field of culture we would not become human beings. We live in bodies permeated by cultural values and meanings, worldviews, internalized in the process of communicating (Vygotsky, 2005). Our semantic vectors are determined both by human culture that is common to us all and by the specific characteristics of a particular culture. Each person develops in a specific cultural environment, rooted in the physical features of the world, its geographical features and the landscape that is seen and felt.[1]

This interplay between nature, culture, and human beings is the subject of several areas of scientific knowledge, such as cultural anthropology, psychological anthropology, ethnosemantics, ethnolinguistics, and even geopsychology. We can say that visible geography creates internal geography, the geography of the soul of the people (e.g., Berdyaev and Podoroga connected the vastness of the Russian soul with the vast landscapes of Russia) (Berdyaev, 1990; Podoroga, 1993, 1995). In a similar vein, Claude Levi-Strauss considered mythological coordinate systems as classification grids, where the dimensions are formed and fixed by specific features of the physical environment, thereby creating a version of the physical world as a text (Levi-Strauss, 1999, p.12).

The problem is that we cannot establish direct contact with nature without the mediation of conceptual "cultural glasses." We cannot go back to primitive thinking or primitive perception, but we can try to look at nature and ourselves as a part of nature, through the prism of ideas that are free from the demands of consumerism and aggressive expansion, and are instead built on the foundation of co-creation. Following Wendell Berry, an American farmer and poet, we can flip the traditional view to one where nature, the surrounding world, or a specific landscape, do not belong to us, but we and our bodies belong to it, and thus move away from anthropocentrism (Berry, 2004, p.143). This co-creative interaction with nature can be experienced through the expressive arts, because they involve a creative act that is inherently renewing and fresh, allows us to go beyond our limited perceptions and establish our own, subjective, poietic contact, not in a conceptual way, but as a living and embodied experience, free from utilitarian purpose.

---

1   Different sources report the many shades of green that people from the Amazon jungle can differentiate, and the many words for snow and white color that people living in the far North have.

Since we cannot get rid of cultural mediation in our relations with nature, why not use it more consciously, by drawing on the experience of those cultures in which different traditions to the body of nature have been preserved? Art forms created in the bosom of similar cultures can act as mediators, and offer a kind of *framing* (Knill, Barba, & Fuchs, 1995, p.89) for understanding the practice of expressive arts and directing the work of consciousness, as any art form does. At the same time, these art forms can allow for a subjective, creative encounter with the *third* (Knill *et al.*, 1995, p.131), a process which involves not conceptual, but bodily, experience.

I want to emphasize the complex and multifaceted nature of the interaction and mutual influence of culture and nature, and to call it "ecopoietic interaction" (Levine, 2012). We can say that the play of ecopoiesis takes place in ourselves, in our consciousness-body, on the one hand, and, on the other hand, in the visible manifestations of culture.

During various stages of the development of humanity, there have existed different relationships between nature and culture. For a long time, there was a kind of invisible contradiction between the culture of civilization—something cultivated and developed—and nature, which was perceived as wild, hostile, chthonic, subject to impulses, and so on.

At the same time, many cultures preserved the myth of a certain Golden Age. According to Mircea Eliade (1994), this myth dates back to the time of the Neolithic Revolution, and can be considered a reaction to the emergence of agriculture. In the myth of the Golden Age, before the beginning of agriculture, human beings lived in complete harmony with nature. Nature was depicted as a garden of Eden, and human beings were natural, innocent, and unencumbered by internal contradictions and social conventions. The people of the Golden Age were imagined to be able to control the elements and animals or to speak to them without feeling separate.

In traditional cultures, the land and nature were perceived as living organisms. Nature was treated as a living body, was revived and personified, and the land and spaces around were endowed with sacred qualities, giving rise to a sacred geography. In Russian traditional culture, characterized by an emphasis on relationships and family ties, Mother Earth and Father Heaven were perceived as a part of a large family. In Indian culture, the entire embodied world was represented in the form of the Sacred Cow.

In many traditional cultures where protoshamanism and primitive animism are not lost (e.g., in the traditional culture of the Indians of

South America and the Indigenous peoples of the North) the land and the nature are perceived as "a gigantic sentient being influenced by the same force that influences us" (Mindell, 2007, p.29). That is why many Indigenous peoples identified themselves with the land they lived in, even taking personal names that reflected natural phenomena or places in the surrounding landscape, for example, "Moving Cloud," "Low Mountain," or "Deep River." In such names, we see an expression of identity that is based on the merging of oneself with the surrounding world. For example, the Australian aborigines of the Yimithirr tribe connected the parts of the body with the cardinal directions, feeling and defining their bodies in relation to the large body of the earth (Mindell, 2007, p.29).

The way of interacting with nature is largely determined by a specific culture. We see differences even in the European view and attitude toward nature. Stephen K. Levine, in his article on ecopoiesis, gives examples of the English and French garden as ways of organizing the space of nature, where, in the first case, a person leaves the possibility of naturalness as part of the landscape, and in the second, forms a garden with greater order and regularity (Levine, 2012). We can also recall Japanese and Chinese gardens, the pinnacle of the human ability to connect nature and spiritual experience, combining man-made and natural things. Europeans and Russians very often make a clear distinction between the spiritual and the material worlds, and consider them total opposites. The material, objective world is perceived as not worthy of much attention. Our research into Russian culture confirmed that this opposition is deeply rooted in the minds of the people (Sidorova, 2012, 2017). There is no such metaphysical opposition in many Eastern countries. The source of the ancient Japanese views of the world, for example, is Shintoism, which is based on pantheism and primitive animism—the idea of the soul of the world living in every object, of the animate nature of things as they are in nature.[2] Hence the astonishingly careful attitude of traditional Japanese culture to the external objective-natural world, the aversion to violence, the refusal to change nature and the cult of the natural, the untouched, that which is not made by human hands.

---

2   Almost all manifestations of nature were represented in the pantheon of Shinto gods. So, in the *Kojiki* "an account of Ancient Matters," we find a list of gods, among which there are: Amatsuhiko—hikonagisatake-ugaya-fu-kinaezu-no mikoto—Heavenly Youth Valiant God of the Cormorant Roof Not Finished at the Seashore; Ame no-sagiri-no Kami—Heavenly God of Mists in the Gorges; Michi-no-Nagatiha-no Kami is the God of the Long Roadside Stones, Suhijinino-Kami is the Goddess of the Settling Sand (*Kojiki*, 2000, pp.64–67).

It is worth noting, however, that the relationship between nature and culture in Japanese culture is not as simple as it might seem at first glance. The traditional consciousness of the Japanese makes a kind of u-turn, from nature to culture and back to nature again (nature—culture—nature). We can say that the main trait of Japanese culture is placing artful emphasis on the natural character of a natural object. Such external and internal work of consciousness gives the natural object a specific cultural content that emphasizes and manifests its nature, without transforming or violating it. Examples of this include Japanese gardens or the Japanese art of admiring suiseki stones. Untouched, uncultivated nature in itself is not an object of interest and admiration for the Japanese, but a Japanese garden, carefully cultivated and conveying the beauty of wild nature in its ideal form, becomes a focus of attention for them.

Cultural attitudes to the body and nature gave rise to a clear division between spirit and matter, which in turn led to the separation between them that we observe in the modern world. Despite all the differences in views of nature, in the modern western world, the dominant attitude stems from the Judeo-Christian worldview. According to this belief system, nature is perceived as matter, which is passive, not feeling, can be subjected to violent manipulation and disregarded and wasted by human beings if it is profitable.

In the modern world, as a result of various factors caused by culture, urbanization, technocratization, and globalization, we can see four main points of rupture. These are: a) broken connections in relationships with our body; b) loss of connection in relation with nature; c) rupture of connection between people (e.g., the loneliness people experience in a metropolis); and d) loss of the connection with traditional cultures. Feelings of separateness and isolation are, in fact, the cause of many mental illnesses and internal conflicts of people living in the modern world. Therapy with expressive arts aims to bring back these lost connections, helping clients to restore subtle contact with their bodies, with nature, with others, with the wisdom of traditional culture, ultimately leading to a renewed sense of co-creativity with the entire world. The pandemic has greatly deepened these aforementioned divisions, but at the same time, it has outlined new trends, such as the need for closeness to nature, which strengthens the processes of attunement to it.

Body of Nature—Nature of Body

We live in bodies that are essentially a bridge between the natural world and the cultural world. The body contains the senses, but the philosophical question remains: what does a rose smell like? Without our senses, we cannot perceive this; and the senses can also be compared to "glasses" that are necessary for perception but are not without their limitations. At the same time, we must remember that our physical body consists of the same chemical elements or the same primary elements as nature, the earth.

In speaking about the body, we first of all speak about "the body felt from the inside, about the mobile, pulsating, changeable element of internal sensations, impressions, excitements" (Vasilyuk, 1993, p.9). The body "turns out to be that space that hosts in its living elements an interference and integration of the external objective world, the world of language, the world of culture and the inner world of man" (ibid., p.10). Many areas of modern psychotherapy (body-oriented therapy, dance-movement therapy, process-oriented therapy, and others) as well as expressive arts therapy, pay attention to subtle bodily reactions and perceive the body as a highly organized entity that stores the memory of all events and is constantly in a state of responsiveness to external and internal stimuli. However, unlike many other forms of therapy, the expressive arts deal with living expressive corporeality, with a body filled with meanings and sense; a speaking, thinking, feeling body; a body that turns into a sounding pipe organ. We look at the experience of creating things here and now, not trying to interpret this language, but simply staying in it, offering a kind of translation into another language that speaks for it. We cultivate this ability of the body to respond, to experience any content of consciousness, to be both feeling and expressing and to give voice to the knowledge of the body.

Our basic ideas about the world are rooted in the body and our feelings. They are formed in early childhood and are based on the experience of the exploration of the physical world, which later becomes material for constructing metaphors and describing the world. For example, an angular, spiked figure will be perceived as dangerous and therefore evil, while a soft and round figure will be perceived as kind (Artemieva, 1980). According to Arnheim, to understand the depth of mind you have to understand physical depth (Arnheim, 1986). Familiarizing herself with the physical world through sensory impressions and experience, the child masters a certain primary language. We return to it while working in the territory of the expressive arts, but at a new level, remembering the polymodal foundations of consciousness and connecting it to our higher functions, the ability to see beauty and to create. Nevertheless, any kind of language or art, be it music, drawing, or poetry, is still experienced at the bodily level. The body is the integrator within which psychic inter-modal life takes place (Vasilyuk, 1993).

Metaphors, however, allow us to identify the features of bodily experience in a cultural context. Metaphors can be mediators and messengers in the therapeutic process; using the methods of intermodal expressive arts therapy, they can give rise to an image or a drawing, and can be expressed, explored, and transformed in dance or music.

The body and the engagement of bodily experience play a substantial role in these psychotherapeutic paths. George Lakoff and Mark Johnson argue that movement and bodily experience are at the basis of cognitive functions as well, such as categorization, metaphor, and mathematics. Primary metaphors (e.g., top = strength, lightness = joy) come from bodily experience (Lakoff & Johnson, 1980). Direct sensory perception is categorized and can subsequently be stored in memory in the form of images, which in turn are the material for creating basic and complex metaphors, as well as new images that can contribute to the "crystalli-zation embodied in an art-work". (Knill et al., 1995, p.31). The body plays a defining role in our understanding of reality, as the body is the key to understanding what is happening to us, while metaphors allow us to identify the features of bodily experience in a cultural context. "The fact that we express our state using metaphors, and that others understand us, is, in fact, a cultural phenomenon and involves the combination of different references, positions and forms of experience" (Lakoff & John-son, 1980, p.16).

Culture shapes physicality as a set of methods of treating the body, its appearance and internal manifestations, the relation to the body and its parts, the placing in space, the interaction of its parts, the nature of the movements, and so on. So we can talk about the culture of the body and of different bodies: the Russian body, the Latin-American body, the Chinese body, and so on. We can talk about the impact that not only cultures, but also subcultures, have on the body; for example, we can examine the post-Soviet body, or urban or rural bodies. The experience of the expressive arts creates awareness of the cultural meanings that fill the body, thus reviving the repressed and colonized body. At the same time, expressive arts offer a different view of our larger Body of Nature.

We can draw parallels between how a person treats their own body and how they treat the Body of the Earth or the Body of Nature. Expressive arts and other modern psychotherapeutic approaches offer a new perspective on corporeality, wherein the body is not inanimate, passive matter, but a living, feeling, and thinking body, filled with cultural meanings while being part of nature (a body-mind approach). This view of the nature of the body causes a tectonic shift in our relations to the Body of Nature and the Body of the Earth: they, too, are no longer viewed as inanimate objects but as living organisms, complex and meaningful, and our bodies are part of them. Stephen K. Levine proposes to move the body out of the control of conditioned attitudes, formed primarily in European culture and subjected to Christian influence, according to which the body is sinful, dirty, and defiled. He asks us to decolonize our own body.

Such action requires great inner work of restoring our integrity and unity with spirit and the matter on the one hand, and on the other hand, the return of a pure view of the body and nature that has been repressed by Christianity. Shaun McNiff called intermodal art therapy a kind of neoshamanism, and shamanism has always played a large role in establishing and recovering connections (McNiff, 1981, p.26). We can say that expressive arts therapy and the expressive arts in all their manifestations are becoming a new anthropological practice, actively using the languages of art and the bodily dimension to return to and maintain the integrity of human existence in the modern world.

Establishing a connection

Art forms and the process of creating a work of art are mediators, conductors, and means of adjusting consciousness that allow one to establish a connection with various levels of external and internal reality, including the body, nature, and others. Art, household items, rituals, ceremonies, language, and etiquette are a set of culture-specific means of tuning in to consciousness. Art, literature, and religion are canonized states of consciousness, internalized by culture's ways of tuning in to consciousness and dealing with one's mental life. Vygotsky, in his book *The Psychology of Art*, regarded art as a "social technique of feelings" (Vygotsky, 1998, p.5).

In virtually all cultures that have preserved the traditions of animism and protoshamanism, the attitude to the Body of Nature and the nature of our bodies is different: they are not perceived separately. The use of traditional art forms, born in the bosom of similar cultures, and used in the context of expressive arts, makes this tuning possible. Such practices can include, for example, talking with nature, the earth, and the elements through natural objects, the practice of exchange, the offering of ritual food, the practice of ritual offerings, and so on.

Working with natural found objects is one of the methods of modern eco-art and nature-oriented therapy with expressive arts, which, in fact, brings back an ancient way of talking with the world. In many traditional cultures, we find this way of speaking through found objects or through the manipulation of objects.

Art from different cultures in its various forms may be made therapeutically within "culture-oriented expressive arts therapy" (Sidorova, 2020, p.267). For example, the Russian round dance, like many circular dances, offers to our experience the cyclical nature of things, their connectedness, unity, movement in a circle, and a culture-specific way of living cosmogonic processes at individual and collective levels. There are a huge number of traditional patterns of the round dance; each of them has a specific meaning and sense. Another example is the traditional Indian drawing of mandalas and patterns on the ground, called *kolam* or *rangoli*. It is an invitation to the deity, serves as a connection with the ground, and, at the same time, helps us to experience volatility and impermanence, as the patterns made with rice flour quickly disappear under the feet of passers-by, are blown by the wind, or are eaten by insects. This art form allows one to live, through dialogue, an experience of unity with the external world.

The art forms of a particular culture used in the context of inter-modal expressive arts therapy become both the *framework* and *the means* of adjusting the work of consciousness, which "expand the range of the play" (Knill *et al.*, 2005, p.79) and allow us to build new relationships with the body, with nature and with others. Any act of poiesis, of creating something new, whether a drawing, dance, or some other art form, becomes a mediator that helps to establish a connection with certain realities through the body. We are not limited to using traditional art forms for such work, but in them we can find collective meanings that seem to be wired and encrypted within us. These meanings begin to be assimilated and experienced on a subjective level, as if discovered again during the act of poiesis, through interaction with the particular art form and co-creation with others.

In the context of expressive arts, the art form itself can also be modified. For example, instead of using a ritual Tibetan drum, where the text of a prayer is written on a round surface and then repeated when the drum rotates, I suggested that my clients wrote poetry on circular sticks, rolled and polished by sea-waves and bleached by the sunlight. The text was written in a spiral; it could be read many times like a mantra or a prayer. I called them "poetic sticks." Paolo Knill gives the example of using sculpture like a sentinel or a guard in the garden, which refers to the tradition of ancient boundary deities, placed at the borders as patrons (Knill *et al.*, 1995, p.40).

In the modern context of expressive arts therapy, we can use art forms born in the bosom of a culture or even subculture, which may include digital culture. We can use photos, Instagram stories or any form of social network presence that represents a modern manifestation of the invisible network of the god Indra, which enables people to feel resonance and contact.

Our experience has shown that distance and separation do not impede such work. For example, one of the ways of ritual tuning in to each other while working on Zoom is to show your ritual meal, a fruit or a sweet. It becomes a kind of offering. The fact that we have mirror neurons and intermodal brain memory ensures that we can taste and smell the strawberries, even if we only see them on the screen, and thus we can experience belonging.

Even more surprising is the fact that others understand us even when we communicate remotely using computers and amplify our verbal language by the language of movement or by making images or drawings that generate an emotional response. The most adequate way we can describe this experience is by using the concept of multiple resonances. In creating resonances on different levels, we can experience a sense of connection and unity, even in online work: "collective resonance" (Rogers, 2011), "aesthetic resonance" (Sidorova, 2020), "interpersonal resonance" (Selvam, 2004), "somatic resonance" (Rand, 2002).

In the pandemic age, modern technology also serves as a conduit that helps to establish a link between our minds and bodies, since any movement of consciousness is experienced on the bodily level. Even when we are sitting at the computer, our body feels the involvement. Here we have a new phenomenon of remote communication, experienced through other means developed in our culture. Digital technologies and means of remote communication are, in fact, instruments of culture that help us to establish the connection both literally and figuratively. In our remote work on the seminar "The Body of Nature—Nature of the Body," we established a connection with nature, with our bodies and with each other. The technical equipment—essentially aspects of our culture—served as a mediator for finding a connection with nature.

Nature and culture exist in the constant interaction of ecopoiesis. A person cannot exist outside their cultural and natural context. We can use cultural mediators and the language of the arts to create a situation of phenomenological presence and a subjective experience of belonging, which removes the neurotic division responsible for many problems of modern individuals. In the context of intermodal expressive arts therapy, we can cultivate the body's capacity for expressive dialogue by postulating the unity of body consciousness. The human body, like consciousness, is saturated with cultural meanings and, moreover, with the meanings of a particular culture. In the context of *nature-oriented expressive arts therapy* (Atkins & Snyder, 2018) we can understand the body as a manifestation of the wisdom of nature, mediated by culture, and restore the connection with the body and nature, proclaiming the unity between the Nature of the Body and the Body of Nature. The way of relating to nature in a particular culture can be used in the context of *culture- and nature-oriented expressive arts therapy* through traditional art forms, which are conductors, mediators, and means of tuning in to consciousness and providing a space for the encounter.

Expressive arts restore our connection with our bodies, with nature, and with traditional cultures, bringing ancient wisdom back in a modern context, using modern forms and the infinite possibilities of consciousness to create something new, even through the medium of modern technology.

References

Arnheim, R. (1986). *New Essays on the Psychology of Art*. Berkeley, CA: University of California Press.

Artemieva, E.Y. (1980). *The Psychology of Subjective Semantics*. Moscow: MSU Publishing House.

Atkins, S. & Snyder, M. (2018). *Nature-Based Expressive Arts Therapy*. London and Philadelphia, PA: Jessica Kingsley Publishers.

Berdyaev, N.A. (1990). *The Fate of Russia*. Moscow: Moscow State University.

Berry, W. (2004). *The Long-Legged House*. Washington, DC: Shoemaker & Hoard.

Eliade, M. (1994). *The Sacred and the Profane: The Nature of Religion*. Moscow: MSU Publishing House.

Knill, P.J., Barba, H.N., & Fuchs, M.N. (1995). *Minstrels of Soul: Intermodal Expressive Therapy*. Toronto: Palmerston Press.

Knill, P.J., Levine, E., & Levine, S. (2005). *Principle and Practice of Expressive Arts Therapy*. London and Philadelphia, PA: Jessica Kingsley Publishers.

Kojiki (2000). *Records of the deeds of antiquity*. Kristall. St-Petersburg, Russia (in Russian).

Kumar, S. (2009). Eco-psychology: An eco-spiritual view. *Journal of Holistic Healthcare*, 6(3), 11–13.

Lakoff, G. & Johnson, M. (1980). *Metaphors We Live By*. Chicago, IL: University of Chicago Press.

Levi-Strauss, K. (1999). *The Savage Mind*. Moscow: TERRA Book Club Republic Publishing House (in Russian).

Levine, S. (2012). Nature as a work of art: Toward a poetic ecology. *Poiesis: A Journal of the Art and Communication*, 14, 186–193.

McNiff, S. (1981). *The Arts and Psychotherapy*. Springfield, IL: Thomas.

Mindell, A. (2007). *Earth-Based Psychology in Shamanism, Physics and Taoism*. Portland, OR: Lao Tse Press.

Podoroga, V.A. (1993). *The Metaphysics of the Landscape*. Moscow: Nauka (in Russian).

Podoroga, V.A. (1995). *The Phenomenology of the Body: An Introduction to the Philosophical Anthropology*. Moscow: Ad Marginem (in Russian).

Rand, M.L. (2002). What is somatic attunement? (somatic resonance). *Annals of the American Psychotherapy Association*, 5(6), 30.

Rogers, N. (2011). *The Creative Connection for Groups, Science and Behavior*. Palo Alto, CA: Science and Behavior Books.

Selvam, R. (2004). Trauma, body, energy and spirituality. *Positive Health*, May: 15–18.

Sidorova, V.V. (2005). Cultural determination of the image of consciousness (on the example of Russian and Japanese cultures). Synopsis of a thesis for the degree of candidate of psychological sciences. Moscow (in Russian)

Sidorova V.V. (2012). *The Culture of Image: Cross-Cultural Analysis of the Image of Consciousness*. Harkov: Humanitarian Center.

Sidorova, V.V. (2017). *The Image Culture: Cultural Determination of the Image of Consciousness*. Kharkov: Humanitarian Center.

Sidorova, V.V. (2020). *Dance of Drawing, Voice of Line, Poetry of Life: Intermodal Expressive Arts Therapy*. Moscow: Genesis.

Sidorova, V.V. & Vasilyuk, F.E. (2009). Cross-cultural study of strategies of the work of consciousness (on the materials of Russian and Japanese cultures). In F.E. Vasilyuk (ed.) *Psychotherapy. Consciousness. Culture*, 2 (pp. 62–79). Moscow: Moscow State University of Psychology and Education/Psychological Institute of the Russian Academy of Education.

Vasilyuk, F.E. (1993). The structure of the image. *Voprosy Pcihologii*, 24(5), 5–19.

Vygotsky, L.S. (1998). *The Psychology of Art*. Moscow: Labyrinth Publications (in Russian).

Vygotsky, L.S. (2005). *Psychology of Human Development*. Moscow: Eksmo, Smysl Publising House (in Russian).

PART 2

Integrating Ecological and Sustainable Development Perspectives in Expressive/ Creative Arts Therapies Practice with Individuals, Groups, and Communities

Chapter 6

Wandering the Beautiful Trail: Ecopoiesis in Ecological Art Therapy

BEVERLEY A'COURT

Abstract

This brief overview builds on previous work (A'Court, 2011, 2016, 2017) presenting paradigmatic, scientific and practice material relevant to ecological art therapy and ecopoiesis. It focuses on a specific expression of ecopoiesis present in my practice of ecological art therapy, based on my several decades' work with traditional stories in conjunction with somatic and nature-based art therapy approaches. These include the interplay between body, art-making, story and landscape, in which stories of complex, archaic lineage act as conduits, guiding us towards core components of 'Earthsense' (A'Court, 2020); 'biophilia' (Kellert & Wilson, 1993) and 'biognosis' (Carter-Quinlan, 2020) faculties developed and enhanced through engagement in ecological art therapy. Specifically, I describe some of my work with the serpentine, an archetypal form present throughout living systems.

I refer readers to the growing body of contextual evidence from ecopsychology, wilderness and nature therapies demonstrating how a more 'ecological self' identity (Macy *et al.*, 1988) supports recovery, well-being and resilience via connection. The human body, the body of the land and the body of stories together enable impressions from the energetic imprints of the ecology, the archetypal lore of the land, human ancestry and the more-than-human world, to enter consciousness through the felt sense and appear as gestures, forms, symbols and

narratives in holistic art works. Traditional narratives – with their epi-
sodes of endurance and often arduous 'passage' achieved in partnership
with the powers of visible nature and its myriad immanent, invisible
beings and forces – demonstrate principles and forms of ecopoiesis that
can richly support and inform the theory, practice and further evolution
of ecological art therapy.

I continue to advocate for the primacy of somatic awareness and
sensory attunement to the field as core skills to ensure the safety and
effectiveness of holistic art therapy and for the inclusion of ancestral
ecological and cultural knowledge embedded and encoded in ancient
stories and earth-based rituals as powerful healing modalities.

The path to a place beyond thinking

Robert Macfarlane, in his wanderings along the ancient paths, roads and
sea trails criss-crossing Britain, describes how walking is also a kind of
unearthing and re-animation of stories and traditions embedded in the
landscape. He quotes the poet Edward Thomas, reflecting on the practice
of beach combing, who noticed how every pebble he looked at seemed
to lead him into a state of being 'beyond thinking'.

Ancient narratives, with their imagery condensed over centuries,
their implicit ontologies, paradigms and magical transformations,
highlight our inescapable intimacy with all-that-is and the relevance
of this embeddedness in nature to mind-body healing, to restoring and
maintaining holistic well-being. These stories, in prose and rhythmic
oral verse, can assist us in recognising and describing forms of knowing
and knowledge acquired by virtue of our body-mind-in-relation to place.
This knowing is itself an interdependent and spontaneous expression
of nature, arising within nature, embedded in a universe of 'unbroken',
'undivided wholeness' (Bohm, 1951, in Nichol, 2003 p.84), a continuum
of being in constant communication with itself. The images and stories
featured in this chapter continue to speak to our deep nature and understanding and point to an embodied awareness of an 'implicate order'
(ibid., p.84) greater than dualistic thought. They display art's capacity
to coax us to see anew, again and again, through the lens of where we
have come from.

Art therapy often includes the art of presence, the ability to find a
point of balance, sometimes called radical acceptance (Hayes, Folette
& Linehan, 2004; Zettle, 2005) a state of being less defined by, and

identified with, one's biographical 'stories' while still able to respect and appreciate them. From here we can risk recognising established patterns, unveil potential possibilities, imagine new personal myths and make space for new paradigms, all the while forging new neuronal pathways to perceive previously obscured aspects of the self, others and the world, and gaining access to more vital ways of being.

The power of return: Looking back, taking in, retracing our steps

Growth, as nature demonstrates, is not linear, and a theme of this chapter is return. Just as in many traditional circle dances, progression forwards is balanced and stabilised by steps backwards, we know ourselves by also looking back – tracing family 'roots', placing our hands over Neolithic handprints or hiking upstream to the river's source; retracing our steps is depicted throughout many spiritual arts and yogic meditative practices. Familiar negative thoughts are welcomed, gently invited to revisit, so that we can observe how they naturally flow by and allow a gradual process of befriending. Like the salmon's upstream leaping to its birth pool, the whale and elephant's pilgrimage to ancestral calving grounds, this faculty of return – the call to not forget where we have come from, to honour legacy but not stay fixed there – is part of our nature and our future and a living part of ecological art therapy.

In every art therapy session, we reflect, we take time to 'take in' the creative journey from its earliest moments in gestures and speech – we look again with the client at the marks made, fully receive them and potentially move into, with and beyond them. Just as in yoga and other body-oriented therapies, time spent lying still following healing movements enables somatic learning and integration, we allow the neurological system to construct new connections, new thoughts.

As outdoor, nature and wilderness therapies have developed, practitioners are remembering, reviving and adapting practices from their own and other cultures' Indigenous, ancestral traditions, both from the ritual activities of daily life and from teachings coded, embodied and transmitted via the arts, in poetry, song, dance, story and ceremony in an ongoing process of reclamation of the deep eco-psyche-soma of the people. I hope to illustrate here a little of how the stories mentioned in this chapter are part of this enriching, holistic healing process.

Transmission, earth-sense and biognosis

Art therapy reveals the inspirited, embodied nature of the artist-client; in their breathing rhythms, in the pace, pressure and intensity with which they handle materials and make marks, the gestural traces of intentional and unconscious movements and the relational dynamic with the body-mind of the witnessing therapist and environment. Every movement, mark and breath exchanged with other life forms, every breath that blossoms into speech, is a 'signature' imprinting the fabric of the macrocosm, disseminating infinite ripples, as suggested in Vedic images of a cosmic dance.

The ability to create art from our experiences as part of nature is an ecopoietic faculty, the function of embodied imagination and an imaginative body. Imaginative making by hand, in attunement with nature, is a cyclical flow of energy and a form of embodied cognition. Inspiration, when nature breathes into and through us and provides material impacts and guidance, is followed by expression, outbreath, that is dependent on, and embodies, aspects of interdependent reality and reveals further knowledge of both inner and outer conditions. This natural form of relational play serves as the medium of 'translation' of earth phenomena into forms of consciousness and reciprocal transmission from consciousness and somatic state back to nature within a shared field of being and communication.

- How does nature communicate with the body-mind when we are engaged in ecological art therapy, when we sense that nature is participating in, and guiding, the process?

Increasingly eco-artists, land artists, body-land artists, eco-dance artists and earth-based arts researchers (Carter-Quinlan, 2020; Morris, 2017) explore such questions in the hope of finding and creating arts practices which empower people to honour their own earth-based life knowledge, traditions and lost or damaged relationships with ancestral lands.

What is received and understood is done so 'by some faculty other than our neocortical thinking, by some function akin to that of connective tissue' (Carter-Quinlan, 2020) that allows direct 'porosity' between nature and our body-mind via imagination. The term 'biognosis' can denote the wisdom of knowing, directly transmitted from one's own biology (and microbiology), and from the biology of other beings, the learning from embodied experience in relation to natural forces and the forms of knowledge derived from relationships with nature internally and externally to the body, uniquely, sustainably adapted to native ecologies. Somatically, the amniotic sac is our first ecology, where we experience the flow of life that is nature. The artist Narelle Carter-Quinlan (2020) has developed an arts practice from her perception of our *embryological origins* in work she calls 'Embodied Ecology'. Already gifted with an ability to somatically experience her 'body's waterways', she has researched how this directly connects her to, and communicates with, the flow of waters outside her body – her local ocean, lakes and rivers. Her long practice of refining sensitivity to the permeability of fluids and fluid patterns and forms outside the body and those within has become a detailed, anatomically sound understanding of the 'interface of spirit and materiality'.

Current cell biology parallels this view of weaving the world into ourselves; the cell membrane, with its receptors, acts as the cell's nervous system, conveying information from the environment to the nucleus, the engine of cell-reproduction, ensuring a constant process of adaptation to conditions (Lelièvre & Bissell, 1998). When we engage in art-making immersed in nature, practising many styles of deep, whole-body listening, we seem to open and enhance the functioning of this channel, linking perception and expression, and our creations appear as utterances from the diverse intelligences of place, with magical gifts or blessings from the forest, whisperings from the shore, warnings in the air...

The forest sees you, the world speaks back:

The Earth is looking at me ...
I, I am happy, it is looking at me;
I, I am happy, I am looking at it.

(from 'When they saw each other', Chant, Dineh Origin legend, see Hyde & Jett, 1967)

Since I began outdoor, nature-based art therapy in the 1980s, one aspect stands out as especially powerful in assisting the transformation of suffering, enabling a reframing of personality and emotional 'disorders' and problems to be 'fixed' in favour of a deeper experience of relational presence. This is a core principle in many Indigenous healing traditions and teaching stories: the shift from 'perception exercised by the self upon the stones, to the perception exercised upon the self by the stones' (MacFarlane, 2013, p.341).

Acknowledgement of nature as a field of diverse intelligences and agency, and inclusion of nature's interventions as expressive communication from a responsive, living system of systems, constitutes a de-centering, decolonising step. David Wagoner invites us in his poem 'Lost' to 'stand still' because 'the forest knows where you are' and 'you must let it find you' (Wagoner, 1999).

Clients come into contact with experiential reminders that they live inescapably woven into the fabric of life, with all the inherent value that implies, and many become able to make, and reflect on, their art in mindful communion with nature. Just as in the great stories, we discover that we share many languages with our animals and other kin in nature.

'... the most powerful (learning) for me has been experiencing nature in the forest seeing me. For the first time I felt this consciousness, how it was aware of me. It has completely changed how I see myself, my life and how I will practise as a therapist.'

'I thought I was doing eco therapy but I have never felt or looked like this before, concentrating on what the forest is seeing, how it is experiencing my presence.

It's always been, What do I see? Where do I want to go? What do I feel? And what I now see was a narrow focus of looking for art materials. This was revolutionary, to see myself walking in the forest and realise all the living things, the whole forest, was aware of me.'

'If I think about it, the smaller the creature, the more aware of my approaching feet it must be. It seems odd that I never thought of this before.'

Respectful practice: Honouring the field of all our relations

As protagonists in old stories approach mountains or enter forests, caves and sacred, secret places, they are observed by beings and 'spirits' of the place. A human presence, with all its embodied ambitions, needs, aggression and desires transmitting loudly, is often registered by wild animals, an elemental guardian or clever trickster character willing to assist, trip or snare the unconscious traveller. To benefit therapeutically from encounters in nature and minimise harm, we must conduct ourselves responsibly in nature, mindful of what we take with us and how nature responds to our presence, and be respectful in how we depart.

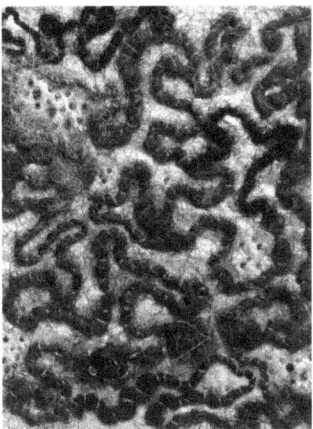

Figure 6.1: Silk river embroidery (artist and photo: B. A'Court)

The following suggested preparatory activities are derived and synthesised from Indigenous practices, teaching stories, somatic and sensorimotor therapies and are constantly informed and updated by evolving polyvagal and neurological approaches to trauma:

1. We acknowledge, as we approach and enter a wild place, that it is already inhabited, that we do not come as colonists but as guests and we announce our presence, our motivation, and request permission and support to conduct art therapy there.
2. We acknowledge the presence of the past and commit to respect the buried traces of events that may surface as embodied imaginative experiences or sensory disturbances in the guests.
3. We prepare the body-mind using somatic self-care exercises to ensure that clients can responsibly and effectively self-regulate if negatively triggered in the wild, and to support open-minded, open-hearted exploration and encounters (Dana & Porges, 2018; Ogden & Fisher, 2015; Rothschild, 2000).
4. We use practices to awaken and sensitise our dormant faculties of body and field awareness, to facilitate attunement to the entire location and life processes there.
5. When we take given materials (fallen wood, stone, drifting leaves, petals, feathers and so on, not live, rooted foliage), we offer thanks, sometimes in the form of a few grains or liquid.

6. On leaving, we take time for appreciation and express gratitude for all that has been experienced. We do our best to depart responsibly and to leave no trace, other than occasionally to leave some biodegradable art in the place, with respect for local culture and religion.

The meandering, serpentine path: Earth-based ritual in art therapy

Ancient stories often speak obliquely, through similes and clues resembling riddles and Zen koans, whose mysterious paradoxes defeat cognition and shift the mind into the pure awareness behind everyday cognition, an experience often described as 'awakening'. In the mysterious story quest with its maze-like twists, traps and turns, its labyrinthine complexity, the protagonist may be unaware that they are, nevertheless, moving towards a destiny with implications reaching far beyond themselves geographically and into both past and future: for the undoing, atoning for or mending past wrongs or the restoration of an eco-spiritual balance which will revitalise land and persons.

In therapy, the initial presenting symptom, life event and 'mission' may turn out not to be the core issue, but a skilfully designed, mythically trickster-like means to propel the characters towards a deeper root and discovery of their more whole selves, including ancestral influences. Painful symptoms are often a manifestation of the body's own immune system responses and psychological defences attempting to suppress or expel a perceived-as-invasive 'toxin', a 'not-me' entity or identity. In traditional stories, the characters' complex sufferings, maze-like challenges and repeated failures seem nevertheless to flow from an inherent and indefatigable drive to restore ecological wholeness and health, which necessitates making peace with, and integrating, many forms of 'otherness'.

The meander denotes both a winding, serpentine landform and a swaying, wavering style of walking, a veering sideways from the straight path, a looping trail that curves round landforms and doubles back on itself, widening or lessening its range, to finally arrive at its destination. The serpent as a symbol and serpentine forms in the arts are among the most ancient and ubiquitous of all cultural images, with richly layered significance in many world cultures across diverse ecologies. In each case, the riverine and mythic serpentine, snakes and wave patterns are associated with the vital forces of the Earth, life, sexuality, fertility, wisdom (and its opposites) and death. Our spine, with its coccyx mirrors the rattlesnake and natural landscape forms shaped by the flow of wind, sand, roots and water. The ascending serpentine spiral around a branch or sword, as a symbol for medicine, echoes its place in yogic spiritual systems as the form taken by our own primordial life energy, *kundalini*, flowing through the body's chakras. The wandering vagus nerve conveys sensory impressions of the world beyond our skin to all body regions and the brain. Thus, the body is a conduit connecting the forces of earth and sky in the same spiral dance as expressed in our models of DNA and plant forms, and in experiences of awakening to transcendent and embodied wisdom.

At the time of writing this, fewer serpentine land forms than spirals and labyrinths seem to have been officially recorded and mapped. However, this absence does not detract from the essence and potential of the serpentine process as an embodied, earth-based therapeutic medium. The word 'meander', whether of a path, or its mode of passage, implies time, akin to the millennia needed for a river to carve its way through rock, eroding atom by atom as it flows, and the qualities of patience and endurance so often central in ancient stories. Serpentine images, of the rippling, undulating snake or the coiled snake in a ringed spiral around its egg, reconcile the apparently polarised linear and cyclical concepts of time and the human life-span that we find in the myths and cosmologies of different cultures.

Tales of princes, princesses, saints, soldiers, children and peasants alike often meander, as characters are lost, swept off course or misled though tangled maze-like forests, returning again and again to the same place or a similar, but more threatening place. The Princes' journeys in 'The Virgin Queen' require them to cross the same three rivers and undergo repeated 'falls' into other realities. Patience and acceptance of repeated failures or encounters is a feature of many stories as nature offers many second and third chances.

This feature of the archetypal serpentine river immediately connects it metaphorically to human life, suffering and therapy. Just as the meandering river reaches its outermost, extending reach, it curves, turning as if back on itself, and appears to be returning almost to its previous position, sometimes only metres further downstream. Much human suffering brought to therapy is expressed in statements like these from my clients over the years:

- 'I can't take any more of the same, not this again, my old enemy, my demon.'

- 'I thought I was over this but the slightest thing reminds and drives me back to it.'
- 'I can't seem to move on, get over it, I can't forgive, I can't find peace, I can't let go.'
- 'I keep finding myself back here again, doing the same thing in the same way.'

Recovery and rehabilitation can feel like travelling a long road yet making interminably slow progress, repeatedly regressing, literally walking backwards, turning back on oneself, compelled to re-face, re-create and re-experience harmful patterns, retracing steps along a familiar old path, to unlearn and relearn. There is a power in looking and walking back; the traditional Heyokah role in some First Nations American tribes was to walk and perform tasks backwards to mirror and satirise profound truths for the collective (Lame Deer & Erdoes, 1972, pp.xxix, 3, 160). Spirals or labyrinths used in ceremonies to celebrate natural cycles and significant life passages repeatedly return us to almost exactly the place we have just passed, while drawing us onwards with moments of circling close to the symbolic centre yet unable to enter. In the serpentine, the meandering river's end – a lake or ocean – is far off, often beyond view. There is no rose garden in sight, no light visible at the end of the tunnel.

The distance between the meanders may be small so we pass close by our recent path or so distant that we do not at first realise we have progressed at all. Where the meander is broad, we may simply feel distracted, led astray, drawn off 'at a tangent' to our conscious purpose, only to find that the path turns again and we are 'heading' back towards our destination. For the protagonists and for earth-based art therapy, each turn in the path often involves a change of pace, a loosening, a letting go, a material or egoic loss.

> 'I slowed down and felt the rhythm of each turn. I took that moment to pause and take stock of where I am. I felt surprisingly good exactly where I was. I wanted to stay there but after a few moments I was ready, excited to set off on the next part of the path. There was a lot in that space.'

These turning points can be experienced as fatigue, disappointment, flashes of insight, or the realisation of something left behind undone, badly done or forgotten that must be returned to and remedied.

'I walked as you suggested, letting my painful, problem knee lead. It led me on a curvy, zig-zag trail. I discussed this with my knee and it insisted we go this way. It felt strange to follow a single body part but I realised how I push myself forward in life, let my head lead me and think I know best even when I am missing so much.'

This mirroring of a tendency within our subjective life in certain states of depression, trauma-induced repetition-compulsion and addiction, makes the serpentine land form and mode of walking a gift for us in art therapy, affirmed by the presence of ancient serpentine landforms associated with astronomical or healing rituals. The nature of the art task and the underlying transmission of the landform work together to create a powerful medium for the transformation of lifelong, self-destructive patterns. Many ancient tales portray an oblique route to truth and freedom, embodied wisdom and mature, compassionate leadership, and an equanimity, mindful of opportunities and able to maintain focus along the way. Long and winding, involving apparently meaningless encounters, pointless tasks and seemingly dead-end trails, the meandering path takes us far from our consciously intended destination and appears to direct us backwards to begin again, over and over, but delivers us transformed.

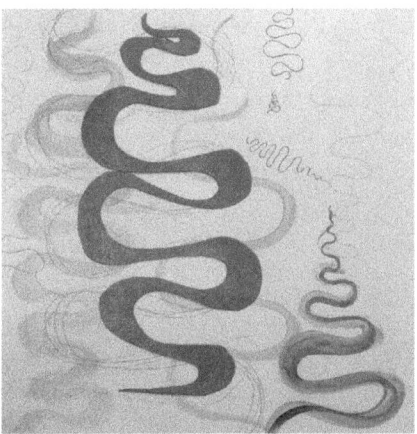

Figure 6.2: Gestural serpentine iii (artist sketch book, B. A'Court)

'I could be kinder to myself and my family, not push everyone so hard. As soon as I set off I felt tears coming and at the first turn the witness looked at me with her kind eyes. Her stillness and silence was calming.

Maybe I don't have to face everything alone, maybe the world is kinder than I think.'

The art of witnessing

As with all sacred ceremonies, the Earth, her beings and elemental forces are already our witnesses and are richly portrayed in the human realm as the all-commentating chorus in ancient Greek drama. This witness role is refined as a compassionate mindfulness practice within the discipline of Authentic Movement (Adler, 1987) and plays an essential role in all the Pathworking methodologies I have developed in collaboration with clients (A'Court, 2011, 2016, 2017). The attentive beings stationed along the way receive the emotional and somatic tone of the walker's passage in their own body-mind, alongside their own impulses and reactions, and witness the resonant environmental ambience and phenomena occurring around them.

'The world is always there. There is always a witness...always someone to look at, be with, talk to.'

'I felt my partner's movements, her walking style, inside my own body. It felt very intimate as if I was walking her soul's path with her.'

Witnesses may play other non-intrusive but anchoring-to-the-moment roles; for example, in one session, witnesses extended a hand slowly, in silence as each pilgrim passed them at the turn in the road, to receive a torn-off fragment of the walker's painted 'problem' to hold in safe-keeping and release the walker of some portion of their burden.

'I wanted him to let it go and hand it to me when he was ready, I didn't want to look directly...expectantly, or influence him at all. I noticed his body change, how he lightened up and looked taller, and I felt as if I was receiving something precious.'

At the end of each walk, these fragments were gathered and later burned in a shared fire ceremony. A single remaining fragment was kept by the walker to be worked on and transformed after their walk. In each case, a deeper truth and beauty was to emerge from these remains, along with transformation, resolution or complete dissolution of 'the problem'.

The ritual animates its own numinous field, inviting and 'magnetising' nature's participation, within which events take on a specific meaning coloured by the participants' embodied realities. In debriefing from these rituals, walkers and witnesses share their experiences and the perceived significance of synchronistic accompanying field phenomena, received as 'gifts' from nature. The healing power of the ritual relies on walkers' and witnesses' trust in their perceptions as valid contributions, however simple, playful or 'extra'-ordinary they seem.

> 'I loved that the rain came just as I was setting out to walk. I felt my walk, my whole life with all my problems, anxiety and stress, was being washed and blessed.'

> 'I appreciated everyone along the way...each seemed to actually become the significant person I needed to communicate with. I was able to say sorry and thank everyone along my path. I feel so much lighter. I made a beautiful flower to wear out of my last "problem" fragment.'

Gifts from the field: Humility, receptivity, gratitude, trust

In 'The Virgin Queen', on the road to the garden of the Queen the Princes notice an old man stitching the parched, cracked earth back together. The youngest Prince is described in terms familiar in stories as simple, dreamy and foolish and riding a scrawny old mare. However, only he, of the three brothers, pauses to dismount and inquire about the old man's well-being and task. In return, the old man offers advice and instructions in riddle form, which the Prince listens to and remembers. Later, the Prince's simple act of noticing seemingly insignificant details immediately around him reveals precisely the moment each instruction is to be applied. There is no struggle with reality, it is a co-ordinated, synchronised weave. When it seems that we have been sent off course, in these stories each 'detour' serves a, usually greater, purpose.

When nature, or a fairy tale character, presents an object, creature or apparent obstacle in our path, there may be a lesson of discernment to be learned. We may also be invited to accept it as a gift: a talisman or possible companion, guide or teacher, however strange its appearance or obscure its purpose may appear initially to our conventional concepts.

In outdoor ecological art therapy we may explore its story, exercising fine attention and minute observation to ask:

- What was its journey to this place, this moment?
- What does this object, obstacle or creature know that I/we do not?
- What news or questions does it bring?

In art therapy, we encourage clients to welcome and accept their unexpected impulses, unedited marks, undisguised images or erupting feelings and to meet them with curiosity, compassion and interest as messages from some part of the self that seeks to be seen and may take a little time to be fully heard. To receive even parts of the self demands humility, openness and receptivity, an acceptance that we do not control everything. This is a challenge and risk in attachment trauma where receiving from others has been shaped by abuse and trust broken or eroded. The strange gifts with special powers remind us of the reality that we are immersed in life's serendipitous, creatively improvisational qualities, and inseparable from all that is and flows towards us.

Each found object mentioned in the old man's riddle-like instructions, 'iron touches iron, grass touches grass, wood touches wood', opens the hero's way into the next phase of the story. Working creatively outdoors we encourage such an attitude of receptivity and gratitude towards surprising natural encounters, giving rise to experiences like the following:

'The garden is pretty but I needed something else, less nice – I found the pile of broken greenhouse glass and knew I wanted it. I thought of the Snow Queen, felt all my hate and anger. I piled it up; it felt really satisfying. Then just by itself I was placing petals onto each piece of glass and arranging them. It was a sweet, slow, careful process. My body filled with sadness, then warmth and I was forgiving and being kind to myself and the whole world. This pleasant feeling washed through me. My tiny flower-windows look like prayers.'

'I wandered the grounds and couldn't settle. ...I found the bonfire...the charred branches and began drawing with charcoal and ash. I was totally absorbed and understood that I have to let [A] have more freedom, make her own choices. I have been trying to control her too much.'

'All day these huge black bees seemed to be following me. I was scared and irritable. Then I decided to watch them, closer and closer...beautiful, shiny, purply-black. I saw how careful they were entering each flower, treading so gently, and someone told me they don't sting. I've reversed my feelings about them. I see how I create tension and irritation in myself again and again on too little information.'

The search for the question

Sometimes the gift is a word, or a mysterious, trick question and having the wit, the presence of mind, to ask the right question is often a feature of the threshold in stories and ceremonial rituals of passages, to gain access to the place beyond the guardian. In many versions of the Russian Baba Yaga stories, the witch's question, 'Did you come here of your own free will?' must be answered with the paradoxical reply, 'Largely of my own free will and twice as much by compulsion.'

Fairy tales often highlight the importance of receiving and asking the right question, precisely when it is required, as critical for progression to the next phase of the story. Correctly, respectfully and intelligently greeting a guardian animal, nature spirit, demon or wise elder with the right question is often more crucial than providing the correct answer (even if with mischievous or cunning intent). The acceptable answer, if there is one, may not even be revealed in the story. This resembles a process in therapy where the art-making is assisting the client to feel their way towards the most honest and meaningful question.

Deena Metzger, journalling about her experience of cancer diagnosis, treatment and recovery, observes parallels between the technologies of environmental violation – mining, factory farming, nuclear and chemical industries – that contribute to causing cancer and the technologies of its treatment – excision, radiotherapy and chemotherapy (Metzger, 1992, p.28). In her search to find meaning in her experience, she voices thoughts expressed by many with cancer and other serious conditions:

'I don't know what questions to ask. I am a woman with feet in two worlds and I dare not slip in either. [And he cautioned me against] bringing the armies against myself, looking for guilt, for culpability, trying to answer the question: "What did I do wrong?"' (Metzger, 1992, p.20)

Suffering is intensified by unkind, self-blaming, self-punishing questions and equally self-harming answers. Compassion-based and narrative therapies aim to counter this by offering alternative forms of inner self-narrative such as asking:

- How would universal love (soul or God) view you, your life, your situation?
- What is the kindest thing you could say or do for yourself right now?

These have the overarching, archetypal quality of fairy-tale questions asked by elders, sages and magical beings in stories, like 'What is it that women really want?', offering a spacious time frame for any potential answer. During installation-building and walking rituals in ecological art therapy, we witness how allowing thought to flow with breath, bilateral transverse motion and walking pace enables tightly focused thought and anxiety to connect with present bodily feeling and far wider fields of space and time, and opens up new, potentially kinder, more meaningful questions to address to ourselves.

The hymn in the bones: Ancestral conditions

The calcium that forms our bones is itself the recycled bone and shell constituents of millions of beings who have gone before us. Embodying the past, when we claim to know something 'in our bones' we feel we know it deeply. Our DNA resembles a winding thread that runs through our inherited line, like the stories that connect us down the generations. The language of thread, spinning and weaving, aspects of a basic ancestral survival activity, pervades both traditional stories and our thinking about cultural and biological inheritance. When we 'spin a yarn' we take the listener on a long, winding journey with broken, loose, knotted or dangling threads that may end far from its geographical and temporal origins.

In my work using somatic and nature-based art therapy with chronic conditions, I have observed a similar long and winding path to the client's current state of body-mind. The science of epigenetics is gradually clarifying how traumatic experiences in one generation impact physiology, gene function and brain structure and function, changes which are then transmitted to, and embodied by, subsequent generations and expressed in physical disease and emotional disposition (Moore,

2016; Yehuda & Bierer, 2008, 2009; Yehuda *et al.*, 2016). I have observed how, during gestural and breath-based art-making and somatic sensing, clients seem to revisit and embody a past trauma in their family line, via a type of somatic empathy, whereby they subjectively experience an ancestor's trauma 'from the inside' in their own body, and relate that to their own current disease in an associated body organ or function. This phenomenon has been most apparent in my clients with cancer, asthma, arthritis, diabetes, Parkinson's and other auto-immune conditions.

Several clients receiving treatment for breast cancer or carrying the BRCA gene and fearful of the disease, entered meditative states during somatic drawing and Authentic Movement, and on emerging from their art works reported that they felt able to sense in their own bodies the presence of a great-great-grandparent's trauma. A vividly arising body memory of shock, restraint or enforced muteness in some dangerous situation is experienced somatically, often as throat and chest tension, compressed, rigid posture, frozen or inhibited gestures and internal organ tension.

The therapy initially involves:

- a journey into the felt sense of the condition or symptom, its precise qualities – identified using sensory inquiry into its colours, shapes, movements, taste, smell
- witnessing its originating moment via further embodiment and somatic sensing, to discover what was embodied in that moment
- allowing this to flow into expressive art-making and then into further embodiment and movement.
- a potentially new embodied state to be intuited or felt as possible, and this can be chosen.

This multi-modal transference or extension of consciousness resembles some aspects of Tamalpa expressive art therapy techniques and the body-mind method pioneered and researched by UK Dance-Movement therapist Professor Helen Payne from 1990 to 2010, both of which similarly work with the body-mind as a unified whole capable of profound 'shape-shifting' connection and identification with other sentient beings.

Similarly, arthritis and asthma-allergy patients have been able to somatically revisit the embodied experiences of their own first experience of a symptom and/or that of an ancestor. Powerfully charged memories may also become associated with ecological features, foods, pollutants or plant and tree pollen. These impacts may have gone unnoticed or been suppressed at the time and held in secret for decades, locked-up words unbreathed in speech, to emerge later as allergies.

Some clients are more easily able to access the felt sense of an ancestor than go directly to their own symptoms. During large-scale somatic and gestural drawing they contact the felt sense of the first appearance of a symptom or condition in the family line, in the form of vivid impressions of how the person breathed, moved and inhabited their body. From here they can proceed towards fully feeling their own symptoms and sometimes move between the two people and their connecting stories. I have come across a number of stories such as the following in historical war zones and areas of socio-political trauma or natural disaster.

The client felt in her own body what she experienced as her grandmother's trauma following a forceful imperative to be silent on a taboo topic for years of her childhood and teens. The client felt the visceral terror which pervaded her grandmother's entire being, but was most energetically present in her chest, heart, lungs and breast areas:

'I feel my chest collapsing, my throat is tight, it hurts, now it's closing. I feel rigid, almost dead. I can barely breathe. Tingling all across my chest and arms, keep them locked-in at my sides. I must not breathe...a word... not let a word slip out or...die.'

At precisely this moment of peak discomfort, a scream shot through our room from the children's playground directly outside. The piercing volume and tone of the young girl's voice was shattering and 'broke the spell' of muteness as it expressed the intensity of what was held inside the client's 'burning breast'. The 'therapeutic intervention', the emergent true expression in the client's 'unoccupied channel' (vocal speech) (Mindell, 1990 p.24) came as an aside, from the margins, just as in wild nature, stories, dreams, flashes of insight and wisdom are catalysed by seemingly peripheral events. Such imperatives to keep silent under duress and in the face of injustice feature in many ancient stories where we witness the protagonist's creative survival strategies, sometimes as despair transmuting into profound inner resilience and self-validation during the course of long, repeated journeys or tasks requiring consistency and endurance. We see how consequences unfold down several generations, always with some positive maturational development in the main characters.

This client, like others, also found dancing triggering; the sexually

expressive exposure of raising her arms had led her to constrain her gestures. She worked on her fears of the disease, internalised prohibitions
and her longing to dance simultaneously, moving between somatic sensing, drawing and moving, gradually extending her range of permitted
moves and emerging with a story, 'The girl who danced herself well'.

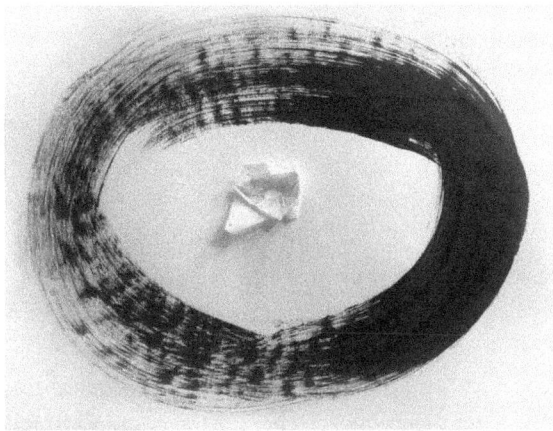

Figure 6.3: Untitled artist workshop participant

The Ancient Egyptian stories of Isis and Osiris and the Greek myth of
Persephone, and many more Indigenous tales globally, emphasise the
unity of the body of the people or the local ruler and the healthy ecology
of the realm. Early in a central story of The Virgin Queen cycle we are
told that the entire realm has fallen into ruin and a cause is hinted at in
the opening line, 'Once there was a King with three sons'. In northern
hemisphere tales, a hunt, for a deer, for a rare white doe, or glimpse of a
shape-shifting animal such as a fox, hare or unicorn is often understood
as a reference to the missing, usually feminine but sometimes masculine, principle, a necessary complementary mode of being and style of
authority, with its own sovereignty, whose presence and powers bring
balance to our psyches, embodied life, societal structures and ecologies.
These stories also often hint at an unaddressed transgression, resulting
in traumatic loss of a beloved person or state of innocence, by one or
more previous generations, and chart the process of repair and renewal.
In therapy, the pervading presence of hidden causes is often reflected
in statements like:

'I don't know where this comes from...'

'After she left she was never mentioned again.'

'I always felt there was something, but I never knew what...'

'My mother/father always seemed sad but nothing was ever spoken about...'

'No one ever spoke about the war/race/religion/suicide/the homeland/ the child that died...but it was somehow always present.'

'I found out in my twenties that I had been named after a sibling who had died in infancy.'

The emotionally charged presence-of-an-absence has the quality of a haunting, neither material nor immaterial. This may loom as an empty space in the sought-for coherent narrative identity and become a somatic abyss that can fill with anxiety, confusing dreams and lonely silence which, over time, may manifest in the body as metaphorical symptoms. Embracing the death and decay part of the life cycle is unavoidable in many old stories, a paradoxical challenge to overcome our instinctive terror and revulsion when the Knight in the tale, 'Dame Ragnelle' agrees to marry a hideous hag whose skin, as the story describes in detail, is rotting and pustulated, too repulsive to touch. His willingness to do this frees not only the woman from the spell but the entire lineage of the story. Wholeness is, once again, arrived at obliquely, paradoxically.

Sedna: Decay, dissolution and reciprocal renewal

Across Nordic Arctic regions, the goddess Sedna was the revered and feared creator-guardian of the seas and sea creatures. Her stories contain threads of many others and can accompany art therapists and their clients journeying through processes of decay, loss and dissolution, descent and recovery. Sedna may begin as a girl who is punished by her father for some unnamed offence, by being flung into the sea where her flesh is entirely eaten away by sea creatures. She descends, becoming a skeleton, and languishes as a jumble of bones being tumbled along the sea-bed by the currents. The oscillation between aversion and tender attention in this story is powerfully supportive in therapeutic exploration of processes of inner and relational healing (Pinkola-Estes, 1992).

'I was struck by the image of the loss of body and as I made my art I felt all the ways in which I "eat" myself, how I let my emotions eat away at myself with aggression and self-recrimination.'

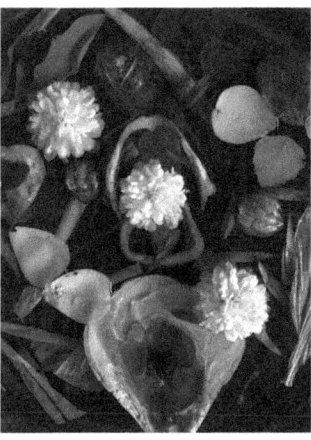

Figure 6.4: Skeleton Woman. Water collage (artist & photo B. A'Court)

As 'Skeleton Woman' she is eventually snagged on a fisherman's line and hauled in a ghoulish tangle to the surface and finally dragged back to his snow-house. Here the process of 'remembering' and the mutual renewal and union of both characters is described in precise, sensory detail. Looking behind oneself, looking and turning back, 'crossing the floor' are repeated images in this story, reminders to turn again towards what needs our care and attention, to not turn away entirely. The story takes time to describe the physicality of disentangling the line and limbs, the contact with the rotting bones, as if we are not to overlook this very physical aspect of healing ancestral trauma. Out of this touch, compassion and intimate care is born.

'I began with a feeling of ugliness and revulsion towards the wet, rotting and stinking flesh and bones but as I worked with the tiny pieces of wood, making her spine (which was difficult!) and limbs, I saw beauty in the broken pieces and finally I really like my Skeleton Woman puppet. She moves, dances, freely and flexibly.'

Working with natural materials allows bodily resonances with the life processes of the story to be awoken and felt.

'As I turned them (a collection of seashells) over one by one I realised I was making the same movements as the fisherman turning the bones and saw how the dirty shells were among the biggest and most beautiful. I had the insight that it can be important to start with things we dislike and as we apply our efforts they become precious.'

'I was most touched by her hand lifting the fisherman's heart out and beating it like a drum. I felt some pulse in the drawing and in my body. It became a movement that led to balance and something new that can happen between a man and a woman – I felt this pulsation as the starting point for birth.'

I have used this story in ecological art therapy with many women's groups and other groups dealing with relationships and gender, family separations and estrangements, loss, grief, illness, and preparation for invasive medical treatments. The resolution arrived at is an image of relational resilience that speaks to many aspects of contemporary experience.

'I felt my great fear of life and anger when Skeleton Woman beat the heart-drum but my painting became a red and black rose which transformed into a heart of two intersecting halves, then became mandala-like, radiating light and I had a feeling of reunion with my husband.'

'I let my fingers spontaneously tear and twist the paper, and when I partly untwisted them they resembled bones, so I made a construction from them and was struck by how life was present in the bones even after years on the sea bed – how even from a tiny spark of life some process can unfold.'

Wandering on...

Many people turn to art therapy to loosen or become free from negative ancestral and biographical stories that dominate and distort their perception and cognition. Psychodynamic and art therapies which have integrated mindfulness techniques help clients to develop skills and habits of:

- sensory awareness, sensitivity to body, materials and situation

- deep listening to the natural ebb and flow of inner and 'outer' phenomena
- self-compassion, acceptance and witnessing
- embodied presence, 'being with' experience to balance cognising 'about' it.

Ecopoiesis is a quintessential form for this; mindful art-making, transforming materials while being transformed, in reciprocal collaboration with nature's beings and forces.

Traditional stories, eroded and layered with sedimentary materials, like a landscape over time, often reach us in concentric circles or cycles. They are not merely 'about' people and events but embody in their structure a mandala-like transmission of profound realities. Looked at closely, they resemble the radiating fractals of chaos theory, where, for example, a single element spirals out connecting to a thousand more. A single medicinal herb, mineral or tree mentioned in a tale may imply not only the affliction for which it is the remedy and its resonances in a body of poetry and myth, but also hints at an originating event, a life-cycle, ecology, and the seen and unseen forces influencing life within that system.

Ecological therapies celebrate this holistic heritage and the shape-shifting, quantumly fluid, nature of living systems; they invite, activate and support inherent systemic self-regulation via processes that realign the person with health-generating forces within the entire field. The client engages with an expanded 'deep ecological self' identity, discerning and attending to authentic experience originating there.

Focusing on body awareness and biognosis or Earthsense as central is a fundamental, paradigmatic principle for developing sustainable and culturally sensitive art therapy that leads us away from the delusion that we can continue to abuse and desecrate nature in our attempts to improve life for humans. The legacy of earth-based healing practices' creative use of land forms – potent archetypal symbols present in the arts of many cultures – contributes to art therapy's development as a co-creative, responsive medium for diverse cultural settings, as it is increasingly called on globally to assist in ecological and other emergencies.

Traditional stories and the earth-based rituals embedded within their narratives present a world of coordinated forces playing out across geography, space and time, in ecologies of body-mind where sensory and poetic truths, universal truths (and their opposites), paradox, contradiction, humour and nonsense all have an active place. As such, these narratives offer a rich basis for ecological art-therapeutic and pedagogical work, a magical, alchemical and compassionate container and channel for the inherited traumas that seem, at least in part, to seed and contribute to ancestral health conditions.

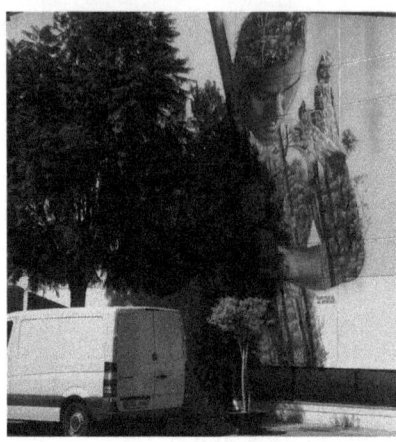

Figure 6.5: Mural, La Palma, Las Canarias
(Artist: Sabotaje L.L. Montaje. Photo: B. A'Court)

Notes: To my knowledge 'The Virgin Queen' story is still not written or published outside the Caucasus region, and continues its life as an orally transmitted tale. I thank Laura Simms (www.laurasimms.com) for her 'Queen of Everything' version and for many years of telling with exploration through art.

Thank you to clients and workshop participants whose experiences are included here. Some comments have been summarised for brevity and confidentiality.

References

A'Court, B. (2011). *The Healing Journey*. St. Petersburg: Rech (in Russian).

A'Court, B. (2016). A Communion of Subjects. In A. Kopytin & M. Rugh (eds), *Green Studio: Nature and the Arts in Therapy* (pp.47–76). Happauge, NY: Nova Science Publishers.

A'Court, B. (2017). The Art of Mindful Walking in Art Therapy. In A. Kopytin & M. Rugh (eds), *Environmental Expressive Therapies: Nature-Assisted Theory and Practice* (pp.123–161). London and New York, NY: Routledge/Taylor and Francis.

A'Court, B. (2020). *Remembering What We Know: Natural Wisdom and Archetypal Sorting Tasks.* Webinar. Short videos introducing this topic are available at www.youtube. com//channel/UCH-KvZpGJfymcrVDSuzUaeA.

Adler, J. (1987). Who is the witness? A description of Authentic Movement. *Contact Quarterly*, 12(1), Interviews.

Carter-Quinlan, N. (2020). *The Saltwater Songlines Project; An Embodied Ecology of Place.* www.embodiedterrain.com.

Dana, D. & Porges, S. (2018). *The Polyvagal Theory in Therapy: Engaging the Rhythm of Regulation.* London and New York, NY: W.W. Norton & Co.

Hayes, S., Folette, V. & Linehan, M. (2004). *Mindfulness and Acceptance: Expanding the Cognitive-Behavioural Tradition.* New York, NY: Guilford Press.

Hyde, P. & Jett, S. (1967). *Navajo Wildlands: As Long as the Rivers Shall Run.* Sierra Club, New York, NY: Ballantine Books.

Kellert, S. & Wilson, E. (eds) (1993). *The Biophilia Hypothesis.* Washington DC: Island Press.

Lame Deer, J. & Erdoes, R.J. (1972, rev. 2008). *Lame Deer, Seeker of Visions.* New York, NY: Pocket Books.

Lelièvre S. & Bissell, M. (1998). Communication between the cell membrane and the nucleus: Role of protein compartmentalisation. *Journal of Cellular Biochemical Supplement*, 30-31, 250-263.

MacFarlane, R. (2013). *The Old Ways: A Journey on Foot.* London: Penguin.

Macy, J., Seed, J., Fleming, P. & Næss, A. (1988). *Thinking Like a Mountain.* Gabriola Island, British Columbia: New Society Publishers.

Metzger, D. (1992). *Tree.* Oakland, CA: Wingbow Press.

Mindell, A. (1990). *Working on Yourself Alone.* London: Arkana, Penguin.

Moore, D.S. (2016). *Behavioural Epigenetics.* https://pzacad.pitzer.edu/~dmoore/publications/2016_moore_behavioral-epige.pdf.

Morris, L. (2017). Out of the Ruins: Australian Sites, Inspirited Landscapes and the Social Sacred. PhD thesis, Deakin University, Victoria, Australia.

Nichol, L. (ed.) (2003). *The Essential David Bohm.* London and New York, NY: Routledge.

Ogden, P. & Fisher, J. (2015). *Sensorimotor Psychotherapy: Interventions for Trauma and Attachment.* London and New York, NY: W.W. Norton.

Pinkola-Estes, C. (1992). *Women Who Run With the Wolves: Contacting the Power of the Wild Woman.* London: Rider, Random House.

Rothschild, B. (2000). *The Body Remembers: The Psychophysiology of Trauma and Trauma Treatment.* New York, NY: W.W. Norton.

Wagoner, D. (1999). *Travelling Light: Collected and New Poems.* Champaign, IL: University of Illinois Press.

Yehuda, R. & Bierer, L. (2008). Transgenerational Transmission of Cortisol and PTSD Risk. *Progress in Brain Research*, 167, 121-135.

Yehuda, R. & Bierer, L. (2009). The relevance of Epigenetics for the DSM-V. *Journal of Trauma & Stress*, 22(5), 427-435.

Yehuda, R., Daskalakis, N., Bierer, L., Klengel, T., Holsboer, F. & Binder, E. (2016). Holocaust exposure induced intergenerational effects on FKBP5 methylation. *Biological Psychiatry*, 80(5), 372-380.

Zettle, R.D. (2005). The evolution of a contextual approach to therapy: From comprehensive distancing to A.C.T. *International Journal of Behavioural Consultation and Therapy*, 1(2), 77-89.

Further reading

Kopytin, A. & A'Court, B. (2007). *Healing Journeys: Techniques of Analytical Art Therapy.* St.-Petersburg: Rech. (Russian).

Levine, P. (2010). *In an Unspoken Voice: How the Body Releases Trauma and Restores Goodness.* Berkeley, CA: North Atlantic Books.

Macy, J. & Brown, M. (1998, revised edition 2014). *Coming Back to Life: Updated Guide to The Work that Reconnects.* Gabriola Island, British Columbia: New Society Publishers.

Merleau-Ponty, M. (1969). *The Visible and the Invisible.* Lingis, A. (trans.) Lefort, C. (ed.). N. Evanston: Western University Press.

Olsen, A. & McHose, C. (1991). *BodyStories: A Guide to Experiential Anatomy.* New York, NY: Station Hill.

Siegel, D.J. (2007). *An Interpersonal Neurobiology Approach to Psychotherapy: Awareness, Mirror Neurons and Neuroplasticity in the Development of Well-Being.* www.ithou.org/node/2730.

Examples: Serpentine paths and mounds

Serpent Mound Park, Adams County, Ohio, USA

Loch-a-Neala, Argyll, Scotland

Otonabee, Ottawa, Ontario, Canada

King, A. (2019) Serpentine: *An Ancient Solstice Monument in Ontario.* https://ottawow.files.wordpress.com/2019/06/secretofthesnake.pdf.

Chapter 7

Making Sense of Solastalgia through Therapeutic Eco-Scenography

ELIZA SWEENEY

Introduction

In the *Poetics of Space*, Gaston Bachelard declares, 'the house shelters day dreaming, the house protects the dreamer; the house allows one to dream in peace' (Bachelard, 1957, p.28). My current doctoral research and art therapeutic practice juxtaposes this optimistic and idealist position to the current socio-political and ecological world context, and I wonder, how can we dream in peace when our home, our world, is falling down around us? For many, our home has lost its protective function which is a root cause for so much anguish and *solastalgia*, a concept signifying the feeling that the environment has abandoned the individual (Albrecht *et al.*, 2007). The dominant anthropocentric worldview, which since the Industrial Revolution has encouraged an ecological separatist vision, seeing human beings as distinct and apart from nature, has culminated in the exploitation of natural resources with little regard to long-term consequences. The crisis of the Anthropocene calls for creative approaches to understand the influence of the arts on mental health and to better comprehend humanity's apparent detachment from its place in ecological systems. The crisis does not represent a direct threat at the individual level for the majority of the developed western world, but primarily affects us by attacking the frameworks on which we have constructed our world. For French psychoanalyst psychologists Alexandre Sinanian and Marco Liguori:

what makes us live the environmental crisis at the stage where we can apprehend it on an individual, social and collective level, seems to be on the side of an anguish of transformation of our environmental meta-setting and a destabilization of the fundamental containers. (Sinanian & Liguori, 2020, p.17)

The unstable external environment is impacting the internal environment, like a disturbance of thought on the scale of humanity (Magnenat, 2019). In addition to the destabilisation of our external space, it has also been suggested that the primary reason for our current state of socio-ecological crisis is the persistent social construct of human–nature dichotomies (Laidlaw & Beer, 2018, p.283). A return to the knowledge that we are a part of and not apart from nature is necessary.

Bertolt Brecht's didactic poem, 'The Buddha's Parable of the Burning House', reminds us that humanity's survival depends on our ability to face the dangers that confront us, coupled with what we do with our home:

Lately I saw a house. It was burning... I went up close and observed that there were people still inside... I entered...exhorting them to leave... but those people seemed in no hurry... I went out again. Whoever does not yet feel such heat in the floor that he'll gladly exchange it for any other, rather than stay, to that man, I have nothing to say. (Brecht, 1961, pp. 31–32)

In responding to Brecht's warning call, 'we must rebuild the house of civilisation under different architectural principles, creating a more sustainable metabolism of humanity and the earth' (Foster, 2017, p.5). The parable alludes to the fact that some 'human beings differ from other biological creatures in that they have the ability to create suitable conditions for themselves using different environmental conditions' (Levine, 2019, p.5). Understanding the reciprocal relationship between the built environment, as a part of nature, and human life is vital, as Winston Churchill reminded us, 'We give form to our buildings and in the end, they form us' (Hall, 1966, p.136).

The work presented in this chapter is framed from my perspective as a scenographer, dramatherapist, philosopher and anthropologist, where 'anthropologists view humans as "meaning-making" beings, and so seek to understand how humans "bestow" meaning on any or all facets of life and the external world, including space' (Aucoin, 2017, p.397). I seek to understand meaning through the interaction and shaping of space using therapeutic scenography. In an ecopoietic way, it is in the shaping, sculpting, imagining and creative abilities of humanity that I look to for solutions to solastalgia. While crisis is a time of instability and insecurity, it can also be a turning point out of which new possibilities arise. The current global crisis can be seen as a liminal space, as a 'time out of time' (Thomassen, 2009), where humanity may be changed, as Van Gennep noted, to shift social status/function as they re-enter the new world. Time being inseparable to space, I propose that we can also provide a liminal 'space out of space' that provides unlimited possibilities from which new structures, frameworks and possible futures emerge.[1]

This chapter unveils the practice of 'therapeutic scenography' (Sweeney, 2014) that is rooted in eco-scenography, ecopoiesis, eco-somatics. As this chapter will attempt to show, therapeutic scenography engages with scenography as a tool for sense-making, for alleviating solastalgia, reclaiming agency over our place in the world, contributing to well-being and mental health and promoting the implicit knowledge that humans are shapers of this world. What I present here is by no means a closed model of practice but an open invitation for shaping, transformation and adaptation in itself.

Solastalgia

According to Australian environmental philosopher and father of solastalgia Glenn Albrecht, there is a correlation between the distress in ecosystems and human distress syndromes. From his phenomenological observations of psychological distress in correlation to the unforgiving Australian climate, Albrecht 'sought a suitable concept to describe the distress people were suffering' (Albrecht et al., 2005, p.42) and proposed the concept of solastalgia to explain the specific role played

---

1   To borrow from my educational dramatherapy colleague Clive Holmwood, the space is void of meaning until the meaning is placed on it, due to its ability to be both amorphous and constantly shifting and an open creative space which can be explored (Holmwood, 2014). For anthropologist Pamela Aucoin, the study of space and place recognizes that landscape, space and place represent important sites for cultural meaning, social and political memory, and public discourse. Space can be used to carry social meanings that are culturally and historically constructed as well as contested, while a sense of place develops out of human relationships, feeling, and imagination (Aucoin, 2017).

by global-scale environmental challenges to 'sense of place' and identity that were impacting human mental health and well-being.

Rooted in 'nostalgia', solastalgia embodies a 'feeling of melancholy caused by grief on account of absence from one's home country' but also a lack of 'solace or comfort derived from [their] present relationship to home' (ibid., pp.42–44). The etymology of solastalgia reminds me of the beautiful Welsh word, *hiraeth*, which signifies a longing for home, the nostalgia for a lost home, but more so, a deep longing for belonging to a symbolic place or a home inside ourselves, a longing for life (Iles, 2019). In this way, if our external environment is crumbling and eroding, then implicit in the experience of solastalgia is the presence of *hiraeth*. For Albrecht, solastalgia is the pain experienced when there is recognition that home is under immediate assault (physical desolation) (Albrecht *et al.*, 2005, p.45). The feeling is manifested in an 'attack on one's sense of place, in the erosion of the sense of belonging (identity) to a particular place and a feeling of distress' (ibid.), which he calls psychological desolation, about its transformation. Alongside this feeling of distress is a sense of powerlessness and 'that environmental injustice [is] being perpetrated' (ibid., p.44) on humanity. Solastalgia could be considered a form of eco-pathology, where the catastrophic effects of the climate crisis (drought, flood, famine, displacement due to extreme weather events, disease) are not only impacting the environment around us but are causing our internal landscapes to erode: isolation, distress, anxiety, depression, grief and melancholy abound. In summation, solastalgia signifies the feeling that the environment has abandoned the individual. (It is noteworthy that solastalgia can also occur in non-climate-related phenomena such as terrorism and war, when the stable environment is equally off-balance.)

Albrecht sees solastalgia as future-oriented, something that produces a counter-feeling to nostalgia, a desire to actively seek and create new things, to engage in collective action, that contributes to solace and offers solutions, where solastalgia can be negated by the natural restoration of the present, to something that is full of creative and productive potential. In this way, solastalgia could be regarded as a positive response in the face of climate catastrophe, as it leads to self-preservation and survival behaviours. This positive consequence to a less than positive feeling is comparable to Sigmund Freud's proposal of the 'anxiety-signal', whereby feelings of anxiety, otherwise experienced as negative, activate the 'fight or flight' response (Freud, 1926). Akin to Foster's call for a world that is constructed on new architectural principles, Albrecht suggests that solastalgia may seek its alleviation of suffering in a future that is redesigned. He suggests that 'the full transdisciplinary idea of health involves the healing of solastalgia via cultural responses to degradation of the environment in the form of drama, art, dance and song at all scales of living from the bioregional to the global' (Albrecht *et al.*, 2005, p.55). Responding to solastalgia involves proposing new ways to take back some agency over the external environment, to find models that put into motion a shift from a passive to active positioning. Overwhelmed by a mountain of feeling about the impending apocalypse, humanity needs a safe place to come to make sense of it all, to image and shape new and possible futures.

The senses

Much *thinking* has gone into understanding the crisis and now is the time to *feel*. Understanding the importance of sensations at the surface of the body, sensations which leave memory traces and contribute to the creation of representations and the constitution of borders between the external and internal environments of bodily interactions, is nothing new. In 1957, British paediatrician and psychoanalyst Donald Winnicott proposed his theory of the transitional object (Winnicott, 1957): the soft, tactile qualities of the object (often a toy or blanket) in contact with the child's skin coupled with the sensorial experience (smell, touch, taste, sight) facilitates the natural process of the development of the child's sense of self and a shift away from co-dependence on the maternal environment towards independence. More recently, French psychoanalyst Didier Anzieu contributed the notion of the 'skin-ego'. Elaborating his theory from Freud's original advocacy of the ego (self) as 'a bodily ego' (Freud, 1923, p.238), Anzieu postulated that supported by external sensations at a skin level, the internal psychic environment continues and organises the individual's internal sense of self. Depending on the type of sensations experienced, the individual will either develop a solid or fragile sense of self and be more or less capable of making sense of the world around them (Anzieu, 1995).

These ideas, rooted originally in psychology, are present in contemporary ecopoietic, philosophic and theatre thought. Amanda Bingley (2003) proposes, in response to Winnicott's theory of potential space, that early childhood experiences of self in relation to other may profoundly influence subsequent perceptions and experiences of landscape as an adult. Stephen K. Levine follows Winnicott, Freud and Anzieu's lead but goes beyond them, asserting that the human being experiences this world through the senses before they are able to understand it intellectually. He reminds us that the senses not only give us bodily impressions, they also make sense and indicate where to take action (Levine, 2019, p.5). Likewise, theatre professor Richard Schechner, in his account of environmental design (1971), takes this thinking a step further and proposes that communication and sense-making come from a relationship specifically to space, 'from within the spaces of the body to within the spaces of the place being explored' (Schechner, 1971, p.388). He goes on to give weight to the belief that space influences emotional experience in his outline of 'rasaesthetics' (2001), where rasa, an emotional or aesthetic response, the juice or taste of an emotional experience, 'fills space, joining the outside to the inside, what was outside is transformed into what is inside' (Schechner, 2001, p.29).

My personal practice of rasa boxes, coupled with understanding rasaesthetics and nourished by readings of the anthropology and aesthetics of the senses by Constance Classen and David Howes, has contributed greatly to the thinking behind the development of therapeutic scenography, which proposes a deeper understanding of the influence of exterior space on internal landscapes.

Therapeutic scenography encourages a direct and sensorial bodily experience with space, the scenographic environment, with the implicit understanding of the body as an extension of that environment. In light of the current climate crisis and dismantling of known and understood external, environmental, political and social frameworks, scenography takes on the symbolic role of a transitional object, a liminal space, providing a sensorial place to meet with dreaming, imagination, creativity and capable of being used as a platform for launching towards future possibilities, maturation and transformation.

Space

My purpose is not to declare that space is significant, which by now is a well-known fact (Warf & Arias, 2009), but to explore the ways in which the understanding of space as a force for change has been neglected and to provide a strong foundation that supports the knowledge that space can be harnessed as a tool for positive change. For Jean Laplanche (1989, p.137), 'space is the terrain where the singular problem of the patient is played out, where he is confronted by the existence, the permanence, the strength of his unconscious desires and fantasies'.

Roger Grainger (1934–2015), a major dramatherapy theorist, contended that the structure of drama has a healing potential in itself, being fundamentally modelled on ritual, emphasizing that in order to understand these processes, the notion of space plays a central role. Space is not simply a passive receptacle, 'an inert figure but is a living and elastic substance' (Serriere, 1959, p.72), in constant 'co-construction with the subject' (Hocini, Le Run & Potel Baranes, 2006, p.6).

Urban planners have specific training permitting them to be designers of the built environment. The very spaces within which we live and work are decided for us. In towns and cities, citizens rarely have much, if any, agency over the built environments within which they live and work on a daily basis and are thus relegated to a position of *spectator*. This phenomenon reinforces the social construct of human nature dichotomies which are at the heart of our current state of socio-ecological crisis (Laidlaw & Beer, 2018, p.283). The very idea that nature is *out there,* that humans are separate from nature, creates an erosion of our implicit relationship with our lived environments. And from this erosion, from this passive positioning, arises, as we have seen, solastalgia. The feeling that we have no agency, and must be spectators to the chaos of the environment collapsing around us, creates the perfect conditions for solastalgia and other eco-related pathologies to grow. Unfortunately, what urban planners have traditionally failed to understand is that space is not simply a physical structure that belongs to a living environment but, rather, quintessentially a phenomenon that possesses the indisputable potential to influence our emotional, sensorial, relational lives as well as our physical and mental development (Hall, 1966).

In response to Hall's proposition, contemporary sociologists, anthropologists, geographers, environmental psychologists and as well as psychotherapists have sought out quantitative and qualitative explanations, providing in-depth studies confirming Hall's proposal (Aucoin, 2017; Foster, 2017; Proshansky, 1976; Shepley, Arch & Danko, 2017; Wells & Donofrio, 2011). Thanks to such studies, urban architects and city planners are thinking more about the potential impact on human mental health and well-being when designing their buildings.

Understanding the interactivity of architecture and psychology comes together in a 'reading of the interior, for both are cultural discourses of the seen and the unseen, the visible and the invisible, of public and private space' (Fuss & Sander, 1997, para. 3). For Richard Schechner, 'articulating a space means letting the space have *its* say. That is, looking at a space and exploring it, not as a means of doing what you want to do in it, but of doing what the space encourages you to do in it' (Schechner, 1990, p.99). Regarding architecture and the built environment from a therapeutic scenographic perspective, I argue that we must better understand how space influences behaviour, in order to build and construct new worlds that encourage healthy, sustainable behaviour and well-being. Further, I argue for the implication of individuals and communities in the design and shaping process of lived environments as a way to increase feelings of agency over an unstable world.

The exponential number of studies inquiring into space and mental health indicates to me that greater importance and weight must be attributed to space in fields that deal with mental health, such as the arts therapies, and, to a further extent, to the influence of scenography, as a space-shaping practice, on well-being and mental health. Levine (2019) talks of our aesthetic responsibility as art therapists, to accompany individuals and groups in finding their aesthetic response by harnessing poiesis, their capacity to shape the world so that it brings about beauty in their lives. Similarly, scenography can be harnessed as an artistic practice through which individuals and communities can project their anguish and feelings of solastalgia into space and see them transformed into something positive, aesthetic, beautiful and hopeful. When we feel that the world is collapsing around us, being able to imagine and stage a scene that embodies a brighter, cleaner, safer, healthier future is vital.

Scenography

Historically, scenography was entrusted to the theatre, concerned with bringing scripted narrative to life in a visual, tangible and sensorial way for the audience. Similar to urban architecture and design, orthodox scenography was defined by the director, designer and writer (Schechner, 1971, p.394), leaving actors and audience with no authority over the spaces they performed in and interacted with. Shakespeare eloquently wrote, 'all the world's a stage and the men and women, merely players'. Both Shakespeare and Schechner support the idea that humanity, like actors and audience members, is passive in the experience and agency of space. Actors have no authority over the space within which they will perform, citizens over the world in which they live – they are 'tenants' (Schechner, 1971, p.394). Coincidentally, Glenn Albrecht informs us that 'connected to powerlessness and a sense that environmental injustice [is] being perpetrated onto them [humanity]' (Albrecht *et al.*, 2007, p.45) is ecologic distress.

Contemporary scenography knowledge goes beyond orthodox traditions, taking scenography into a 'beyond' (Hann, 2019) where scenographics are situated outside 'conventional roles and sites of theatre' (Hannah, 2015, p.128) and have the potential to enact speculative worlds that afford new insights (ibid.). Scenography is harnessed not only as a tool of 'human action' (Hann, 2019, p.22), but is considered an interrelated phenomenon that breaks down the binary of human to non-human distinction and proposes something more comprehensive where human and non-human forms encounter one another in a harmonious relationship (Beer, 2016). This theory calls to mind Rachel Hann's approach to scenography as 'an act of place orientation' (Hann, 2019, p.19), where 'orientations emerge from how bodies relate to objects...relate to other bodies, and how objects relate to objects' (ibid.). Hann postulates that 'To speak of orientation is to recognize the multiplicities of phenomena that situate bodies *within and with place*, oscillating between internal (symbolic, embodied) and external (experiential, proxemic) influences' (ibid.). Contrary to orthodox scenographic scholarship, Hann invites us to 'consider how scenographics move spectators and performers emotionally as well as physically' (Hann, 2019, p.5). Such ideas are rooted in the ancient Japanese philosophy of *Keshiki*, a philosophy that denotes that space is felt and not seen (Sasaki, 2013) and is incorporated into the philosophical roots of therapeutic scenography.

Scenography implies something more than creating scenery or costumes or lights. As Arnold Arronson notes, 'It carries a connotation of an all-encompassing visual-spatial construct as well as the process of change and transformation' (Arronson cited in Hann, 2019, p.39). I propose that imagining and creating new and possible futures through scenographic sculpture spaces can provide a creative and symbolic space that encourages individuals and communities to reconnect with land, discover safety and solace, reclaim their identity, and bring about a form of unification and community that ultimately leads to improved well-being and transformation. Not only does scenography offer a model of artistic and design practice that promotes the creation of space, it is an art form imbued with sensory experience and aesthetic power.

Therapeutic scenography

At the very heart of combining psychology with scenography is the understanding of the interface between human design and human well-being. For the past six years, I have defined and refined the application of scenography for therapeutic and wellness outcomes. This practice came to be named 'psychoscenography' or 'therapeutic scenography', neologisms that I use to denote that practice of understanding how scenography (more particularly eco-scenography), influences human psychology, behaviour and relationships. Similar to Schechner's environmental theatre, therapeutic scenography promotes the principle that 'the performer is the chief designer of environmental theatre spaces' (Schechner, 1971 p.397; 1990, p.98). In the same way, clients should be the chief designers of the spaces in which they play, explore, learn and live in the dramatherapy space, as communities need to have agency over the built environment in which they live, in cities across the world.

While the intentional application of scenography for therapeutic outcomes is new, indications of scenographic practice in therapy settings can be traced back to the birth of Freudian psychoanalysis when in 1913, Freud spoke of the psychoanalytical space in *The Psychoanalytic Technique*. Freud presented his understanding of the importance of space when he attributed a conscious and precise function to the couch, with the intentional placement and orientation of the couch in his office: 'its objective is to prevent the contamination of the body transfer by associations of the patient, of isolating and withdrawing the transfer' (Freud, 1913, in Strachey, 1958, pp.133–135). For Hann, the placement, the *situatedness* of an object, speaks volumes, where its orientation 'can articulate as much as the object itself' (Hann, 2019, p.28), creating what Hann calls 'place orientation' and 'worlding' (Hann, 2019).

To put a complex notion in simple terms, the placement of an object transforms the space into something or somewhere else. Taking the couch from a therapeutic scenographic perspective, the object is therapeutic in its containing and holding function, in its promotion of reverie but equally in its sensorial qualities that evoke sensorial experiences in the patient, leading to shaping or finding form for their experiences. It is scenographic in its place orientation and worlding. In providing the space for reverie, the Freudian couch becomes a 'stage-life', an *outer landscape* where the inner story of the patient is played out. Though the term 'scenographic' was undoubtedly absent from Freud's mind at the time, his choice of aesthetics calls to mind '[a] mysterious lion's den or Aladdin's cave of treasures' (Fuss & Sander, 1997, para. 27). Evoking a dramatic aesthetic, his decision to position the couch in such a particular way is undisputedly scenographic.

The connection between psychotherapy, drama and space is not a new idea. In his article, 'A psychoanalytical model for the stage', George Balassa (1978) presents initial elements of a psychoanalytical theory of theatre from a spatial positioning, drawing specific attention to the more than remarkable coincidence that theatre director Jerzy Grotowski and Scottish psychiatrist R.D. Laing 'found themselves compelled to define, almost simultaneously, theatre and psychotherapy' in spatial terms (Balassa, 1978, p.36). In *Towards a Poor Theatre* (1965, p.20), Grotowski wrote, 'theatre needs a specific space, organised and created by the actor and the audience member'. In *The Politics of Experience* (1967), Laing wrote, 'psychotherapy needs a specific space organised and created by the therapist and patient'. In recent years, Richard Schechner has reiterated the importance of space for agency in his extensive publications on space, theatre and the environment (1968, 1971, 1990). Both theatre directors and psychotherapists acknowledge the need for an explicit understanding and use of space for both theatrical and therapeutic purposes and affirm my belief in an important overlap of space, drama and psychotherapy that has been undervalued for too long. Therapeutic scenography brings together Schechner, Laing and Grotowski's proposals in one space, where therapy, scenography, drama and space offer a specific paradigm for agency, well-being and creativity. Therapeutic scenography provides a sensory-based process to explore internal landscapes through the creation of external scenographic spaces, through which the suffering of solastalgia can be eased, and a reconnection and a healing with the external or non-human environment can occur. It provides a sensorial space to imagine and stage new scenarios of possible futures and then encourages these discoveries to be taken out into the real world, moving from possibility to existence.

Early in my career as a dramatherapist, I had the opportunity to observe how children in a paediatric psychiatry setting engaged with the built environment as a tool for support: throwing their bodies up against walls, ripping curtains, enveloping their bodies in the fabric, hiding and reappearing behind walls, creating cubby houses or tents under tables, and so on. These movements and sensorial interactions with space suggested to me a need in these children for spaces that were malleable and flexible, as well as solid enough to contain their fragile internal landscapes. It was not through role play or puppetry that they were finding solace, structure or transformation, but in their relationship to the built environment. Based on these observations, I constructed programmes that intentionally utilised space, scenography and the built environment as tools for therapeutic outcomes. My understanding of the therapeutic implications of the built environment and mental health, coupled with practice-based research, led to the establishment of a paradigm and practice of 'therapeutic scenography'. As with all practice, it is evolving and I increasingly feel a professional and artistic responsibility to apply this practice in response to the environmental crisis. Consequently, I have been drawn to exploring deeper applications of eco-scenography, as a specific scenographic paradigm that can be applied for therapeutic and wellness outcomes.

Towards a therapeutic eco-scenography

Understanding that we are inextricably a part *of* nature and not apart *from* nature is key to understanding and resolving psychological anguish and unsustainable behaviours. Drawing from eco-scenography, I try to engage individuals and communities with a process of imagining, shaping and making natural, strong, beautiful scenographic spaces, as a way to gain back agency over the failing external world and as an avenue to reconnecting to the implicit understanding that *we are* nature.

Eco-scenography is a burgeoning field that proposes a new paradigm for the performing arts. For award-winning ecological designer Tanja Beer, 'like ecology, scenography is concerned with interrelationships – the interactivity between architecture, light, sound, bodies and the senses; a metaphor for the "ecosystem" of total theatre experience'. This perspective extends the potential of scenography to influence human health and well-being in the face of an ecological crisis. The concept of eco-scenography recalls Schechner's outline for environmental theatre and 'the need for taking into account the relationship between body space and theatre space' (Schechner, 1990, p.100). Beer defines eco-scenography as 'the integration of ecological thinking into all stages of scenographic production and aesthetics' (Beer, 2016, p.18). She proposes that 'embracing scenography for a thriving future will require a strong desire to seek out meaningful relationships, opportunities and abundance with readiness to respond, adapt and evolve to changing circumstances' (Beer, 2016, p.195). Furthermore, eco-scenography applies the idea of *Keshiki,* that space is felt and not seen and provides more opportunities for individuals and communities to engage with the design-making process with all their senses: touch, smell, sight, sound and even taste. Beer's seminal project 'The Living Stage' is an example of a bold experimentation with stage design, permaculture and community engagement. Part theatre, part garden, the multisensory aspects of scenography engaged its audience on a haptic, olfactory and gustatory level (the set was edible) (Beer, 2013) bringing from theory to practice Schechner's view that 'all space senses are to be included in planning an environment' (Schechner, 1971, p.397).

I did not always define myself as an eco-scenographer. Thanks to personal exchanges with Tanja Beer, I have come to understand that my design work was always very much in line with eco-scenographic principles: creations were made by available (recycled, repurposed) materials as opposed to materials being sourced to achieve a particular design, there was the intention for an 'after-life' of the sets and costumes, and I always felt that my designs embodied a form of implicit social or environmental activism.

I adopt Beer's eco-scenographic values as a form of engaging with ecology and human health that takes into consideration the creative process as an explorative territory, that 'encourages exploration and research for personal and creative development' (ibid.). Beer argues that 'ecoscenography works from the premise that there is nothing more fulfilling than connecting to the living world in a way that is fundamental, positive and inspiring'. Therapeutic scenography practice integrates this philosophy by encouraging re-thinking, re-imagining, restoring and regenerating in the face of a degenerating world. It offers a model of artistic practice that engages the senses, whether it be through colours and textures, shapes and space configurations of an immersive scenic space, the feeling of a particular fabric against the skin when wearing a purposefully designed costume, or tasting the fresh herbs straight off the walls of Beer's 'Living Stage'. It encourages embodiment, movement and the expression of emotions and can contribute to the process of making sense. Combining eco-scenographic principles (Beer, 2016) with psychology is based on the explicit understanding of the interface between living systems, human design and human well-being.

Practice example

In 2018, I was invited to Utrecht in the Netherlands by the Dutch Drama-therapy Association (NVDT) and was privileged to provide an explorative workshop on my model of therapeutic scenography for dramatherapy professionals working with trauma. Entitled The Metamorphoses Project, this practice was scored by the metaphor of the life cycle of the butterfly. Before becoming a butterfly, the beautiful insect must be egg, cocoon and chrysalis. It is an exact example of metamorphosis and perfectly embodies the philosophy and process of therapeutic scenography: the client enters the liminal dramatherapy space in one form, immersing themselves in sensorial explorations with the built environment (cocoon, costume, set space) and emerges transformed, thus recalling Van Gennep's (1960) and Turner's (1969) vision of liminal space.

Ted Hughes' adaptation of Ovid's *Metamorphosis* text contributed sensorial imagery to support the scenographic creations. Ovid's text is rich in thick and descriptive language that invites an embodied exploration of its central themes: metamorphosis, identity, transformation, the victim and the hero, the body, the soul, the psyche, power and weakness, fear, mourning, loss and the future. The text was initially explored through dance, free movement and human sculpture, putting into form a sensory experience of 'bodies changed into new forms' (Hughes, 1997, p.1). Participants explored the limits of their physical selves in the play space, creating striking visual physical landscapes that formed aesthetically beautiful physical poetry. I consider movement and embodiment of text or emotions as vital to the creative therapy process, informed by Schechner's positioning that 'theatre space is derived from body space' (1971, p.388). Furthermore, the work is framed by theories and practices of eco-somatics where the direct sensory relationship of the body with space in nature and as nature creates new knowledge and understanding. In an attempt to unveil ourselves *as* nature not *in nature*, an embodied exploration of the images embedded in Ovid's narrative contributed to a reconnecting of human and nature: 'blood as sap, arms as boughs, fingers twigs, skin bark'. Nature is commonly framed as something out there, beyond the city – when it is in fact everywhere, in us and all around us (Laidlaw & Beer, 2018), as Ovid's text demonstrates.

From this physical reconnection to nature, this awakening or rebirthing of self as a part of nature, participants engaged with set and costume making. In the first instance, creating a cocoon space from recycled sleeping bags, fabrics and craft materials, and in the second, forming a costume space, a second skin that visually represented the transformed internal state of the individual.

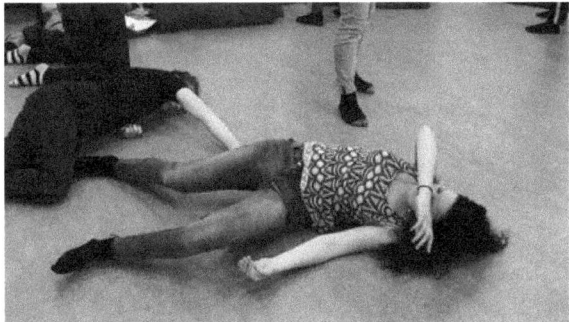

Figure 7.1: Some are transformed just once, and live their whole lives after in that shape (Hughes, 1997)

Ovid's narrative text can be understood, from an orthodox theatre perspective, as the departure point for scenographic design. On the contrary, I encouraged participants to embody the words in the first instance, and in the second, to connect with the emotions and subjective imagery generated by this experience and the materials provided, as the departure points for scenographic creations. The design brief was short: to create a cocoon that signifies (for the individual) a safe, protective and 'home-like' space, and a costume that represents rebirth and a projection of self after metamorphosis (transition from post-crisis self to post-therapy self).

Participants and clients always take great care and express pleasure in the creation of their spaces, nurturing their creations similarly to how they have experienced nurturing in the art therapy process, affirming the idea that 'we find happiness in our capacity to shape the world so that we can bring beauty into being' (Levine, 2019, p.5). The costume space acts as a second skin, becomes a part of the client, and so in the creation of their costume, they are bringing to life a part of themselves. The costume design symbolises the transition, embodying the transformative process of art therapy, arriving in the therapy space in one form, and leaving as another. The wearing of the costume demonstrates in a visual way the crossing of the threshold from the liminal space back into the reality of the everyday space, but now changed. It marks the final transition from one form to another, encapsulating in one final scenographic creation, the move from the therapy space out into the world. It signifies a celebration, a rebirth into new forms, a shift into colour and beauty.

In this practice-led example, the cocoons, symbolic of a transitional space and even a literal liminal space, remained surprisingly simple in design, almost in keeping with the sober style of a true chrysalis (Figure 7.2). The costumes, however, were bright, colourful and vibrant, and took the form of butterfly wings (Figure 7.3). In this way, I see my aesthetic responsibility as therapist to be guiding clients towards metamorphosis, and a new aesthetic form, encapsulated in the form of the butterfly.

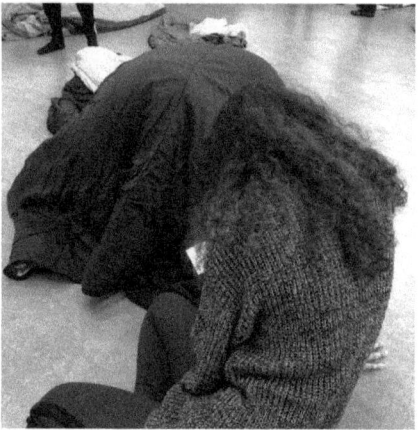

Figure 7.2: A participant prepares inside the safety of her sleeping bag cocoon

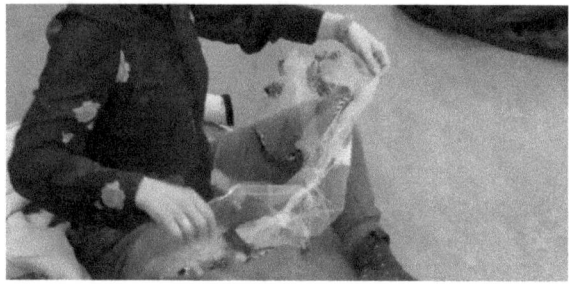

Figure 7.3: A participant in the midst of creating her wings

The process of shaping the cocoons and the wings not only provided an artistic support for the group to sew and weave their personal stories into creation but simultaneously furnished a storytelling community, an invaluable tool for sustainable development. Sharing experiences serves as 'an emotional mortar where participants form layers of meaning that activate personal, aesthetic and ecological sensibilities'.

Once the participants were satisfied with their scenographic creations, they played in the dramatic space, orating lines from Hughes' text, forming physical sculptures and dance as dramatic supports to tell their stories, before gliding inside their sleeping bags to rest, breathe and connect with arising emotions. In their own time, they emerged from their safe space, their chrysalis, donning their costumes. Their bodies unfolded, limbs stretched and extended into a final statue (Figure 7.4). We were met with something aesthetically beautiful at the end of this process: the body holding an open sculpture, arms outstretched, a peaceful expression across the individual's face, and the colour, shape and texture of their costume creation wrapped around them. Finally, the caterpillar, having completed its journey, was transformed into the beautiful butterfly ready to fly out into the world.

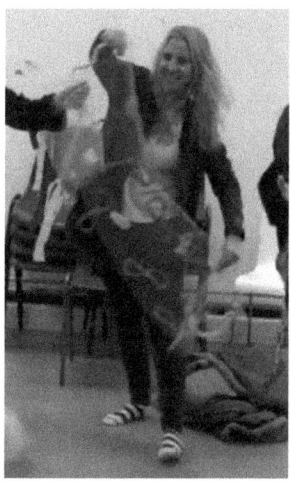

*Figure 7.4: Taking a final statue at the end of the
process, the participant spreads her wings*

Conclusion

Housing can be safe, and housing can be dangerous, depending on your socio-economic situation; in certain circumstances, it can lose its protective function (Nemet-Pier, 2006). I came to appreciate this idea during the Covid-19 lockdowns in Paris through my interactions with children and families in precarious situations. In response to the crisis, I implemented a therapeutic scenography programme within a French national programme for childhood protection and educational support. The programme was elaborated around the immediate need to *get out of the house,* to take space from family members and from the reality of the crisis, without actually leaving the building. Via an online platform, I supported children in the construction of scenographic sets and costumes. In line with eco-scenographic principles, the children were encouraged to use materials found around the home (old bed sheets, pillows, recycled egg cartons, cereal boxes and milk cartons, paper and colouring pencils and special treasured objects).

The costumes – astronaut helmets – provided creative distancing from the oppressive reality of the surgical masks worn outside the home. When coupled with enacting or role-playing astronauts, children were better equipped to manage a mask, wearing without it causing as much fear and anxiety. Compared to the sterile, cold blue and white masks, their creations were beautiful, and the children wore them proudly. Appropriating the dining room table (in most cases), the children set about using bed sheets, pillows, toys, and treasured objects to make a 'space ship' set space. By appropriating these common home spaces, they not only created a scenographic space that encouraged imaginative and dramatic play, but in homes where personal space was rare, it simultaneously offered them a chance to develop agency over their built environments, as well as providing some rare private space (Hall, 1966; Nemet-Pier, 2006), beneficial to well-being. This experience illustrated to me how eco-scenography can be taken further, beyond private practice and applied in real-life situations.

In late 2021, I had hoped that therapeutic scenography would be explored for the COP26 (Climate Change Conference) meeting in Glasgow, Scotland, where in collaboration with local eco-scenographers, we had planned to provide a therapeutic and artistic scenographic space for people to gather and contribute to the design and construction of an eco-scenographic therapy house. It was intended that this eco-therapeutic space would be open to the public in a permanent installation in a local garden in Glasgow, embodying a place that invites community gathering to open up discussion, to sense and feel about the climate crisis, to face solastalgia and find collective solutions. Unfortunately, our proposal was not accepted this year, but the project is being reconsidered for another event or social cause.

Therapeutic eco-scenography is an evolving practice and continues to grow in the face of the catastrophic climate crisis. It is undeniable that the built environment on the one hand evokes aesthetic and emotional responses, and on the other hand, can influence behaviour, relations and well-being. The shaping of space offers a potential that engages clients actively in the creation and construction of built environments that are intended to facilitate paths to well-being. Inspired by Buddhist Monk Matthieu Ricard and astrophysicist Trinh Xuan Truan's *The Quantam and the Lotus* (2001), I am reminded that humanity rarely sees the world exactly as it is. Our experience is filtered through the screen of our longings, our *hiraeith,* and our fears, our *solastalgia,* onto which we project the interpretation of what we call reality. If what we take to be true is our reality (Bohm in Ricard and Truan, 2001), then in the face of the environmental crisis, we must as artists, therapists and change agents offer up to humanity the possibility to view the world with a new perspective, and to imagine and create new and possible futures and discover new truths. Embracing *Keshiki,* inviting individuals and communities to understand that space is felt and not simply seen, may be a way to guide a new perspective. What has been presented in this chapter is an opening for ongoing inquiry into the importance of built environments, the climate crisis, well-being and community engagement.

References

Albrecht, G. (2020). Negating solastalgia: An emotional revolution from the anthropocene to the symbiocene. *American Imago, 77*(1): 9–30.

Albrecht, G., Sartore, G.M., Connor, L., Higginbotham, N. *et al.* (2005). Solastalgia: The distress caused by environmental change. *Australasian Psychiatry*, 15(1), 41–55. doi:10.1080/10398560701701288.

Anzieu, D. (1995). *Le Moi-Peau*. Paris: Dunod.

Aucoin, P.M. (2017). Toward an Anthropological Understanding of Space and Place. In B. Janz (ed.), *Place, Space and Hermeneutics: Contributions to Hermeneutics*. Berlin: Springer. https://doi.org/10.1007/978-3-319-52214-2_28.

Bachelard, G. (1957). *La Poétique de l'Espace*. Paris: University Press.

Balassa, G. (1978). A psychoanalytical model for the stage. *Performing Arts Journal*, 3(1), 35–39.

Bingley, A. (2003). In here and out there: Sensations between self and landscape. *Social & Cultural Geography*, 4(3), 329. https://doi.org/10.1080/14649360309081.

Beer, T. (2013) *The Living Stage*. https://ecoscenography.com/the-living-stage.

Beer, T. (2016). Ecoscenography: The Paradigm and Practice of Ecological Design in the Performing Arts. PhD thesis. Faculty of Architecture, Building and Planning and Victorian College of the Arts, The University of Melbourne, Australia.

Brecht, B. (1961). *Tales from the Calendar*. London: Methuen.

Foster, J.B. (2017). The Anthropocene Crisis. *The Jus Semper Global Alliance: Essays on Building the New Paradigm of People and Planet* (pp.1–6). Adapted from the foreword to I. Angus (2016) *Facing the Anthropocene: Fossil Capitalism and the Crisis of the Earth System*. Monthly Review Press.

Freud S. (1923/1981), *"Le Moi et le ça"*, Essais de psychanalyse, Paris, Payot, p.238. (Freud 1887, p.157)

Freud, S. (1926). Inhibition, symptôme et angoisse. *OCF XVII* (1992, pp.203–286). Paris: University Press.

Fuss, D. & Sander, J. (1997). Berrggasse 19: Inside Freud's Office. *Stud: Architectures of Masculinity*. London: Routledge. http://joelsandersarchitect.com/berggasse-19-inside-freuds-office-with-diana-fuss.

Grotowski, J. (1965). *Vers un Theatre Pauvre*. Lausanne: Editions L'Age d'Homme.

Hall, E. (1966). *The Hidden Dimension*. New York, NY: Doubleday.

Hann, R. (2019). *Beyond Scenography*. London and New York, NY: Wiley.

Hannah, D. (2015). Constructing barricades and creating borderline events. *Theatre and Performance Design Journal*, 1(1–2), 126–144.

Hocini, F., Le Run, J-L. & Potel Baranes, C. (2006). De l'Espace avant toute choses. *Enfances & Psy*, 4/6 (33), 6–7.

Holmwood, C. (2014). *Drama education and dramatherapy – exploring the space between disciplines*. London and New York: Routledge/Taylor and Francis.

Hughes, T. (1997). *Tales from Ovid*. London: Faber and Faber.

Iles, H. (2019). *Hiraeth: Out Longing for Belonging*. Simple Living Project.

Laidlaw, B. & Beer, T. (2018). Dancing to (re)connect: Somatic dance experiences as a medium of connection with the more-than-human. *Choreographic Practices*, 9(2), 283–309. doi:10.1386/ chor.9.2.283_1.

Laing, R.D. (1967). *The Politics of Experience*. London: Routledge and Kegan Paul.

Laplanche J. (1989). *Traduire Freud*. Paris: University Press.

Levine, S. (2019). *Philosophy of Expressive Arts Therapy: Poiesis and the Therapeutic Imagination*. London: Jessica Kingsley Publishers.

Magnenat, L. (2019). Le propre de l'homme à l'âge de l'Anthropocène: Homo sapiens demens. In *La Crise Environnementale sur le Divan*. Paris: In Press.

Nemet-Pier, L. (2006). Investissement et aménagement de l'espace dans la dynamique familiale. *Imaginaire & Inconscient*, 2(18), 215–224.

Proshansky, H.M. (1976). Environmental psychology and the real world. *American Psychologist*, 31(4), 303–310.

Ricard, M. & Truan, T.X. (2001). *The Quantum and the Lotus*. New York, NY: Crown Publishers.

Sasaki, K. (2013). Perspectives East and West. In *Contemporary Aesthetics*. https://contempaesthetics.org/newvolume/pages/article.php?articleID=670.

Schechner, R. (1968). 6 axioms for environmental theatre. *The Drama Review: TDR, Architecture/Environment*, 12(3), 41–64. www.jstor.org/stable/1144353.

Schechner, R. (1971). On environmental design. *Educational Theatre Journal*, 23(4), 379–397. www.jstor.org/stable/3205747.

Schechner, R. (1990). Behavior, performance, and performance space. *Perspecta*, 26 (*Theater, Theatricality, and Architecture*), 97–102 www.jstor.org/stable/1567156.

Searles, H.F. (1972). Unconcious processes in relation to the environmental crisis. *Psychoanalytic Review*, 59(3), 361–374.

Schechner, R. (2001). Rasaesthetics. *The Drama Review*, 45, 3 (T171).

Serriere, M.T. (1959). *Le T.N.P (Theatre National Populaire) et Nous*. Librairie José Corti. p.72.

Shepley, M., Arch, D. & Danko, S. (2017). Design as healing: The next generation of research informed practice. *Journal of Interior Design*, 41(1), 5–7. https://doi.org/10.1111/joid.12090.

Sinanian, A. & Liguori, M. (2020). Prolegomena of a psychoanalytic psychology on the environmental crisis. *In Analysis*. Revue Transdisciplinaire de Psychanalyse et Sciences, France.

Strachey, J. (1958). On Beginning the Treatment. In *The Standard Edition of the Complete Psychological Works of Sigmund Freud. Vol. XII (1911–1913)* (pp.133–135). Standard Edition. London: Hogarth Press.

Sweeney, E. (2014). Introduction to Therapeutic Scenography. MA thesis. Faculty of Artistic Creation and Psychology, Paris V La Sorbonne University, Paris.

Thomassen, B. (2009). The uses and meaning of liminality. *International Political Anthropology*, 2(1), 5–28.

Turner, V. (1969). *The Ritual Process*. Chicago, IL: Aldine.

Van Gennep, A. (1960). *The Rites of Passage*. London: Routledge.

Warf, B. & Arias, S. (2009). *The Spatial Turn: Interdisciplinary Perspectives*. London: Routledge.

Wells, N.M. & Donofrio, G.A. (2011). Urban Planning, the Natural Environment, and Public Health. In J.O. Nriagu (ed.), *Encyclopedia of Environmental Health*, volume 5 (pp.565–557). Burlington, MA: Elsevier.

Winnicott, D.W (1957). *Playing and Reality* (second edition). London: Routledge.

Chapter 8

Ecological/Nature-Assisted Art Therapy with War Veterans: How Nature Can Heal the Trauma of War

ALEXEY LEBEDEV AND ALEXANDER KOPYTIN

Introduction

Against the backdrop of military campaigns that involve many countries across the globe, the challenges that medical, therapeutic, and other helping professionals face in their work with veterans can be considered universal. As our awareness of the mental health and psychosocial issues facing veterans increases, we can observe a growing interest in programs and services that can effectively address the holistic well-being of ex-service personnel. Empirical experience and research findings related to art therapy programs adapted for veterans and other military members support the implementation and further improvement of these programs.

There are currently many different ways that art is used therapeutically with military personnel that vary depending on the professional background and theoretical orientation of practitioners, as well as the particular settings providing services, and other contextual factors. The range of existing approaches and models of art therapy applied with military and veteran populations is impressive and includes unstructured studio and gallery experiences (DeLucia, 2017; Haeseler, 1998; Lobban, 2014), group interactive art therapy/art psychotherapy (Backos & Mazzeo, 2017; Howie, 2017a, 2017b), along with individual and family art therapy (Howie, 2017b).

The social group known as war veterans comprises individuals who present a broad spectrum of mental disorders. Although a certain percentage of them have been identified as suffering from post-traumatic stress disorder (PTSD) and other stress-related disorders, some veterans reveal behavioral and mood disorders, addictions, and even psychotic states. Many of them are characterized as having high levels of emotional tension and instability, low impulse control, difficulties in interpersonal relations, distorted reactions to others, ambivalent and inadequate self-perception, and difficulties in securing existential meaning (Apchel & Tsygan, 1999; Faber-Taylor & Kuo, 2009). They may have a retrospective orientation towards life, or may organize their lives around those values and norms that were acceptable in combat situations while feeling lonely and unsafe in civilian life (Apchel & Tsygan, 1999; Kolov, Ostapenko, & Krivtsov, 2005).

Therefore, it would be impossible and ineffective to use certain unified models of art therapy with military and ex-service personnel. Specific characteristics of the particular clinical subgroup and the context of therapy should be taken into account in order to develop useful interventions for the therapy goals and conditions.

Environmental and ecological factors of veterans' health and well-being

The use of the therapeutic potential of natural objects and environments with different categories of clients, including war veterans, is relatively well known and is taken advantage of in multiple therapeutic interventions. These factors were often a part of treatment and rehabilitation programs with client groups such as war veterans long before trends like environmental psychology, ecopsychology, and ecotherapy entered the mainstream, along with their concepts and practices.

During World War II, gardening was used as occupational therapy for US veterans. This eventually led to the development of the horticultural therapy profession (Simson & Straus, 1998). At present, with the growing need for effective mental health services, many veterans are turning to alternative forms of "green" treatment in outdoor settings. Since camaraderie, physical challenge, and personal growth are characteristics of both military service and of many of the ecotherapeutic programs cropping up in different parts of the world, it makes this "green" treatment a relevant therapeutic modality for veterans struggling with post-traumatic stress and other mental disorders.

In the last two decades, a significant increase in the use of various ecotherapeutic/nature-assisted and environmental therapies applied with military populations and other groups of post-traumatic stress sufferers has been observable. Ecotherapy, an umbrella term to encompass many outdoor therapy approaches, can include adventure therapy, wilderness therapy, horticultural therapy, walk-and-talk therapy, and numerous other nature-oriented programs.

Challenging themselves physically and mentally and striving to attain a goal are familiar tasks for most individuals with a military background. Some veterans report being more willing to engage in an active form of treatment than conventional modes of therapy. Many veterans who engage in outdoor recreational activities have begun to rediscover their resiliency and have tapped into leadership skills they learned during military service. The aim of these ecotherapy programs and services is to help veterans reconnect to nature in a way that will conjure positive emotions and elicit a sense of confidence when reintegrating into the civilian world. This form of treatment is a way to garner the benefits of supportive therapy while being out in the wider environment. It encourages veterans to get out, connect with others, both humans and the more-than-human world.

Some of the research themes that are relevant to veterans and occur in parallel to health issues are as follows: psychological and physical healing from trauma, improving self-esteem and social skills, finding meaningful work, making sense of previous life experiences, and distraction from pain. Findings from numerous studies support the premise that contact with nature is beneficial for human health and well-being (Burls, 2007; Faber-Taylor & Kuo, 2009; Fleming, 2015; Heerwagen, 2009). Burls' (2007) research links human interactions with nature to human growth and development in the cognitive, emotional, spiritual, and aesthetic domains. Although not specially developed for military personnel, Burls' theory is compelling because it identifies human growth and development areas that speak to the experiences of both active military personnel and veterans. These include coping with adversity, heightened awareness (during combat), physical and mental fitness, and critical thinking skills.

Research by Batt-Rawdon and Tellnes (2005) reveals that outdoor activity for rehabilitation can provide stimulation, empowerment, and creative opportunities that can distract people from their social and health problems for short periods of time, contributing to their making sense of experiences by providing a feeling of continuity and coherence in their lives. Research by Groeneweggen and colleagues (2006), and others, indicates that human needs can be met through interaction with nature, including mental stimulation, socialization, and fulfillment, as well as a sense of usefulness, self-worth, love, and nurturing (Nebbe, 2006; O'Brien, 2005).

An increasing number of creative arts therapists/expressive therapists also strive to implement "green" and environmental practices in their work with military populations and other client groups who suffer from post-traumatic stress (Berger, 2008, 2009; Berger & Lahad, 2013; Haeseler, 1998; Kalmanowitz & Lloyd, 2011). Creative and expressive arts therapists are beginning to pay more attention to a complex "field of interactions" established not only by the client, the therapist, and an art object, but by many other objects and processes both inside and outside the therapy room.

Treatment setting, brief group art psychotherapy program, and procedure

Group interactive art therapy has been used at the specialized psychotherapy department at Volgograd Regional Clinical Hospital for War Veterans, Russian Federation, since 2003. The hospital belongs to the Ministry of Public Health and provides holistic treatment for war veterans. The psychotherapy department was established there in 1997, in accordance with "The Law on Veterans" and Order #373 (07.01.1997) to provide high-quality medical and psychosocial support to war veterans residing in Volgograd city and the Volgograd Region, who were involved in the military campaigns in various "flash point areas," and whose emotional disorders could not be treated outside the hospital setting due to their severity.

The staff of the psychotherapy department includes psychiatrists, psychotherapists, clinical psychologists, and nurses. Art therapy (art psychotherapy) is provided by a clinical art psychotherapist, who trained as a psychiatrist and psychotherapist and later took art therapy training over a period of two years. He is a member of the multi-professional team working at the hospital. The team provides patients with a combination of medical and psychosocial interventions including occupational therapy, counseling, individual and group therapy and group interactive art therapy (art psychotherapy) in order to enable not only a reduction of symptoms, but to provide multifaceted psychological and social support and the chance for veterans to work through their personal issues. Since 2006, art therapy remains the only expressive therapeutic modality applied at the department.

Group interactive art therapy sessions take place three times a week (every two days) in the afternoon and last for two and a half hours. They consist of warm-up activities, a main art-based activity with a discussion, and an ending. The beginning of each session includes some warming-up and introduction to the theme of the session, after which participants are involved in art-making, usually for 45–50 minutes, with the remaining 30–40 minutes reserved for discussion. Participants are encouraged to interact with each other through the use of materials and the process of discussing their artwork.

The process of the art therapy program involves four stages that materialize naturally in the group interactive context and synchronize with the phases of group dynamics ("forming," "storming," "performing," and ending). Groups are usually formed of five to eight patients. The group art therapy program lasts for one month and includes 12–14 sessions. Various art-based activities are used throughout the course of art therapy in connection to the stage of treatment and group dynamics, and are aimed at achieving different therapeutic goals. The therapist suggests a topic or theme as a directive for patient participation in the group. However, after the particular theme or directive is suggested, the group can discuss and suggest alternative themes or expand on a given directive.

Case example 1: Making natural objects special

This work was done during the 13th session of the art therapy program which lasted for one month and included 14 sessions. Initially there were eight participants in the group, but three of them had already been discharged from the hospital. The remaining part of the group included four men and one woman. Though all other patients were staying in the hospital for the first time, one client (Gregory) had previously been hospitalized and had participated in group art therapy several times. He had more experience of participating in different groups as compared to other members and was often very active in art-based activities.

During the 12th session, participants made their "personal coat of arms." This session was quite resourceful and helped patients to express inner strengths and created some link to the 13th session. The 13th session was the first one in which the therapist encouraged the participants to use found natural objects within an art-based activity. Between the 12th and 13th sessions, participants were involved in an outdoor activity, during which they searched for natural or discarded objects as a part of their art therapy program.

The idea was that through the use of some environmental assignments, the patients could be facilitated to go through a termination phase of therapy and move to a more open space as a new symbolic ground of their more autonomous functioning. This activity could also help the patients to frame and reframe their self-perceptions, to find meaning in the environment, appropriate it and personalize it (Heimets, 1994). This assignment could also lead to more active participation in the design and management of the inhabited spaces on the part of the patients.

The therapist believed that though the condition of this activity was new and somewhat perplexing, the patients could, however, find enough resources to cope with the situation and solve this creative task due to their previous involvement in art therapy. The participants indeed had had multifaceted experiences during the process and had felt safe enough being in the therapy room, but they had not yet taken part in any outdoor activity.

In order to help participants prepare for the 13th session, the therapist suggested a piece of "homework" during the 12th session. He invited them to look for some natural objects while outdoors on the hospital territory between the sessions and bring them to the art therapy room. The therapist encouraged the participants to either work with an open-ended format with no particular topic chosen beforehand, spontaneously responding to the environment and choosing any natural objects that they found attractive or meaningful, or on the basis of a theme, such as "self-image object." While walking outdoors they could ask themselves: Is there some natural object (objects) in the environment I feel connected to, have some affinity with, or which can represent my personality?

When they arrived for the 13th session, there was a selection of natural objects, such as sticks, branches, cones, stones, and wire present in the room. However, the spectrum of objects was rather limited. The more "experienced" patient (Gregory) demonstrated the two marble stones with cleaved sides that he found at some distance from the hospital building (Figure 8.1). He perceived these stones as a symbolic representation of some of his personal traits.

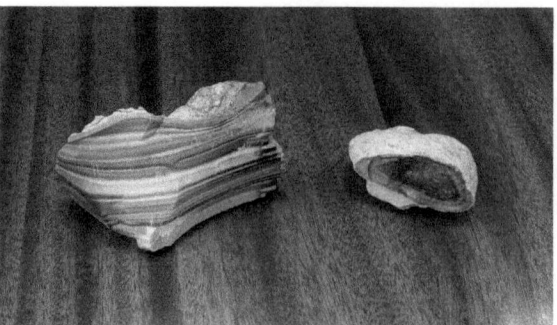

Figure 8.1: The two stones brought by Gregory that
represent his perception of himself

When the therapist invited the participants to show and comment on their findings, Gregory said that he liked the stones very much and associated them with himself, his reliability and endurance, the ability to steadfastly cope with difficult, stressful situations. The life history of this patient was indeed full of stressful situations, in particular due to his chronic physical illness which had required several serious surgeries.

The patient said that the two stones, though similar, signified somewhat different sides of him. There was a natural sequence of light and dark lines that the patient associated with sea waves on the top of the first bigger stone. He also associated the whole stone with a ship steadily going to its destination. The patient suggested that this object could serve as a symbolic cornerstone of his stance in life, which included his will and ability to strive for his place in life despite many challenges and limitations. He also declared that his optimism and belief in a "better future" helped him to go on a journey through "the turbulent sea of life." He found that the alternating light and dark lines on the edge of the stone could represent "his life credo": "There is the sun behind any dark cloud." His observation was that, though he had intuitively followed this life credo for quite a long time, his participation in the art therapy program helped him to recognize it and even consciously use it on a daily basis, not only for the sake of himself, but for the sake of the people who surrounded him.

He recognized the stone with its delicate layering of blue and white shades as a representation of a significant personal "discovery" which he made as a result of his participation in art therapy program. He explained that he came to a more balanced and nuanced perception of reality, which he developed through his experience of artistic self-expression and communication with other people. When he noticed this stone during his outdoor walk, he instantly realized that it was very special and could be his metaphorical self-portrait, a representation of his new perception of himself as a result of art therapy.

The second stone was also very special to him. He noticed that this stone had a dark blue "heart" surrounded with a lighter peripheral zone. He associated these two structural parts of the stone with different emotions and feelings related to different aspects of his personality. He associated the dark "heart" of the stone with some "core" feelings that he could not control, while the peripheral zone of lighter colors was associated with social, interpersonal skills and positive emotions, sense of humor, in particular, that he could use in order to effectively regulate his state of mind and relationships. Gregory also showed a third, bigger, brownish stone, which, unlike the two other stones, had no clearly defined meaning for him. He only said that the stone resembled him: "a horse with a smiling muzzle."

Andrey hadn't found any interesting object during his walk, but Gregory's findings and explanations evoked a strong reaction and inspired him to continue his search until the next session. He brought his art-object, a combination of the three natural creations, to the 14th session. His art-object consisted of a whale's vertebra, a small figure of a crab made of a walrus' bone, and a part of deer's horn (Figure 8.2).

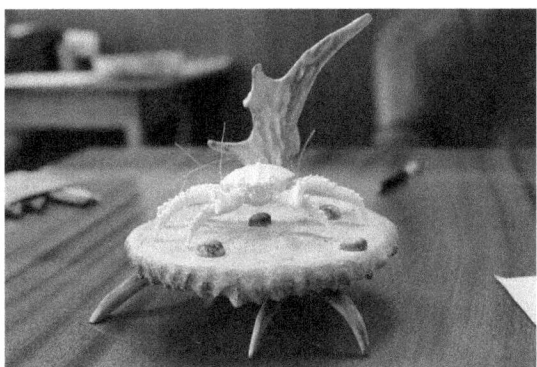

Figure 8.2: A combination of the three natural creations with the central small figure of a crab made of a walrus bone which was brought by Andrey as a representation of himself

Andrey said that the small figure of a crab was the central part of the composition. It caught his attention when he first noticed this object at the market place and he decided to buy it, though it appeared to be quite expensive. When the therapist asked him what was special about this object, Andrey answered that he was impressed with the skillful elaboration of the figure of the crab and that it could serve as a symbolic representation of himself. He felt an inner "attunement" to this figure and it implied some meaning and strength. Andrey became very emotional when he was commenting on his reactions to this figure.

Andrey explained that a crab was "nice and slow," but could be a "safeguard for his family." He associated the platform made of the whale vertebra with his family. Andrey added that the crab was very strong and it could not be "easily crushed like a crayfish." He even recalled that his comrades had given him the nickname Crab when he was in the army. He was often behind them due to his sluggishness. However, his comrades found him to be a trustful and reliable person. When the therapist asked Andrey which of his other personal characteristics the crab could symbolize, he emphasized such qualities as courage, good temper, safety, and the ability to defend his family and territory. It could also be very steady and fast if needed.

Other group participants wanted to support Andrey. They joined the discussion and noticed that crabs are indeed very interesting and resourceful creatures. Some participants even touched the figure and appeared to be impressed with the composition and Andrey's comments.

Case example 2: Environmental photo-taking assignments leading to resilience discovered in natural objects

As a continuation of environmental activities initiated in the previous sessions (see the above example), the therapist invited the participants to use cameras to take a series of photographs while walking outdoors. This activity was introduced as their homework. He invited them to look for some natural objects or landscapes when they were outdoors in the hospital grounds between the sessions. They were encouraged to either work with an open-ended format with no particular topic chosen beforehand, spontaneously responding to the environment and choosing any natural objects that they found attractive or meaningful, or on the basis of the theme "self-image objects/landscapes."

He explained that they must later make their selection of most meaningful or interesting photos. He suggested that they select, in particular, those photographs that had some affinity to them, symbolically illustrated their personal issues or personality, or presented their "healing" or emotionally loaded experience during their walkabouts.

In order to motivate the participants to use phototherapy as a means of eco-art therapy and facilitate self-expression, the therapist used a literary quote from *Hadji Murad*, a novel by Leo Tolstoy (2006). The therapist perceived this quote to be an eloquent illustration of how environmental objects, a plant in particular, may express meaningful human experience and relationships.

He explained to the participants that Leo Tolstoy was inspired by a crushed but still living thistle he found in a field. It became a symbol for the main character of his novel *Hadji Murat*, about an Avar rebel commander who, for reasons of personal revenge, forged an uneasy alliance with the Russians he had been fighting. The plant resonated with Tolstoy's memories of being in active service during the military campaign in the Caucasian region. Though he was ill when he was writing the novel, his later letters suggest that this work gave him a brief, final moment of vigor. Just as the author was struggling with his near death, his extended meditation on the concept of the individual refusing to give in to the demands of the world helped him to complete the book. Although it was written about 50 years after the events of the story actually happened, Tolstoy paints a picture of Russian civilization at the time. Tolstoy portrays the differences between bureaucratic decay and the healthy passionate life of a mountaineer.

By reading and explaining this quote, the therapist encouraged the clients to perceive the environment for their photo-taking assignment from a new perspective, as "a creative arena" and to "connect" the objects, which were loaded with emotional content, by taking photographs of them. This potentially enabled the participants to engage with the process of photographing meaningful natural objects/landscapes as a medium which helped to mend broken connections in the inner world.

Photographs and comments made throughout this form of environmental activity by one group participant (Gregory) illustrate some phenomena and therapeutic effects achieved during this process. However, these effects should be considered in the context of the whole group art therapy program, as a result of participants' previous involvement in various art-based activities and their interaction with each other and the therapist. At this stage of therapy, the group was "mature" and able to work together effectively on core personal issues. The phenomena and effects observed throughout the environmental photo-taking activity demonstrated the group's contribution to resolving the main therapeutic goals.

After completing his environmental photo-taking activity, Gregory brought some photographs to the next session. He printed them in an A4 format and added a few photographs that he had taken earlier on his own initiative as a response to various elements of the environment which attracted him. He fixed them on the wall, creating a kind of a personal exhibition, and he explained that some of his photographs had been taken spontaneously, with no particular topic chosen beforehand, while he was unconsciously responding to the environment and natural objects. At the same time, he also made two photographs on the basis of the theme "self-image objects/landscapes."

He then explained why he chose the objects and answered the questions the group and the leader asked him. Most of the photographs he made were related to the animals whose images he recognized while meditating on the trees that were abundant in the hospital grounds. He mostly concentrated on parts of the trees such as tall broken branches and stumps. As he explained, his preoccupation with these parts was evoked by the first natural object that he met right after he left the hospital building. This was a tall branch that was cut, but gave life to young shoots. For Gregory, it evoked an illusory image of a deer with horns (Figure 8.3).

This image signified a central theme of the whole series of Gregory's photographs, related to his perception of himself as a person who was able to cope with life's challenges and traumatic experience. This theme was already well represented in the example describing Gregory's found objects.

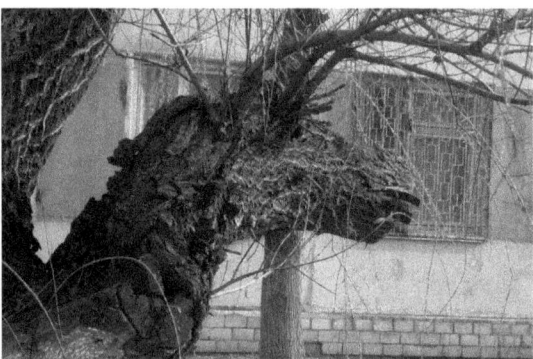

Figure 8.3: A tall cut branch with young shoots which Gregory perceived as a deer with horns

Initially, Gregory spontaneously responded to this object without any relation to himself. When he concentrated on the image, he noticed that the creature had "a smiling muzzle" and, though its head was connected to the fixed body, the creature appeared to be comfortable and friendly to the world around it. At this moment, Gregory realized certain associations between this image and himself. He discovered a complex meaning in it, which embraced both dramatic, painful, life-affirming, and positive sides of his life.

Gregory became sympathetic toward "the creature" that he recognized in the image and accepted a considerable similarity between the deer's and his own qualities. Like him, the creature was damaged, but survived and was still full of life. As already mentioned, beside psychological trauma, Gregory suffered from severe physical illness and had undergone several serious operations, but he did not let despair and pessimistic feelings dominate him. Even during the most painful and dramatic periods in his life, he searched for sources of positive feelings and relied on his sense of humor, connections with his family and friends, and even physical exercises. His life-affirming philosophy had proved to be helpful in coping with the challenging situations with which he had been confronted and this was eloquently illustrated by the image of the deer.

Some other group participants actively supported Gregory's stance in the world during their discussion of his photographs. They found it similar to their own perception of life and themselves. Thus, Gregory's photographs enabled the group to feel even more coherent and emotionally involved in each other's photographs.

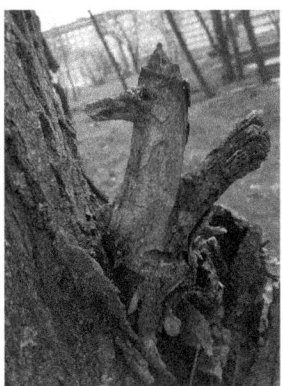

Figure 8.4: The tree trunk which Gregory associated with a woodpecker

Another of Gregory's photographs represented a part of a tree trunk with a chaotic combination of cut branches. He associated it with a woodpecker and not only identified the type of the bird, but mentioned its name, a "large variegated woodpecker'" (Figure 8.4). He later explained that this bird was very special and that he felt a certain affinity to it. He even demonstrated a photograph that he had taken earlier and brought to the session from home (Figure 8.5).

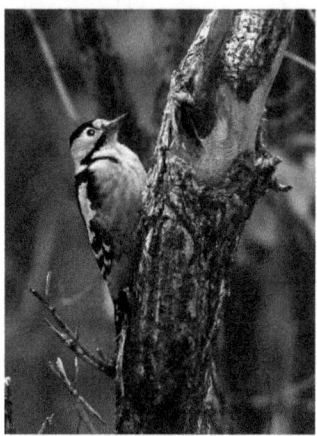

Figure 8.5: A photograph representing the real large variegated woodpecker

Gregory said that it was difficult to take a photograph of the large variegated woodpecker, since this bird didn't like people's attention. He explained that this kind of woodpecker was very cautious and intuitive and did not let people approach it. Gregory was very proud since he had made many unsuccessful attempts to take a photograph of this bird in its natural environment, but eventually had managed to take a good one. He believed that the woodpecker noticed him, but was trusting this time and let him come closer.

Gregory also said that he shared with this bird characteristics such as intuition, diligence, and a sincere wish to do good things for society. He believed that the woodpecker benefitted the environment when it "healed" the tree by clearing it from pests and that this could serve as a metaphor for his own public activity, motivated by his wish to make the world better. He said that he did that naturally, following his inner need and responding to the world around. He explained that intuition for him was not so much about caution, but rather a quality such as attention to the environment and people around him, their needs and feelings and that it was impossible for him to live without being "intuitive" in this sense of the word. He presumed that as a result of his participation in the art therapy program, he had been able to recognize such an altruistic and active position as being very practical and helpful for him in improving his well-being and health.

Discussion and conclusion

Based on the experience of using ecological/nature-assisted art therapy techniques with war veterans who are treated at the psychotherapy department of the hospital, the following observations and conclusions can be made. Though the sample was relatively limited, certain observed phenomena and effects seem to be valuable and enable us to understand why such therapy can be relevant with ex-service and military populations.

The 13th session can be considered a good illustration of how group art therapy with the use of found objects/ready-mades works, if participants are able to playfully experiment with objects and symbols in order to therapeutically work through some core personal issues and traumatic material and reveal their resilience through their "dialogue" with nature.

Some clients were frustrated when they were encouraged to go outdoors in search of found objects or take photographs. Such assignments appeared to be unusual for the clients and broke their habitual patterns of interaction with the environment. Some patients were frustrated in having greater freedom of choice and felt that the instructions were too wide and there were several options of what to do.

The specific mental attitudes of the military populations with their reliance on external control should be taken into account here. As Berger (2008) puts it, if the therapeutic process takes place outdoors, "in nature, in a place that does not necessarily have human-made boundaries; which is open to the world's influences, not owned by the therapist… basic issues that influence the therapeutic contract and the therapeutic relationship" (p.27) will be involved. He continues that "it seems there is a potential for people with an extreme need for clear boundaries, hierarchy and a high level of control to be hurt by the overwhelming experiences in nature" (ibid., p.27).

It is possible that some patients' resistances and frustrations in response to the therapist's suggestion to look for and work with found objects or take photographs of the environment were also related to their traumatic material. Natural damaged or discarded objects they were confronted with during their walks around the hospital building (fallen pine cones and branches, discarded parts of stone and wire, etc.) could be perceived as evoking difficult feelings. As Bat Or and Megides (2016) explain, collecting such objects:

> may evoke identification with their wounded aspects within clients. As a result of trauma and/or loss, the individual literally experiences themselves as damaged, wounded. On a metaphoric level, it can be said that those broken objects may give voice to the injured and painful parts in us that were caused by the trauma. In the realm of mental functioning, they also serve as representations of those elements, which the traumatized person tends to dissociate, repress and/or mute. (p.12)

At the same time, according to Shapiro (2005), there is an inherent message in inviting clients to use broken, useless, or ruined objects as raw materials for creative work. Specifically, it communicates non-verbally that deconstruction holds the potential to create the new (p.13).

The therapist's hypothesis—that through the use of an environmental assignment the clients could be facilitated to go through a termination phase of therapy, assume a new symbolic ground for their more autonomous functioning and learn a valuable lesson about how to create the new out of deconstructed or damaged material—proved to be correct. The use of environmental activities helped the clients to appropriate, personalize (Heimets, 1994) and find meaning in the found and photographed environmental objects. Patients were able to get involved in the "subjectification" of natural objects with the following basic functions: a) providing patients with an experience of their own personal dynamics, b) acting as an intermediary in a person's relationship with the world, and c) acting as a subject of joint activity and communication (Deryabo, 2002).

As Kopytin puts it (2020):

> ecopsychology, and the eco-human approach in general, justifies the specific subjective mode of perception of the surrounding world often defined in ecopsychology as the "subjectification" of the environment and natural objects (i.e. the perception of the environment and objects as having their own subjectivity), which in turn is based on the *ecopoietic* function of the soul. (p.10)

The patients were involved in the act of environmental personalization and subjectification, which implied selecting and taking either real objects or their photographs and later combining them in some cohesive constructions/ready-mades, or photographic series. Through scanning and/or collecting the found objects or taking their photographs, clients participated in sensory, kinesthetic, perceptual, and emotional exploring activities. Some emotional responses as well as specific memories (some of which may have been painful) could have been evoked. But by choosing the objects, the clients might have experienced their control capability through making choices. This phase of outdoor activity is basically offering a choice, which is a significant therapeutic aspect of art therapy and can be seen as counter-traumatic since the traumatic state is one of psychic helplessness.

The main process was connecting and integrating objects, either real or represented in the photographs, into a new construct and elaborating on a personal narrative. Traumatic events and later problematic life situations of the clients had affected their systems of attachment and meaning. By actually connecting the objects and creating narratives, which were loaded with emotional content, the medium enabled the mending of broken connections in the patients' inner world. This phase inherently consisted of combining the objects to create a new construct, which can be seen metaphorically as the opposite of the psychological splitting and fragmentation that are well-known reactions to trauma (Fonagy, 1991).

As Bat Or and Megides (2016) explain, "Finding the right words for describing the subjective meaning in the ready-made art may thus be a real therapeutic challenge and achievement for the client, similar to finding meaning in their suffering as the only thing that helps them bear it" (p.19). The case examples demonstrate that the group explored different perspectives on how a life situation could develop according to their story. As a result of their joint activity, they experienced many new insights.

The therapist's role in the process was mostly to facilitate patients' moving from one phase of working with found objects to another. His careful phenomenological observation assisted, according to Bion's (1962) concepts, "first in detecting the beta elements—those raw, unprocessed, and unrepresented elements—and second in containing and transforming the client's nonverbal communication of implicit memories into Alpha elements" (Bat Or and Megides, 2016, p.21).

The therapist, however, did not always remain in the witness role, but also participated in the ready-made process, especially taking into account the group dynamics. He directed his attention to the relational, immediate, emerging experience during the process of creating ready-made art.

During the discussion, the leader's role was mostly to facilitate group members' spontaneous reactions to the artwork and photographs and to help them create personal narratives. He supported multiple narratives/interpretations to explore and integrate alternative perspectives. He didn't comment on their adaptive potential, but emphasized the importance of coming out of rigid mental schemas.

Some positive outcomes observed through the use of environmental, nature-assisted practices included improved interpersonal communication, greater appreciation of underlying themes of psychological trauma and recovery, hope, enjoyment in utilizing new art media, successful completion of projects that reflected personal meaning for clients, and recognizing personal resilience revealed through clients' relationship to the environment.

Clients learned to use the restorative, healing potential of their interaction with the environment and natural objects and the power of art-based environmental activities to express themselves and uncover important underlying themes. The environmental and nature-assisted activities facilitated additional benefits for the war veterans, such as sensory and emotional stimulation and the experience of joy and pleasure as a result of their immersion in the "green" space. They were able to mobilize and effectively use their creative resources during their acts of personalization and subjectification of the environment as a significant resilience and coping strategy.

Based on the outcomes achieved through ecological/nature-assisted art therapy intervention with the use of found objects/ready-mades and photographs, it would be pertinent to develop a special program of ecological/nature-assisted art therapy with war veterans in order to more fully realize the potential of this therapeutic medium with this particular client group.

Please note that all names of participants in the art therapy program in this chapter have been anonymized.

References

Apchel, V.Y. & Tsygan, V.N. (1999). *Stress I sovladanije so stressom* [Stress and coping with stress]. St. Petersburg: Peter.

Backos, A. & Mazzeo, C. (2017). Group Therapy and PTSD: Acceptance and Commitment. Art Therapy Groups with Vietnam Veterans with PTSD. In P. Howie (ed.), *Art Therapy with Military Populations: History, Innovation, and Applications* (pp.165–175). New York, NY: Routledge/Taylor and Francis.

Bat Or, M. & Megides, O. (2016). Found objects: Readymade art in the treatment of trauma and loss. *Journal of Clinical Art Therapy*, 3(1). http://digitalcommons.lmu.edu/jcat/vol3/iss1/3.

Batt-Rawdon, K.B. & Tellnes, G. (2005). Nature culture health activities as a method of rehabilitation: An evaluation of participants' health, quality of life and function. *International Journal of Rehabilitation Research*, 28(2), 175–180.

Berger, R. (2008). Building a home in nature. *Journal of Humanistic Psychology*, 48(2), 264–279.

Berger, R. (2009). Nature Therapy—Developing a Framework for Practice. PhD thesis. School of Health and Social Sciences. University of Abertay, Dundee.

Berger, R. & Lahad, M. (2013). *The Healing Forest in Post-Crisis Work with Children.* London: Jessica Kingsley Publishers.

Bion, W.R. (1962). *Learning from Experience*. London: Karnac.

Burls, A. (2007). People and green spaces: Promoting public health and mental well-being through eco-therapy. *Journal of Public Mental Health*, 6(3), 24–39.

DeLucia, J. (2017). How the Studio and Gallery Experience Benefits Military Members and their Families. In P. Howie (ed.), *Art Therapy with Military Populations: History, Innovation, and Applications* (pp.30–40). New York, NY: Routledge/Taylor and Francis.

Deryabo, S.D. (2002). The Phenomenon of Subjectification of Natural Objects. PhD thesis. Moscow State University of Psychology and Education, Moscow (in Russian).

Faber-Taylor, A. & Kuo, F.E. (2009). Children with attention deficit concentrate better after walk in the park. *Journal of Attention Disorders*, 12(5), 402–409.

Fleming, L.L. (2015). Veteran to farmer programs: An emerging nature-based programming trend. *Journal of Therapeutic Horticulture*: American Horticultural Therapy Association, 25(1), 27–49.

Fonagy, P. (1991). Thinking about thinking: Some clinical and theoretical considerations in the treatment of a borderline patient. *International Journal of Psychoanalysis*, 72, 639–656.

Groeneweggen, P., van den Berg, A., de Vries, S. & Verheij, R. (2006). Vitamin C: Effects of green space on health, wellbeing and social safety. *BMC Public Health*, 6, 149–159.

Haeseler, M.P. (1998). Crossing the Border: Cultural Implications of Entering a New Art Therapy Workplace. In A.R. Hiscox & A.C. Calisch (eds), *Tapestry of Cultural Issues in Art Therapy* (pp.327–346). London: Jessica Kingsley Publishers.

Heerwagen, J. (2009). Biophilia, Health and Wellbeing. In L. Campbell & A. Wiesen (eds), *Restorative Commons: Creating Health and Wellbeing through Urban Landscapes* (pp.39–57). Pennsylvania: USDA Forest Service.

Heimets, M. (1994). The phenomenon of personalization of the environment. *Journal of Russian & East European Psychology*, 32(3), 24–32.

Howie P. (2017a). Family Art Therapy Treatment at Walter Read. In P. Howie (ed.), *Art Therapy with Military Populations: History, Innovation, and Applications* (pp.53–63). New York, NY: Routledge/Taylor and Francis.

Howie, P. (2017b). Group Art Therapy: The Evolution of Treatment and the Power of Witness. In P. Howie (ed.), *Art Therapy with Military Populations: History, Innovation, and Applications* (pp.64–74). New York, NY: Routledge/Taylor and Francis.

Kalmanowitz, D. & Lloyd, B. (2011). Inside-Out Outside-In: Found Objects and Portable Studio. In E.G. Levine & S.K. Levine (eds), *Art in Action: Expressive Arts Therapy and Social Change* (pp.104–127). London and Philadelphia, PA: Jessica Kingsley Publishers.

Kolov, S.A., Ostapenko, A.V. & Krivtsov A.G. (2005). Psuhologicheskoje issledovanije posttravmaticheskogo stressovogo rasstrojstva [Psychological study of the Post-Traumatic Stress Disorder]. *Vestnik Psychotherapii*, 13, 23–35.

Kopytin, A. (2020). Archetypal psychology in the context of the eco-human approach. *Ecopoiesis: Eco-Human Theory and Practice*, 1(2), 6–16.

Lobban, J. (2014). The invisible wound: Veterans' art therapy. *International Journal of Art Therapy*, 19(1), 3–18.

Nebbe, L. (2006). *Nature Therapy: Handbook of Animal-Assisted Therapy*. San Diego, CA: Academic Press.

O'Brien, E. (2005). Publics and woodlands in England: Wellbeing, local identity, social learning, conflict and management. *Forestry*, 78(4), 321–335.

Shapiro, J. (2005). Destruction as Raw Material for Creation. In *Adolescents and Self-Injury: Symposium Papers*. Jerusalem, Israel: Summit Institute: Association for Treatment Services, Psychosocial Rehabilitation, and Welfare (in Hebrew).

Simson, S. & Straus, M. (1998). *Horticulture as Therapy: Principles and Practice*. Binghampton, NY: The Hawthorne Press.

Tolstoy, L. (2006). *Hadji Murad*. New York, NY: Cosmo Classics.

Chapter 9

Walking the Common Place of Commemoration

PAMELA WHITAKER

A place of beginnings and departures

This chapter presents a proposal for art therapy to align with commemoration in the landscape of the commons. The commons is a shared landscape that can exist as a park, community garden, nature sanctuary or as an open access public space. It is a location for gatherings and happenings and assembles people in connection to a shared living environment or common place. It can be a place to find serendipitous objects (natural or otherwise) that allow for commiseration and commemoration. The word commemoration relates to acts of ceremony, remembrance, observance and tribute. It can be a forming of place for compositions that are personal, collective and civically minded. The commons is a space for aesthetic connectivity, and a social sculpting of landscape for personal and collective creations. It may be found in every community, neighbourhood and region as a space for reparative metaphor, imagination and rituals of passage (Till, 2012). The commons can become a terrain for enacted assemblage with associations to physical and emotional memories, affects and shared communal stewardship. It is shaped by multiple forms of design, authority, resistance and cultivation, and its materiality can be adapted according to the aesthetic preferences of the many – the multitude of participants, who make it their own.

The chapter will explore rituals of care and agency within nature-informed public spaces incorporating the metaphor of the herbarium (as a public archive of remembrance) and examining the potential for art therapists to become walking celebrants with those who wish to commemorate through public acts of walking. The herbarium is highlighted in relation to the artistry of collecting (foraging) while walking through landscapes and habitats. A herbarium is both a scientific archive of plants and a celebration of life, place, habitats and how humans interact with landscapes. It is a recording of nature charted through plants that have been preserved for research and memorialisation. There is an association with loss and a recognition of the importance of documenting the memory of habitats. A herbarium chronicles the materiality of place as a composition of what has grown within a specific location. It is an archive that maps discovery and natural history and a person's own journey within place and time.

I consider a herbarium to also be relevant to art therapy as a memorialisation through the gathering and display of botanical materials. Whether through book artefacts, or installations, the gathering of nature specimens also shares a personal story of foraging for consolation and inspiration. The life of the plant has been preserved, as a record of both a search and a revelation. The collection of nature specimens may relate to specific timeframes and life narratives. There is an association to nature therapy, whereby people find solace, regeneration and artistry within nature as a *psychoecosocial* foundation for being with nature's ephemerality and metaphors of change (Berger, 2017). 'The morphological qualities of place are the material and social environments that nurture inhabitants and offer support through familiarity, routine, aesthetically comfortable spaces, and a sense of belonging and security' (Till, 2012, p.10). Creative placemaking is a term that describes the crafting of spaces for aesthetic engagement and documenting narratives within environments of impact (Clarke, 2017; Creative Placemaking, 2016). Creative placemaking can enhance art therapy's capacity to accompany a personal mapping that binds connections to landscape. It can also suggest leaving something behind that someone else can take away in terms of its intention to make a coordinate or situation of reflection.

Installing commemorations along the walking routes of the commons creates places to pause and reflect on the significance of a memorial for personal and collective loss (Figure 9.1). The security of knowing these constructed places are steadfastly present speaks to the impact of the material and natural landscape combining as a kind of meta-subjectivity. A landscape can be both biographical and sociological. These locations are metaphorically restorative and are places of social and botanical engagement and commemoration. 'As inhabitants of the world...[humans] are *wayfarers*, and that wayfaring is a movement of

self-renewal or becoming rather than the transport of already consti-
tuted beings from one location to another' (Ingold, 2016, p.132).

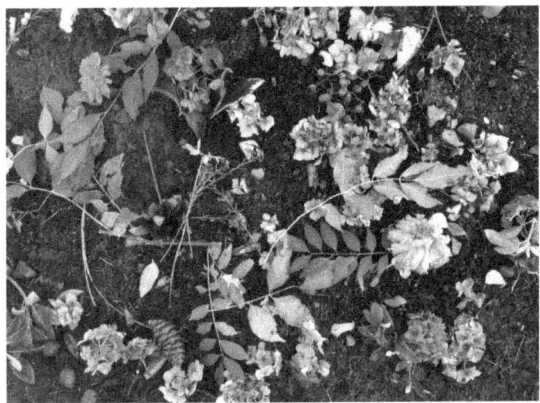

Figure 9.1: A Passing Tribute [flower display]
by Whitaker, 2017. (Dublin, Ireland: personal collection)

As a walking celebrant, an art therapist accompanies the pathways of
commiseration as a companion and witness. The witnessing relates to
what is collected and displayed along the way as milestones and turning
points. The park as commons has been a featured landscape in my own
art therapy practice, in relation to collecting the specimens of nature that
comfort experiences of loss – particularly flowers which can be gathered,
displayed and preserved at home, and also displayed in situ for others
to discover as a kind of impromptu herbarium that links a certain place
to memorialising.

The herbarium: An archive of preservation

Whereas found objects are recognised as having significance in art
therapy, found plants can also relate to human histories and cultural
traditions. In other words, plants can have associations for people and
ecologies of nature. The herbarium acknowledges botanical times past,
and the anthropogenic impacts of habitat wounding, but it is also a
preservation of memory which can evoke a past and a future of care in
both botanical and human terms.

A herbarium is an archive of plants collected as specimens to preserve
a record of botanical life. A plant specimen is collected to represent
a distinct species for scientific research related to habitat change and

human impacts on the environment (or an anthropogenic history of human interactions). The herbarium located in the National Botanic Gardens of Ireland is a scientific and artistic resource for researching the life of plants that showcases a national and international botanical heritage (National Botanic Gardens of Ireland, 2021). The legacy of these plant collections is preserved as a repository that is both a botanical and social history of collections. Details of who collected the plant, where and when it was collected, and the plant's characteristics are documented in archives that are in themselves artistic artefacts. These legacies are curated art collections stored as botanical testimonies to a particular time and place. A herbarium is an organic metaphor for keeping a memory alive in a biography of a site that can 'analyse how transgenerational encounters, performances and rituals transmit and circulate understandings about the past across historical and lived times and through social spaces' (Till, 2012, p.7). A biographical landscape is a terrain of subjectivity that both inherits and performs rituals of care, signifying transitions as a form of human geography.

The botanical and social traditions linked to plants in Ireland form associations to customs, cures, artistry and celebrations. Wild plants are harvested for specific remedies along with foraged curative plants that offer restoration from a wide variety of ailments. Botanical specimens transmit transformative potentials in relation to traditional Irish celebrations marking the cycles of the growing season. As such 'the specimens are snapshots in time' (National Botanic Gardens of Ireland, 2021), and can be considered memorials to historic botanical and human environments that also implicate life in the present day. The herbarium is a living inquiry into botanical and social histories (MacCoitir, 2006). The metaphor of the herbarium could also relate to the grieving of habitats lost and to the loss of customs associated with how plants can benefit human life. As such, it can be considered a plant community that retains a legacy to a human community. As a collection it relates to memories, ways of life, traditions and social and cultural heritage. The herbarium, as a legacy of plants, is maintained as a memorial. The associations with each plant specimen are contextual and cultural in relation to the impact of anthropogenic and environmental relations (Botanical Society of Britain and Ireland, 2021).

Kopytin, Bockhorni and Zhou (2019) highlight the significance of botanical arranging as an *ecotherapeutic* form of artistry that informs therapeutic practice with a biophilia impulse – a focus on nature as a life-affirming form of restoration. The cultivated or foraged materials composing botanical arrangements can ignite ancestral memories associated with domestic and public gardens, parks, places in the wild and also with home-based botanical displays where we evoke connections to personal and cultural lineage. 'Plants enter a spectrum of experience through colour, symmetry, scale, texture, scent, and shape whose attributes merge with an individual's own history' (Kopytin *et al.*, 2019, p.100). The botanical arrangement is a memorial to a particular encounter with nature, often occupying a place at home, as a way to observe and embed elements of nature into everyday life. As an artistic installation, nature enacts a transformation that can be witnessed in relation to our own psychological processes of change.

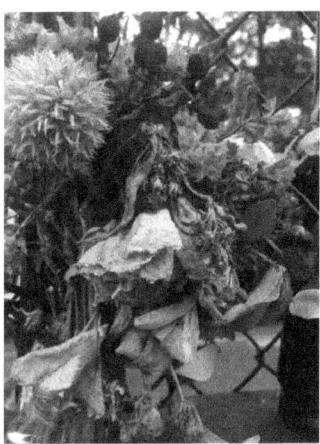

Figure 9.2: A Memorial in Passing [floral display]
by Whitaker, 2019. (Dublin, Ireland: personal collection)

Floratherapy recognises the significance of flower and botanical arranging as a way to reflect on milestones, tributes and life occasions (Perryman & Keller, 2009) (Figure 9.2). Flowering plants inform multiple areas of perception through colour, shape and smell. They contribute to embodied aesthetics and environmental rituals, due to their links with significant life events. The autobiographical nature of flowers facilitates our tending to their care, and the observance of their passing can be a documentation of a personal transitioning (Huss, Yosef & Zaccai, 2018). The displacement and uprooting of a living species brings into focus ways in which dislocation can also impact our own identity, security and belonging. 'Colour, scent, symmetry, imperfections, petal-count, and texture all [acknowledge] feeling' (Lagreze, 2019, p.5). Flowers mark events and passages, and as displays they resemble the preservation of memory, not unlike a herbarium keeps alive the memory of times past through its collections.

> The embodied sensory level of flowers seems to be connected to the positive elements of relationship...as well as to general positive, social interactions... From this, we can surmise that the aesthetic experience of flowers leads to the embodied and socially embedded experience of feeling connected positively to the world. (Huss *et al.*, 2018, p.38)

The art of commemoration

The commons, as a collective landscape, is oriented towards shared occupation, shared natural resources, and the sharing of goodwill (Menatti, 2017). As a form of communal nature, it is based on the customs and history of a specific region both in terms of a bioregion and as a social territory. It is also the sharing of an emotional landscape, a place for experiences to be made with passers-by. The role of consolation and ritual within the commons can be considered a form of public practice art therapy (Timm-Bottos, 2006, 2017), where art therapy enters the common place with therapeutic intentions. I am proposing the commons as a shared place for personal commemoration. Attachment to place informs connections to human geography, as a participatory engagement with the shared common grounds of daily life and vernacular culture (Mackey, 2010). Local distinctiveness evokes the idea of habitats of people and nature forming a bioregionalism that represents the particularities of sharing a common territory of life (Common Ground, 2020). The social network of a commons brings people together so that the land is subject to associations by individual and collective intentions. Bioregionalism also includes an awareness of 'myths, legends, folklore and...the rituals and practices that sustain local diversity and resilience' (Wahl, 2017). These associations to culture evoke a sense of bioregionalism as a complex cultural repository.

The commons as a physical and cultural landscape has a relationship to experiential geography. A commons is an immersion into a shared place and the placing of one's narratives into a community terrain. Each person enters the region with their own circumstances, which engage with the nature of the place and the nature of those who also dwell within it. The commons encourages participation in both the environment and the human condition as a 'place based ethics of care' (Till, 2012, p.3). The idea that a commons can incorporate the woundedness of people in nature and within communities can be aligned with the art of walking in art therapy. The sorrows of people can find psychosocial relief in their performance through walking and social gatherings. The social ecologies of the commons are the ways in which people mediate losses within the ephemeral nature of the outdoors, where temporality is felt by the passing of light, weather, seasonality and environmental conditions (Till, 2012). The commons may also be considered a social sculpture composed through societal inputs which have bestowed a collective authorship of place. This appropriation of landscape into a *humanscape* of interventions is a form of connective practice for a representation of communal aesthetics – a place where we come to our senses, form social sculpture, and where our creative practices re-imagine and reshape the places where we live in community (Sacks, 1995).

Art therapist as celebrant

The commons as studio has the potential for 'expressive cooperation' (Sennett, 2012, p.17) and the negotiation of social complexity. It may also be considered a threshold that incorporates social concerns and adds ingenuity to art therapy practices that combine personal and collective agendas. A commons grows a community along with it, as a combined aesthetics of biodiversity that is contemporaneously varied. It is a resource for living art materials that can be foraged for home displays or outdoor artworks. The commons exists as a liminal zone, where one can be at home in an environment that is also home to others, as a public home place (Timm-Bottos, 2006).

A commemoration can be a recognition of shared history that dates back to legacies of land occupation and also to collective and personal histories finding their representation. The commons declares multiplicity with civic contributions that are both anticipated and improvised. Here an art therapist can be a curator of gatherings, celebrations, festivities or memorials. Each is performed as an assemblage of influences that are freely chosen as an encounter by each contributing artist-producer (Whitehead, 2003). As celebrant, the art therapist assists with the composition of location and facilitates the construction of a place apart to come together. This is a relational art encounter, where 'artworks begin to assume a living reality – an evolving continuity in the space and time of their articulation' (Whitehead, 2003). A ceremonial gathering is not unlike a material enactment of social media, a sharing of artistic content that extends ideas and practice outwards with an immediate and multiplying effect (Magee, 2020).

Ceremony and commemoration can extend the practice of art therapy, so that 'rather than being fixed in one place, art therapy flows through landscapes of meaning and context' (McLachlan, 2017, p.8). In this regard, art therapy can enact celebration as an opportunity for social mixing, pride of place and being present to each other through shared art-making. A park, as commons, offers gifts of refuge, shelter and retreat and it can be a place for human regeneration. A park, as an open source landscape, is conducive to community repair in terms of its availability for re-creation. Botanical interventions can be a subtle form of land art which can relate to either planting or creating with botanical elements of display (Kellhammer, 2020). Commemorations exist for a variety of reasons, as both planned or spontaneous markings of time and place, with specific references to themes and meaning. I propose these created experiences to be artworks that inscribe a distinguishing effect. Commemoration provides a structure that also performs a sense of recognition. It can be considered 'an intermedial form that subtly challenges the lines that would demarcate where an art object ends and the world begins' (Jackson, 2011, p.28).

A commemoration is a rhizome of experience that exists between participants and locations. A rhizome 'denotes a system of three-dimensional growth with multiple entryways and exits that can be approached through many different vantage points' (Whitaker, 2012, p.345). Ingold (2016) asserts that the commonality between walking, observing and storytelling is lines. A rhizome is a network of lines, or paths, that cross over each other as routes of inquiry that mark out connecting narratives. A walk in itself is a line made by footsteps that marks a personal geography and lines of thought – the writing of a story that also traces contemplative gestures (Ingold, 2016).

> As with the line that goes out for a walk, in the story as in life there is always somewhere further one can go. And in storytelling as in wayfaring, it is in the movement from place to place...that knowledge is integrated. (Ingold, 2016, p.108)

We walk our storylines and we re-trace the storylines of others – both are connecting thoroughfares (Ingold, 2016). This is a kinetic landscape that moves, extends and re-locates. The nature of assembling is a tactile expression and an interaction with the physical material of the world and with people (Skaife, 2001).

> For people inhabit a world that consists in the first place, not of things but of lines. After all, what is a thing, or indeed a person, if not the tying together of lines – the paths of growth and movement – of all the many constituents gathered there? (Ingold, 2016, p.21)

Deleuze and Guattari describe a line of flight (2004) as a generation of new territory, a new mapping of experience that marks out new psychological dimensions, the extending out of a rhizome, not unlike adding another direction (detour) that embarks on an unexpected journey. The rhizome is composed of lines that extend in all directions, as choices for making. These lines take us somewhere, and a new line of passage marks out another territory to pursue.

A commons is an open studio that is available for different forms of commemoration. It is a place for impromptu occasions and encounters with people on routes of passage. According to Moon and Shuman (2013), the art therapist, as social mediator, extends art therapy into public participation, by utilising a professional toolkit composed of 'relational sensitivity, observational skills...knowledge about art materials and practices...knowledge of local resources, and how to create psychologically safe and nurturing environments' (Moon & Shuman, 2013, p.302). Adding event coordinator, celebrant and curator to this repertoire of professional practices enhances the role of an art therapist and their artist identity. Within the act of celebrancy, the art therapist enables community members to create their own artistry – forging relationships out of the ordinary with themselves, others and the supporting landscape (Warner, 2001). This offers an added dimension of professional capacity, and duty of care on a larger scale of reference – reaching out and being present where people naturally gather is a civic consciousness towards relationality, empathy and responsibility.

In terms of celebrancy, the outdoors can facilitate life reterritorialisation that creates re-positioning (Spindler, 2010). As a horizon of potential, the expanse of a commons offers the environmental scaffolding for intensive events that move us on into becoming or transitioning between life places (Spindler, 2010). In the 'passing present' (Deleuze & Guattari, 1994, p.113), we become in alignment with 'what already we are ceasing to be' (Deleuze & Guattari, 1994, p.112). A commemoration as an event horizon is a re-orientation from established life locations to curated life spaces, as occasions that are created in the 'play of movement' (Lorraine, 2006, p.174). The relational aesthetics of commemoration, gathering and installing an arts-informed celebration of life can generate defining moments that are punctuations, transitions and landmarks (Heath & Heath, 2017). As a form of resilience, commemorations can create a scene to construct positive social encounters that make special the composition of milestones. Often a botanical display in nature stops us in our path; it is an installation that assembles a place of reflection and observation for not only the maker, but everyone who finds themselves in the same place.

Civic remembrance is typically installed within the commons, as either a monument or a ceremony. Personal memorials are an assemblage of symbols that represents a person's life, but also resonates with those who find the memorial representative of their own loss. The herbarium here is the passing away of flowers left in a particular place. In the passing of these floral arrangements, there are revealed aesthetics related to grieving. 'Bunches of flowers...fade, as no one removes them from their temporary shrines... Personal memory, too, is adapted until what did happen, and what might have happened, begin to fuse' (Miles, 2016, p.153). Shrines are forms of public art and visually represent grief in public spaces. In material and psychological ways, commemorations in the commons are an interface and a collision of rites of mourning (Miles, 2016). These handcrafted shrines are a form of artistic production (legacy art) and also a gathering place for the connectivity of grief.

Rituals of sustenance (Brucker, 2017) can be restorative and an abiding routine during periods of distress and loss. They can be considered threshold ceremonies 'acquiring new skills for the path ahead' (Brucker, 2017, p.230) and the result of accumulating experiences that prepare for a public declaration witnessed by others either simultaneously or within their own time of discovery. A sanctuary space within the commons can be revisited and added to over time (Figure 9.3). Ritual is a series of steps, or actions, that lead to an enactment of symbolic meaning that is designated through its intentions and arrangement.

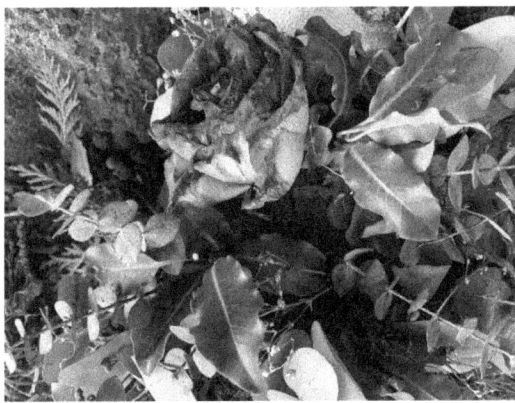

Figure 9.3: Sanctuary Passage [flowers]
by Whitaker, 2021. (Dublin, Ireland: personal collection)

Moving towards closure

A pilgrimage characterises routes taken for the purpose of salvation, redemption or release. It is a term related to exile within pathways of devotional intention. The pilgrimage route is one that is accompanied by others seeking the same determinations of intent, retrieval and humility (Gros, 2015). One seeks regeneration and the discovery of symbols of remedy along a pathway that finds solace within ritual and the placement of offerings. The pilgrimage is itself a working through of misery into reconciliation and sanctuary, with the quest to be altered (Gros, 2015).

Neuroscience confirms that walking is restorative and facilitates revitalised attention to ourselves and human welfare. The benefits of walking and gathering thoughts and materials in the commonplace is a form of neurogenesis. The art of movement enables activation in extended regions of the brain, and the rhythm aligns and relates to behavioural synchronisation with features of the environment (O'Mara, 2019). Commemoration is an immersion in time and history and the characteristics and specimens of the environment that declare significance and sanctum. The commons within nature can bestow conviviality and representational spaces that are significant in bringing all our walks of life together as accumulative productions (Lefebvre, 1991). The making of memorials to commemorate loss is a navigational point of reference within public places, a marker that references a particular loss and the experience of loss as common ground. A making of commemoration is a chance to perform repetitive acts of consolation. These social works offer an aesthetics of support for fragilities. The assembly of materials, environment and public engagement bestow a shared practice of supportive relations that sustain purpose and living (Jackson, 2011).

Commemoration is a spatial practice that is totalising in the way it combines human and site-specific ingredients that enunciate geography and actions into legibility (De Certeau, 1988). The art therapist can accompany people to places as a celebrant witness, and it is this act of commemoration and incorporation of human geography that sets into motion a living herbarium of landscape meeting a collection of stories that want to relate.

References

Berger, R. (2017). Nature therapy: Incorporating nature into art therapy. *Journal of Humanistic Psychology*, 60(2), 244–257.

Botanical Society of Britain and Ireland (2021). *Herbaria*. https://bsbi.org/herbaria.

Brucker, S. (2017). Digging Bones and Crossing Thresholds: Healing Individuals and Communities Through Nature-Based Expressive Arts, Ceremony and Ritual. In A. Kopytin & M. Rugh (eds), *Environmental Expressive Therapies: Nature-Assisted Theory and Practice* (pp.226–245). New York, NY: Routledge.

Clarke, M. (2017) *Field Guide for Creative Placemaking in Parks*. San Francisco, CA: The Trust for Public Land.

Common Ground (2020). *Local Distinctiveness*. www.commonground.org.uk/local-distinctiveness.

Creative Placemaking (2016). Editorial. *Journal of Art for Life*. https://journals.flvc.org/jafl/issue/view/4260.

De Certeau, M. (1988). *The Practice of Everyday Life*. Los Angeles, CA: University of California Press.

Deleuze, G. & Guattari, F. (1994). *What is Philosophy?* London: Verso.

Deleuze, G. & Guattari, F. (2004). *A Thousand Plateaus: Capitalism and Schizophrenia*. Minneapolis, MN: University of Minnesota Press.

Gros, F. (2015). *A Philosophy of Walking*. London: Verso.

Heath, C. & Heath, D. (2017). *The Power of Moments: Why Certain Experiences Have Extraordinary Impact*. London: Bantam Press.

Huss, E., Yosef, K.B. & Zaccai, M. (2018). Humans' relationship to flowers as an example of the multiple components of embodied aesthetics. *Behavioral Sciences*, 8(3), 32–42.

Ingold, T. (2016). *Lines: A Brief History*. New York, NY: Routledge.

Jackson, S. (2011). *Social Works: Performing Art, Supporting Publics*. New York, NY: Routledge.

Kellhammer, O. (2020). *Botanical Interventions: Open Source Landscape and Community Repair*. http://oliverk.org/publications/non-fiction/botanical-interventions-open-source-landscape-and-community-repair-essay.

Kopytin, A., Bockhorni, R. & Zhou, T.Y. (2019). From Ikebana to botanical arranging: Artistic, therapeutic, and spiritual alignments with nature. *Creative Arts in Education and Therapy*, 5(2), 96–108.

Lagreze, K. (2019). Art Therapy Blossoms: Developing Floral Design in Art Therapy for Adults with Anxiety. Unpublished MA thesis. Lesley University, Cambridge, Massachusetts.

Lefebvre, H. (1991). *The Production of Space*. Oxford: Blackwells.

Lorraine, T. (2006). Ahab and Becoming-Whale: The Nomadic Subject in Smooth Space. In I. Buchanan & G. Lambert (eds.), *Deleuze and Space* (pp.159–175). Edinburgh: Edinburgh University Press.

MacCoitir, N. (2006). *Irish Wild Plants: Myths, Legends and Folklore*. Cork: Collins Press.

Mackey, C. (2010). *Random Acts of Culture: Reclaiming Art and Community in the 21st Century*. Toronto: Between the Lines.

Magee, J. (2020). Personal communication, 16 June.

McLachlan, C. (2017). Art therapy caves: Linking community art to a therapeutic space. *Canadian Art Therapy Association Journal*, 30(1), 4–10.

Menatti, L. (2017). Landscape: From common good to human right. *International Journal of the Commons*, 11(2), 641–683.

Miles, M. (2016). Civic Remembrance and the Politics of Place. In J. Vickery & M. Manus (eds), *The Art of the Multitude: Jochen Gerz—Participation and the European Experience* (pp.153–171). Frankfurt, DE: Campus Verlag.

Moon, C. & Shuman, V. (2013). The Community Art Studio: Creating a Space of Solidarity and Inclusion. In P. Howie, S. Prasad & J. Kristel (eds), *Using Art Therapy with Diverse Populations: Crossing Cultures and Abilities* (pp.297–307). London: Jessica Kingsley Publishers.

National Botanic Gardens of Ireland (2021). *The National Herbarium*. http://botanicgardens.ie/science-and-learning/the-national-herbarium/.

O'Mara, S. (2019). *In Praise of Walking: The New Science of How We Walk and Why it's Good For Us*. London: Vintage.

Perryman, K.L. & Keller, E.A. (2009). Floratherapy as a creative arts intervention with women in a retirement home. *Journal of Creativity in Mental Health*, 4(4), 334–342.

Sacks, S. (1995). Joseph Beuys' pedagogy and the work of James Hillman: The healing of art and the art of healing. *Issues in Art, Architecture and Design*, 4(1), 52–60.

Sennett, R. (2012). *Together: The Rituals, Pleasures and Politics of Cooperation*. London: Allen Books.

Skaife, S. (2001). Making visible: Art therapy and intersubjectivity. *Inscape: Journal of the British Association of Art Therapists*, 6(2), 40–50.

Spindler, F. (2010). Gilles Deleuze: A Philosophy of Immanence. In J. Bornemark & H. Ruin (eds), *Phenomenology and Religion: New Frontiers* (pp.149–163). Huddinge: Södertörn University.

Till, K. (2012). Wounded cities: Memory-work and a place based ethics of care. *Political Geography*, 31, 3–14.

Timm-Bottos, J. (2006). Constructing creative community: Reviving health and justice through community arts. *Canadian Art Therapy Association Journal*, 19(2), 12–26.

Timm-Bottos, J. (2017). Public practice art therapy: Enabling spaces across North America. *Canadian Art Therapy Association Journal*, 30(2), 94–99.

Wahl, D.C. (2017). Bioregionalism – Living with a sense of place at the appropriate scale for self-reliance. *Medium*. https://medium.com/age-of-awareness/bioregionalism-living-with-a-sense-of-place-at-the-appropriate-scale-for-self-reliance-a8c9027ab85d.

Warner, D.A. (2001). The lantern-floating ritual: Linking a community together. *Art Therapy: Journal of the American Art Therapy Association*, 1(1), 14–19.

Whitaker, P. (2012). The Art Therapy Assemblage. In H. Burt (ed.), *Art Therapy and Postmodernism: Creative Health Through a Prism* (pp.344–366). London: Jessica Kingsley Publishers.

Whitehead, D.H. (2003). Poiesis and art-making: A way of letting-be. *Contemporary Aesthetics*. https://quod.lib.umich.edu/c/ca/7523862.0001.005/--poiesis-and-art-making-a-way-of-letting-be?rgn=main;view=fulltext.

Chapter 10

Re-Imaging Art Therapy in the Global Crisis: Storm Clouds and Silver Linings

MONICA CARPENDALE

Introduction

Expressive arts therapists all over the world are working to re-imagine creative and therapeutic possibilities and ways of working in the context of current global dilemmas. Art therapy has generally been more focused on the internal individual emotional issues pertaining to mental illness, physical health, and social challenges such as attachment, loss, trauma, and developmental disabilities. There have been an increasing number of art therapists working in areas of environmental arts therapy, social change, restorative justice, and community development (Carpendale, 2010; Kopytin & Rugh, 2017). Art therapy has always been a studio-based physically engaging process, which has had to change considerably due to the need for physical distancing and concerns regarding the spread of the Covid-19 virus. We are now providing art therapy online and in nature.

Eco art therapy, environmental arts therapies, environmental expressive therapy, environmental education and therapeutic art, land-based healing, nature-based therapy, art for community development and social change are all different ways to refer to the combinations of integrating nature, art, therapy, and education (Berger & Lahad, 2013; Carpendale, 2010; Cohen, 2007; Kopytin & Rugh, 2017; Macy & Brown, 2014; Macy & Johnstone, 2012). In essence, whether we are talking about art therapy or environmental education, we are always talking about the wonder and mystery of nature and the wonder and mystery of the creative process. Art-making and being in nature can attune our senses, restore our spirit, and engage a deep appreciation and gratitude for the earth and all its multispecies kin. Telling and creating stories in nature and about our experiences in nature reframes our understanding of the earth and provides an opportunity to envision new paths forward (Carpendale, 2010).

Donna Haraway speaks of how we need to "stay with the trouble" and the importance of our ability to be responsive: "response-able" (Haraway, 2016). A core aspect of all expressive art therapies is training in imaginative and creative processes and the ability to be responsive and empathic. These are important skills in uncertain times. Our creative imagination is one of the most important gifts that we bring to the world in crisis. Our ability to respond in crisis, to repurpose materials and ideas, is invaluable in recreating our future. The storm clouds wash the landscape clean, leave the air fresh, and the world shining and new. Staying with the trouble in the present allows us to move graciously and gratefully into the future.

Davenport (2017) talks of living in the era of climate change in which during "this dark and painful time there is a surprising gift available, a radical invitation to a profound transformation. We can aim to go beyond protecting the environment to creating the kind of world where the environment is no longer in need of protecting" (p.19). She goes on to speak of the need for a true understanding of interdependence and "interbeing" (p.20). Haraway talks of our multispecies kin (2016), and Indigenous people affirm that we are all related to the four-legged, two-legged, crawling, flying, and swimming creatures/beings.

Environmental education

At the center of my thinking about education are the words of the philosopher David Orr, and his claim that "all education is environmental education. By what is included or excluded, students are taught that they are part of or apart from the natural world" (1994, p.12). And by this, he means that when we do not consider our immediate environment and acknowledge what we are experiencing environmentally, we are doing bad environmental education. I have taken this statement very seriously. When my husband died, and I was immersed in the grief of one individual, I thought also about the dangers of losing our planet, and what we were leaving to our grandchildren and great grandchildren. I found that life decisions became very simple when living with the constant awareness of death. What was hard to understand was that if we knew what needed to be done to address the climate emergency, why were we not doing it? One of the things that the global pandemic precipitated was the awareness that we could stop what we were doing and make a radical change very quickly. We could, metaphorically speaking, press a reset button.

With my awareness of the need for a paradigm shift in awareness I focused on our internal relationship to nature and the environment, our ecological identity (Carpendale, 2010; Parker, 2008; Thomashow, 1995). Ecological identity refers to our relationship to nature; it develops through engaging in creative and self-reflective processes. Around the same time, my son, Will Parker, was writing his thesis on the development of an ecological identity (2008). Our work and dialogue with nature, with each other, with the participants/students, evolved into many of the ideas and projects introduced in this chapter.

In the art therapy training program that I created at the Kutenai Art Therapy Institute, I teach via the circle. By this I mean that we start the day in a circle, with reflections, metaphors, and story. While I have always been engaged in earth art and environmental issues, I have brought a new awareness of our relationship to nature to the circle in many ways. Sometimes I bring a basket or collection of natural objects for participants/students, telling them to choose one to introduce themselves and how they are feeling that day. In the basket might be shells, stones, moss, seeds, bark, branches, leaves, and feathers, as various possibilities. Sometimes it is a collection of different kinds of seeds, or different colours, or stones from the lake or river (Macy & Brown, 2014).

Each of the four semeters of the two-year program has an element: earth, air, water, and fire. We explore the elements metaphorically and with story. I always introduce it in a dialectical way: reflecting on the positive/creative aspects and the negative/destructive aspects. Stirring the pot, so to speak. Invariably, the metaphors and insights are deep and meaningful, both personal and profound. Then I start to give each month a tree for reflection; for example, January is Birch month, and the birch tree sheds its skin in beautiful and generous ways, February is Maple month, and maple trees have inner sweetness and are very beautiful in their transitional time.

At the beginning of the year, I might suggest that the students describe the landscape they have come from or where they feel a strong sense of belonging. During a particularly intense winter immersion, when several students had been seriously impacted by the bad weather conditions and were unable to fly in for days, when they finally arrived, we told stories of powerful experiences with weather.

I also use old maps as a base for collage and for creating "self maps" (Carpendale, 2009). I believe that it is important to explore both metaphors and real materials. Our art shelves include art materials plus found and recycled objects (Siano, 2016), as well as various assorted natural materials. In the spring, I collect the Canada geese feathers that are spread on the ground during molting time. I collect all kinds of natural things like pinecones and chestnuts. A ground rule is to not take anything that will die if brought into the studio and to not hurt a living creature or plant. Eco-art therapy is both about going into nature to do art therapy and bringing nature into the studio.

During the pandemic when we had to suddenly move our classes online, this practice of the circle became even more important. But how could we feel the circle? I started to see the Zoom screen as a mosaic and referred to it as such. I also changed the practice of having the mute and unmute always centered on the host and asked each person to pass the reflection on to the next person with their name and sometimes a mark of gratitude. This contributed to building connection in our virtual circle. I became very aware of the need to resource the students being on Zoom screens for too long, and I structured breaks for walks and nature-based art activities and reflections.

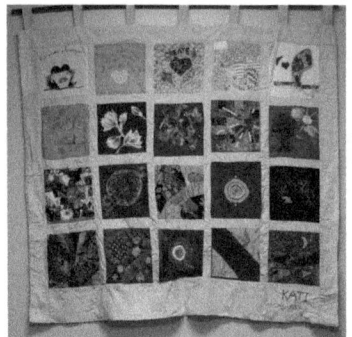 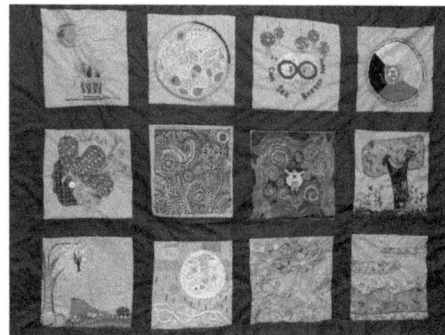

Figure 10.1: The quilts

A few days after our first lockdown, I started the quilt project as collaborative community art to co-create with materials that could be washed and then brought together as a whole. Students were working on their quilt square during Zoom class time and this appeared to ease the stress of extensive screen time or Zoom fatigue. Figure 10.1 shows two examples of "quarantine" or "compassion" quilts created by the students and faculty at the Kutenai Art Therapy Institute.

"Under the umbrella" is a project of painting umbrellas to symbolize the need to protect oneself from the coronavirus and to socially distance. Umbrellas physically protect us from rain and weather, and they also create a "bubble" of space around us. Umbrellas were painted in virtual open studios and "bubble" studios. This can be a way to express gratitude for the planet. This initiative by the Kutenai Art Therapy Institute engages community in an intergenerational project. We had children, parents, grandparents all painting umbrellas, both at open studio and in various placements. We hosted an outside "umbrella" painting day and then took all the umbrellas up to the seniors' assisted living home and created an outside installation for them to enjoy.

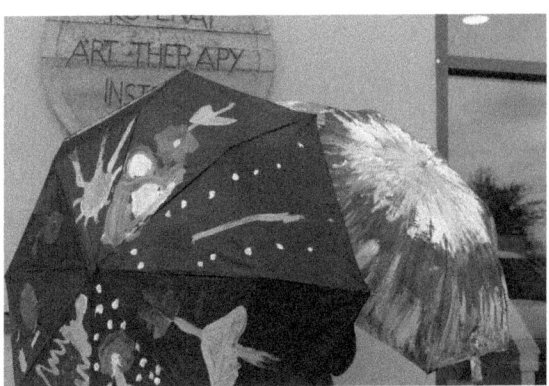

Figure 10.2: The umbrellas

Parzival and the Fisher King

Our land and country are in trouble, dying, just as in the Parzival story of the quest for the Grail. The question that Parzival initially fails to ask the Fisher King is, "What ails thee? What has happened to wound thee?" There is a long time of waiting in the castle until he is willing to ask the question. The first time in the castle, Parzival does not ask the question (Shaw, 2014). We need to think about the parts of ourselves that may be waiting to be rescued and that feel wounded and caught between life and death. "What ails thee? What has happened to thee?" are the essential therapeutic questions that precipitate the therapeutic process.

Sometimes we do not know what ails us nor what ails the land and country, and we are adrift in extremely uncertain times, living in a global pandemic, with an ongoing climate emergency, escalating racism and social justice issues, while facing the potential of a full-scale economic collapse. It is a "perfect storm," and whether we are struggling or not, it is all around us; we witness widespread distress and physical health needs, with escalating mental health issues.

We have learned that kindness can become a mantra, a value, an ethic, and a practice. We have learned the importance of a sense of belonging and compassion for each other and ourselves. We have learned about kin and connection. We are all in this together, and we are all interconnected. We now know without a doubt that our health and well-being depend on the health and well-being of others.

Nature is essential and restorative—the safe place to be. Nature can press a reset button if given half a chance to breathe. Wildlife will return to places they have not been in a long while, the waters will clear, and pollution will go down. We have learned that we can stop and do not need to rush around and go everywhere all the time. This ability to stop, wait, reflect, and take care of each other as a priority has become evident.

This is a perfect time to inspire creativity with art-making/poiesis, as a place of playing with uncertainty, of imagination, of possibility, of wonder, of exploration and expression (Levine, 2019). Creativity can find expression in the home, in the garden, in nature, in words, and in music.

Re-imaging art therapy

People often do not realize that the arts as well as environmental education can function to develop critical cognitive skills, observation, classification, and imagination (Cohen, 2007; Eisner, 2002). The arts provide a place for rehearsal and to try out new ideas safely. Creative and critical thinking skills are utilized in all aspects of the creative process. The studio can provide an experiential safety net. The use of unusual materials provides an opportunity to engage in creative problem-solving and flexible repurposing (Eisner, 2002). Aesthetic experience increases perception and the ability to notice and see the world in new ways. Different tactile and sensory experiences serve to expand horizons and promote self-regulation. Art-making encourages the development of empathy and the ability to "step into the shoes of the other." An artwork is a personal expression that speaks back to the artist and communicates to the viewer as well. The arts are a way to explore our own internal landscape—our emotions, experiences, and responses (Carpendale, 2009).

Art allows what has been "said" to be seen. All of this occurs in environmental education through exploration, play, and the creation of worlds (Berger & Lahad, 2013). The therapeutic and educational focus is to encourage an emotional connection to nature, enhance a sense of belonging, and release imagination with the awareness that one can create and re-create with all the materials one finds or is given (Carpendale, 2010; Cohen, 2007; Parker, 2008).

Rethinking art materials in the pandemic precipitated many changes in the art studios. Separate art bins of tools and materials were created for students and participants. Assorted recycled and natural materials were placed in "mystery bags" for creative projects, as we could not have artists grazing through our shelves filled with collections of recycled and natural materials. Natural materials were gathered outside that were free of contaminants. Nature was abundant and provided prolific opportunities for creativity and "safe" places for therapeutic engagement. Online virtual art therapy sessions focused on simple home art materials, digital art-making, collage, and available natural and recycled materials. It was important to consider accessibility and ease of creative engagement. The use of natural materials, found objects, and unusual recycled materials helps in building skills in flexible repurposing, innovative thinking, and imagination (Eisner, 2002).

Poiesis and sympoiesis

Poiesis is about making and bringing into being something that did not exist before (Levine, 2019). Sympoiesis refers to "making with"—collaborative art-making, community art-making, co-creating, and storytelling (Haraway, 2016). In poiesis and sympoiesis, the engagement with creating and co-creating awakens awareness of how small change can precipitate big change. This is the genesis of hope. The pandemic and the climate emergency bring so much uncertainty into our lives that it is sometimes difficult to keep hope active and hold a positive vision for the future. The importance of empowerment and choice, expression and creativity cannot be over-emphasized. Through the process of poiesis, we can work and play with uncertainty, making and re-making, discovering and transforming, re-imagining materials, and we can give expression to feelings and find words to give voice to our internal life and respond to the world unfolding.

The arts are an invitation to pay attention and to give expression to the environmental experience: to imagine and be able to create. The stimulation of imagination refines the senses and enhances subtle awareness to give form to feeling. Increasing perception increases awareness, imagination, and the interconnectedness of the world around us. Constructing worlds in nature, as in the secret garden activity, is like creating dioramas or drawings in art. There is ongoing metaphorical interpretation through the creation of story and possibilities. The artist is always responding to the unanticipated; this promotes flexibility in thinking and the repurposing of materials and ideas. The creative process always involves taking risks and tolerating uncertainty, ambiguity, and impermanence (Eisner, 2002; Grudin, 1990).

The importance of story

Martin Shaw (2020, p.3), British mythologist and storyteller, writes:

> The business of stories is not enchantment.
> The business of stories is not escape.

The business of stories is waking up. We need new stories, new eco-tales like the stories in *Dancing with Trees* (Galbraith & Willis, 2017). I particularly like the "Magpie's Nest" in it. The Magpie goes around trying to make the perfect nest; each time something is not quite right, but each time another bird has been observing and finds this method to be perfect for them. This works metaphorically to illustrate how we need to go forward, to try new things, to try others' ideas, to share experiences, and to create new stories.

We are telling our stories and retelling our stories. The multispecies kin and other-than-human beings have been included in stories throughout all cultures. Hayward (2012) considers storytelling as "one way we can help young citizens learn to create shared spaces for conversation, and enhance their skills for radically decentered democratic listening, to improve public deliberation across different world views" (pp.121–122). Dr. Seuss has the Lorax speak for the trees. Bronwyn Hayward (2012, p.5) writes of the importance of fostering in children the development of a "democratic imagination and ecological citizenship." She talks of rethinking environmental education and moving on from recycling and energy consumption to the larger critical social justice and political issues.

Fairy tale structures are helpful in establishing a pattern where the least likely, the smallest, the youngest, the "dumb" one is going to be successful. Stories with magic break through patterns of bias, assumptions, and "taken-for-grantedness" (Van Manen, 2014). Small steps and insignificant creatures and people can change the tide of events. Playing Dungeons and Dragons provides older teens with a process of storytelling that engages imagination and creativity in envisioning hope and possibility.

Environmental education

The field of environmental education has the challenge of supporting existing educational perspectives as well as differentiating itself from them (Van Matre, 1999). To my mind, environmental education is most simply described as the appreciation of connections and cycles in nature. It involves emotional connections and personal experience. It reframes environmental questions into a metaphorical story of connections in the complexity of interconnectedness. By listening to each other's stories and valuing their experience, we allow them to value the experience in a new way, and we can all appreciate a new aspect of nature. Appreciating nature seems to be deeply interconnected with telling stories. To appreciate all our experiences of nature does not mean that we must like or want to repeat them. We can appreciate our selves, diversity, and the innate value of nature with a great amount of respect. Some things you teach because you know the answer, but other things you teach because you hope to inspire. Appreciating nature is the first step to becoming an environmentalist.

Teaching creative ways to think about cycles in nature is a simple way to dive into nature appreciation. We use our senses and experience of nature to appreciate its complexities. A tear from my eye is on its way to the ocean. Nature appreciation is also a great approach because it is often politically or culturally insensitive or inappropriate to teach specific environmental agendas. The environmental movement needs to set root in every heart and appreciate the experiences of everyone. Appreciating nature is the most universal and powerful aspect of any environmental education program (Van Matre, 1999).

I like to teach about the ecopsychologist Michael Cohen's 53 senses

(2007). He says we do not just have the usual senses of taste, touch, sight, sound, and smell. Cohen talks about the sense of gravity, of light, of warmth, of balance, and so forth. Attuning to our senses and moving to what attracts us in nature can enhance perception in many ways.

I tell students to never underestimate the value of a well-used prop. Use your imagination to become smaller or go back in time. A magnifying glass is a new experience of the world lived by an insect that can be shared by several people. A small segment of string can create the boundary around a special area that encourages active imagination and storytelling. Sometimes we call this making "secret gardens." When trust is given over to nature, something amazing can happen as people start to play with things and find a strong place for their emotional connections. The intention in sparking play is to increase perception and sensory exploration. Resiliency, imagination, and inner resources are strengthened with creating magic, mystery, and story.

Trash monsters and power insects

In the construction of trash monsters and power insects, we talk about creatures that existed in the past or might exist in a future world that we can barely understand. We encourage ideas about how these creatures might have super-powers or eat different things in a future world. There is also the possibility that a creature might have a weakness or a power place that they might need to go to recharge their energy the way a superhero does. We generally use recycled materials, found objects, tape, wire, and glue. We take apart old electronics and mechanical things to add exciting new possibilities of modified robot creations. The intention of this activity is to increase inventiveness, work with flexible repurposing, build skills in problem-solving, and encourage story-making.

We suggest beginning with a body that limbs and sensory organs can be attached to. That could mean noses or heads, or mouths, or eyes, or whatever students think their creature might need to interact with the environment. They can use a mixture of natural materials and found objects to create stick puppets or creatures for an interactive set. We encourage the development of character and story and provide a place and space for sharing of an art tour.

Creating art is an act of construction and deconstruction. Let us think about the value which using deconstructed materials can have on the psyche of the artist. The metaphor of taking that which has been thrown out or handed down, and seeing it anew in different configurations, increases the ability to perceive spatially, to reinvent and to see patterns and human characteristics in the non-human and animal forms. Judith Siano writes of the value of "lost, found, and rejected objects in art therapy" (2016).

Circle reflections from a single day experience

As part of the art therapy program, we integrated environmental education with art therapy and ecological identity work in a day-long workshop that included activities like the secret garden, finding the extraordinary in the ordinary, and making creatures and stories with both natural and recycled materials. In the closing circle at the end of the day, workshop participants spoke of what they had valued in the day and the themes and benefits that emerged.

Participants spoke of the feeling of safety in being in nature, of not feeling isolated. They experienced the reassuring and stabilizing aspects of nature and named the security of simple steps: collecting, gardening, balancing, repetition, and meditative time. Self-regulation was evident in the talk of feeling creative but not flooded with emotion, of the value of play and how it relaxed the nervous system. Participants spoke of the pleasure in being outside, how it calmed their anxiety. They experienced quiet joy and deep absorption.

They spoke of enjoying the large play space and the creativity. Imagination abounded in the play, story, and character development. Objects were transformed into new forms. The use of unusual materials disrupted conventional ideas and approaches to art-making, increasing invention and multiple repurposing with different kinds of thinking and creating.

Nature teaches patience and reflective introspection as well as the creative aspects of surprise with making and finding meaning. Spirituality and elements of the sacred were named as coming with the meditative quality of making art and making special or sacred spaces. Working with earth and nature became a pathway of connecting to ancestors and a yearning for depth and aloneness. The elements of the day provided tranquility and were experienced as nurturing and reassuring. The memory of place and a sense of belonging were significant in the symbolic garden, creating a memorial with the expanding story.

All spoke of increased self-awareness and inspiration, with enhanced perception and a movement from the small to the large. There was increased sensory awareness and stimulation from being outside: light, sound, texture, image, scent, physical interactions, and engagement. All participants expressed gratitude for and appreciation of nature.

Closing musings about wonder and imagination

Art-making, play, nature, and storytelling go hand in hand. The intention of weaving together environmental education with art therapy is to develop mindfulness, responsibility, imagination, and citizenship. The creative process engages the creation of imaginary and parallel worlds and of creating kin with animals, insects, trees, and stones. Hayward emphasizes the importance of imagination and creativity to engage children and youth in developing skills in citizenship and leadership (2012).

Creativity, art-making, metaphor, and storytelling are key aspects of art therapy and environmental education. They all interweave and function to increase self-awareness and a positive sense of self, and develop an ecological identity or the ecological self that Joanna Macy refers to (Carpendale, 2010; Macy, 1991; Parker, 2008; Thomashow, 1995). This way of working is accessible to everyone and provides much wisdom and many thoughts to follow up on everywhere, but most of all it highlights the need for creativity, critical thinking, and trusting the healing possibilities of connecting with and even just talking about nature. I am committed to working with respect and compassion for justice and health for humanity and for an ecologically respectful relationship to the natural world. It is my hope that this chapter becomes part of the dialogue, inspiring new ideas and adaptations—a small contribution to the creative and transformational work that is needed in the world.

References

Berger, R. & Lahad, M. (2013). *The Healing Forest in Post-Crisis Work with Children: A Nature Therapy and Expressive Arts Program for Groups*. London and Philadelphia, PA: Jessica Kingsley Publishers.

Carpendale, M. (2009). *Essence and Praxis in the Art Therapy Studio*. Victoria, BC: Trafford Publishing.

Carpendale, M. (2010) Ecological identity and art therapy. *Canadian Art Therapy Association Journal*, 23(2), 53–57.

Cohen, M.J. (2007). *Reconnecting with Nature: Finding Wellness through Restoring your Bond with the Earth*. Lakeville, MN: Ecopress.

Davenport, L. (2017). *Emotional Resiliency in the Era of Climate Change: A Clinician's Guide*. London and Philadelphia, PA: Jessica Kingsley Publishers.

Eisner, E. (2002). *The Arts and the Creation of Mind*. London and New Haven, CT: Yale University Press.

Galbraith, A. & Willis, A.J. (2017). *Dancing with Trees: Eco-tales from the British Isles*. Cheltenham: The History Press.

Grudin, R. (1990). *The Grace of Great Things: Creativity and Innovation*. Boston, MA: Ticknor & Fields.

Haraway, D. (2016). *Staying with the Trouble: Making Kin in the Chthulucene*. Durham, NC and London: Duke University Press.

Hayward, B. (2012). *Children, Citizenship, and Environment: Nurturing a Democratic Imagination in a Changing World*. New York, NY: Routledge.

Kopytin, A. & Rugh, M. (eds.) (2017). *Environmental Expressive Therapies: Nature-Assisted Theory and Practice*. New York, NY: Routledge Taylor and Francis.

Levine, S. (2019). *Philosophy of Expressive Arts Therapy: Poiesis and the Therapeutic Imagination*. London and Philadelphia, PA: Jessica Kingsley Publishers.

Macy, J. (1991). *World as Lover, World as Self*. Berkeley, CA: Parallax Press.

Macy, J. & Brown, M. (2014). *Coming Back to Life*. Gabriola Island, BC: New Society Publishers.

Macy, J. & Johnstone, C. (2012). *Active Hope: How to Face the Mess We Are in Without Going Crazy*. Novato, CA: New World Library.

Orr, D.W. (1994) *Earth in Mind: On Education, Environment, and the Human Prospect*. Washington, DC: Island Press.

Parker, W. (2008). The Development of an Ecological Identity. MA thesis. Dalhousie, Halifax.

Shaw, M. (2014). *Snowy Tower: Parzival and the Wet, Black Branch of Language*. Ashland, OR: White Cloud Press.

Shaw, M. (2020). *Courting the Wild Twin*. London and White River Junction, VT: Chelsea Green Publishing.

Siano, J. (2016). *Lost, Found and Rejected Objects in Art Therapy*. Toronto: Caversham Booksellers.

Thomashow, M. (1995). *Ecological Identity: Becoming a Reflective Environmentalist*. Cambridge, MA: MIT Press.

Van Manen, M. (2014) *Phenomenology of Practice: Meaning Giving Methods in Phenomenological Research and Writing*. Walnut Creek, CA: Left Coast Press.

Van Matre, S. (1999). *Earth Education: A New Beginning*. New York, NY: Earth Institute for Education.

Wilson, S. (2008). *Research is Ceremony: Indigenous Research Methods*. Halifax: Fernwood Publishing.

Chapter 11

Coronavirus as a Rite of Passage: Finding Cures for "Colonialvirus" through Expressive Arts-Based Research

GRACELYNN CHUNG-YAN LAU

Prologue

Once we cross the threshold, there is no going back.

The coronavirus arrived in Canada in mid-March of 2020. In a surge of cancellations, physical distancing, panic buying in grocery stores and death tolls in global news, I began to wonder: if the coronavirus is a rite of passage sent from the more-than-human world, guiding humanity into a collective future with the Living Gaia, what is it we are to understand in all this?

Pandemic narratives frame viruses as malevolent instead of integral to the interdependent web of life in which humans and viruses must co-exist. Charles Eisenstein noted that, soon after the coronavirus began spreading in North America, if there is one thing our civilization is good at, it is fighting an enemy: "We manufacture enemies, cast problems like crime, terrorism, and disease into us-versus-them terms, and mobilize our collective energies toward those endeavors that can be seen that way" (Eisenstein, 2020). Since the European co-opting of North America, the colonial powers have introduced separation and control to Indigenous soils and ways of being, in the name of "security," "progress," and "health." Let's just call it "Colonialvirus" as a thought experiment:

The Colonialvirus is a highly contagious virus that has been around for centuries. When conditions are right, the Colonialvirus multiplies in the host's body, sometimes killing the host. The most common symptoms of Colonialvirus disease are the mindset of separation (us versus them), domination, control and desire to individualize; it affects the heart-spirit-mind connection, and causes difficulty in the capacity to relate to others. Early symptoms also include the loss of imagination and a sense of belonging in the larger-than-human world. Unlike the novel coronavirus, not much expertise has been put into containing and combating the Colonialvirus; and none of us has ever successfully flattened the curve. But we have seen cases of antibodies from recovered patients rooted in some Indigenous and Indigenous-led communities...

What does it mean to decolonize the Earth and how could it be answered through expressive arts-based research (EABR)? Would the creative process in EABR help humanity to re-member ecological identity and to participate in the ongoing creative process of the Living Gaia? Could play and imagination inform us about decolonizing and healing ourselves as we heal the Earth?

In this chapter, I will document a research process that took place from March 15 to May 30, 2020 in Kingston, Ontario, Canada. The process started four days after the World Health Organization declared a global pandemic, and two days before the Ontario government declared a state of emergency in response to the coronavirus outbreak.

I will follow the basic tenets of EABR outlined by José Miguel Calderon (Calderon, 2020) to structure this inquiry into three sections, "Filling in," "In studio," and "Harvesting," in accordance with the "architecture" of an expressive arts session (Knill, Levine, & Levine, 2005).

In "Filling in," I will elaborate the research questions in the context of our "habitual worlding," that is, everyday experiences of the researcher and their academic relationship with the research questions. "In studio" designates the transition wherein the researcher will leave the research questions temporarily to enter into an art-oriented de-centering process, in which they will access the "alternative worlding" (imaginative experiences) by engaging in multisensory intermodal art-making. This de-centering process takes the inquiry into "liminality," a state similar to a rite of passage process, where one is capable of receiving deep knowing that comes from an awareness of one's limitations and possible resources (Levine, 1992). "Harvesting" is the last section wherein the researcher will return to the research questions, and weave between those images, surprises and findings emerging from the "Studio" in order to present the results.

Filling in

My personal and academic relationship with decolonizing the Earth is intertwined intimately with my faith, my worldview's evolution and my career path for the last 13 years. As a child growing up in the concrete jungle of Hong Kong, I developed a severe animal phobia and a deep-seated aversion to most forms of activities in nature. In 2006, at the Institute for Christian Studies in Toronto, I discovered ecofeminist theology. My Judeo-Christian religious foundation underwent an earthquake for the first time.

Ecofeminist theologians have challenged the predominant anthropocentric and androcentric tendency in Christian theology, in terms of which human beings dominate the rest of Creation. The image of God, as well as humanity's relational experience with the Divine, has been limited to a masculine father/son figure (Gebara, 1999; Ruether, 1992). Ecofeminist theologians also have criticized the Cartesian dualistic assumption in the formation of theology, which fundamentally polarizes chaos-order, nature-culture, body-mind, material world (earth)-metaphysicial world (heaven), contriving an ecologically disembodied Christianity that is "not earthly enough" (Berry, 2002). The ecofeminist lens has opened up biblical imagery in perceiving the Divine as an ongoing creative process, a mystery, and including non-masculine elements in Creation (2003). This new approach has also proposed metaphors to experience God as mother, lover, and friend, and also has envisioned the evolution of the Universe as the embodiment of God (McFague, 1993). In Hebrew, *Adamah* means earth and is a feminine form. While the biblical name for human beings, *Adam*, literally means *earthling* (one formed from the earth), the biblical name for the first woman, *Eve*, means "the mother of all living beings" (Berry, 2002; Lal, 2017).

This reshaping of the human-divine relationship turned my biblical worldviews "downside up," challenging me to reconsider the human role in relation to the rest of all creatures sharing the Earth and in our participation in the creative process. The lack of Christian literature in deepening these questions has brought me toward deep ecology and Gaia theory. The work of Brian Swimme and Thomas Berry has offered an intellectual and scientific articulation to understand the 14 billion years of evolution of the Universe as a self-regulating complex system and a living process (Swimme & Berry, 1992). Berry proposes that the Universe is not understood as a collection of objects, but a communion of subjects (Berry, 1999). Thomas Berry famously lamented humanity's "autism towards the world," the fact that we have lost "our great conversation" with the more-than-human world. The powerful metaphor of Gaia, the Greek goddess, employed by James Lovelock and other Earth system scientists to convey the scientific understanding of Earth as a living system with cultural understandings of human society as a continuum of that system, was helpful intellectually. But in terms of our experience, how is it possible to have "a great conversation" with Gaia, the Living Earth?

Joanna Macy created "The Work that Reconnects" (WTR) (Macy & Brown, 1998), a participatory theoretical framework attempting to widen the sense of identity to include the planetary self through the "Great Turning" and "the Greening of the Self" (Macy, 2007). Along similar lines, the work of ecopsychology pioneer Theodore Roszak calls for interdisciplinary collaboration between traditional psychology and environmental studies, and a holistic view of connection between the environment and the human soul. The Buddhist root of Macy's model, and the ecopsychology literature, have helped me to embrace the suffering of all living beings and to view environmental issues from the perspective of the more-than-human world. I have, since studying these works, become a facilitator for WTR. I also acquired professional training in horticultural therapy in 2014. Yet, as someone who grew up with animal phobia and has had symptoms of what Richard Louv calls "nature deficit disorder" (Louv, 2005), how could I hope to embody this ecological identity in a felt sense in lived experiences, let alone participate in and create with the Earth as God's body.

Nine years after I first learned of ecofeminist theology, I became a permaculture teacher and nature-based therapist at an ecovillage on Vancouver Island. I immersed myself in the cycle of seasons by tending seven acres of annual vegetable gardens and food forests, living with domestic and wild animals for almost five years. Pioneered by Bill Mollison and David Holmgren in the 1970s, "permaculture" is a set of ethics and design principles for whole-system thinking and regenerative design, based on observing and mimicking the patterns found in nature. This is by far the closest empirical practice to embody my ecological identity with integrity, but nonetheless the ontological concept of human partnering with Gaia in co-creation remains, to some degree, disembodied and distanced.

In the face of the global pandemic, climate disruption and looming ecological collapse, the question of decolonizing and healing the Earth and ourselves has become increasingly significant to our species and future generations. The question arises, could expressive arts-based inquiry illuminate a path to re-member our ecological membership in the interdependent web of life, so that we as a species can participate differently in our embodiment on this shared living Earth?

In Studio
1. De-centering process—water: Lake Ontario
The world went mad within days. Classes were cancelled. The Canadian dollar dropped. Universities closed campuses. Students were packing to go home. People were fighting over toilet paper and hand sanitizer. Everybody was ordered to stay at home. I did not know what to think about this pandemic, but I knew that water was my resource; I decided to turn to Lake Ontario.

I met an Anishinaabe woman in Peterborough at the Canadian Indigenous and Native Studies Conference in February 2020, who told me that water was my helper and I should offer tobacco to it. Now that nature has pressed the pause button on our civilization, I have begun visiting the lake every other day, recording the sounds and shades of the water. Every time I offer tobacco, I feel a sense of, "Listen, the water is speaking. Listen to what is."

Sometimes I take a book to read by the water. That particular day I came upon Craig Chalquist's essay on terrapsychology and Lauren Schneider's eco-dreamwork. Chalquist explains that by exploring a place's myth, history, and the recurring motifs in the infrastructure, and by tracking our moods and dreams while there, we can hear the geographical "discourse" of the living landscapes we inhabit (Buzzell & Chalquist, 2009). Schneider argues that attending to dreams collectively may help a society through critical issues (Buzzell & Chalquist, 2009). I began to wonder about dreams, ecological identity, and the pandemic.

I took this wondering to an expressive arts session. My supervisor Dr. Stephen K. Levine asked me to go to the kitchen sink. "Follow your impulse and see what comes." I played with a bowl of water, the water tap and a stainless-steel pot, sliding water back and forth, drumming with water in the pot to create soundscapes. When the sound play came to a pause, I put some water on my face and stayed in stillness. A moment came wherein I felt strong impulses to shake first my hands then my whole body, as if I were a water droplet, an amoeba, or currents hidden in the water. The shaking turned into a slow dance, where my hands found their way to my womb, as if the source of water, the ocean in me, is where I am from and who I am. I placed my hands on my womb in silence. As my body gently swung, I heard my womb saying, *"You are water, water is you. You are air, air is you. Don't be afraid, all of creation is going through a birthing now."* The following poem emerged from this water dance:

THE INVITATION
We are from the ocean
of our mothers' womb;
to the earthy womb
of soil we shall return.
Nothing to be afraid of,
this is a birthing yet again.
Let us all take a deep breath
and return to the sacred.

The phenomenological relationship between dreams, the pandemic, and ecological identity began to be illuminated. The spaciousness and intimacy created by the simplicity of playing with the water in shaping soundscapes took me to a place of dreaminess, where I could "hear" differently. The creative process in the imaginal held that space, where there seemed to be unrealities revealing and connecting themselves to the seemingly more real realities.

2. "The Third"—the ocean of mother's womb

To deepen the exploration, I further shaped "The Third" (according to EABR, this is the powerful images that arise in the creative process) by taking "the ocean of the mother's womb" image into embodied sound and poetic inquiry.

In one such session, a sea creature, butterflies, and a new born baby emerged from a two-hour intermodal movement-soundscapes exploration. The movement brought me to the myth of "Lu Ting," a half-fish-half-man creature recorded in the Hong Kong Indigenous Tanka people's legend. I heard about "Lu Ting" during a family visit last year. In our oral history, this mermaid-like creature is the ancestor of the people of Hong Kong. With all the images arising from that process, I wrote this story:

> Lu Ting wakes up from a dream. In the dream, she was waiting to dance with the whales. But she has forgotten that she is a horse. Can a horse dance in deep water? No. She runs with the horses. A new herd isn't her own. Lu Ting is a lone horse in this herd. She doesn't go as fast as the rest of them, because she loves watching butterflies. It's the butterflies' season now. Many leave their cocoons at last.

> Today, when she stops to listen to the woodpecker and the decaying leaves, she hears a vague voice moving through the thin air in the dark soil. She isn't sure what it is. It sounds like a prayer but also like an electrical frequency; something not of this planet, at least not of this era. It sounds like a muddy murmur, as if someone was struggling to send a rescue message:

> "Help... help us... we don't want to be here. But they trap us here.

> We aren't from here. We want to go home..."

> Lu Ting instinctively knows that this old voice is from the ancient viruses. As old as the voice of the roots, ancient in time. Lu Ting doesn't know what to do, so she asks,

> "Hey, I hear you. Can I do something to help?"

> The voice responds, "Please, wake them up from the dream. When they wake up from this dream, we'll be free."

> Lu Ting replies, "But how? How can I wake them up?"

> The voice says, "Sing. Sing your songs with the ocean. Sing the ocean songs. The water will teach you."

In another session, I improvised a dance response to the 34 minutes *Songs of the Humpback Whale* album, and recorded a video. In the dance, a little floating transparent creature emerges from the movement sequence, like a delicate and flimsy new-born of some sort, dancing with my hands. It seems expandable, light, and intricate. After the movement, I wrote a dialogue with this emerging image:

Me: What's your name?

Little creature: Fluffy Crystal. I am a flying creature that lives in the water too.

Me: Can you tell me more about yourself, Fluffy Crystal?

Fluffy: I am the air when I'm in the air, I am the water when I'm in the water. I move, expand or contract depending on more or less air in me. I am transparent and I move between solids.

Me: Are you bacteria? Or a virus?

Fluffy: Yes, viruses are my relatives. Some of them aren't like us floaty fairies. They are trapped. You have the word "genetically modified," right? Some of our relatives are like that, having been mixed with something else in your world. They're crying for help, because they don't want to be trapped in human bodies. That's not where they want to be.

Me: Fluffy Crystal, why do you come to me?

Fluffy: Because you listen. Because I am your relative.

Me: What? I'm a horse, how can you be my relative?

Fluffy: You are in this body, made out of us fluffy crystals. Learn the whale songs. Their songs communicate with all the microorganisms in everybody. They will help you to remember your song.

These images and stories guided me to another spontaneous embodied inquiry, in response to the sound of a gong, with this poem arising as an ending:

GRANDMOTHER'S PRAYER
Become river
you're the water
never ever stop
folding
just illusion
unfolding
just illusion
you are the water
step in

Later, I discovered that Lake Ontario is a proglacial lake. For thousands of years, most of Ontario was covered in ice. Ancient whale bones have been found in the Ottawa Valley (Kennedy, 1977). At the end of the last ice age, the glaciers retreated, creating the Great Lakes in their wake. At this stage, Lake Ontario was known as "glacial Lake Iroquois." Around 12,000 years ago, the waters receded significantly and fell back to sea level. Water from the upper Great Lakes bypassed Lake Ontario, heading directly to the St. Lawrence river via the Ottawa Valley. Five thousand years ago, water flew through the lower Great Lakes, and Lake Ontario almost reached its current level, indicating that the earliest evidence of people in the area is now mostly underwater (Fiddes, 2014).

3. Loom/Blanket—my aesthetic responsibility to the pandemic

In expressive arts theory, "poiesis" entails poetry and art-making, but, more, refers to a fundamentally human way of being-in-the-world. Poiesis is a sensitive, sensible, and sense-making process to what has been given to us by making something new, as our "aesthetic response-ability" in the world (Knill *et al.*, 2005).

As I continue to weave these images and stories emerging from the creative processes and the theme of inquiry, I ask myself: What do I do with this information? Does it inform me about my own response to the pandemic? What is my poietic action and my aesthetic response-ability to the pandemic?

> "Listen, listen, don't ask what you can bring, ask the water:
> What is needed? What is asking to emerge?"

To my surprise, the weaving resulted in a decision to offer multiple groups online! In spite of my resistance to and lack of confidence in online facilitation, I seemed to hear the call and went with it. The interrelated birthing of these online groups has come to be another "Third", in which I have found myself witnessing groups unfolding, as I continuously shape and work with what was asking to come to life.

Together with my colleague Sara Anderson, I decided to offer "expressive arts practices for holding turbulence," a four-week online group beginning in early April. Neither of us had created online workshops before. We resolved the inevitable technology hiccups with clumsy grace. The group gathered for one and a half hours each week; in between sessions, participants would engage with "home play" to deepen their relationships with a "nature being" who chose and called to them. Here is an extract from the group online promotion:

> *In this four-week group we'll hold space together by tapping into our innate creative, imaginal abilities. We will carry each other, while exploring how to be held by nature through this time of turbulence. We will draw from our capacity to recognize and witness beauty amid chaos... Deep connection is our resource. May we return to what is sacred.*

This initial impulse led us to hosting three online groups. The first group started on April 3, and the third group was to end on May 29. We were deeply surprised and moved by the spaciousness and sense of connection co-created by the participants and the natural elements participants brought to the work. The work went far beyond "therapy" in a limited sense, but was restorative to our creative beingness as humans.

I have also created grief ritual online circles specifically for people in Hong Kong. In one two-hour ritual, I asked participants to prepare a bowl of water, a candle and some salt. As we lit the candle to begin, I asked them to connect with the fire in them to the fire burning in the forests, and to connect their tears to the rain. As each person held the "bowl of tears," we took turns sharing our grief by saying: "My tears are for..." We paused to remind ourselves that we were witnessing the true condition of the human heart in the midst of political, economical, and ecological crises, that our tears were Mother Earth's tears.

As I am writing this chapter now, these groups and circles are evolving. Invitations to facilitate other group experiences with this poietic approach are knocking at the door...

Harvesting
Are there cures for "Colonialvirus"?
Expressive arts practices as treatment
Exiting the art-based de-centering "studio," we will now return to the questions set forward in this chapter: how do play and imagination inform us about decolonizing/healing the Earth as ourselves? Can expressive arts-based inquiry help us to re-member our ecological identity and to participate in the ongoing creative process of the living Earth in embodied and lived experiences?

With centuries of Eurocentric colonization which has been exploit-ing the rest of the world for economic gain, Indigenous peoples across continents have to a great extent lost their lives, languages, sacred land, and cultural practices. Non-Indigenous peoples in industrial growth (and globalized) societies have been equally separated from their pre-modern ancestral cultures, traditional worldviews, and their own imaginations. The colonial mindset of separation, domination and individualism has taken away our interrelating capacity and our sense of belonging to the more-than-human world.

While decolonization should mean repatriation of Indigenous land and ways of being to Indigenous peoples (Tuck & Yang, 2012), I propose that there should also be work done among non-Indigenous peoples to reverse and heal the colonial way of being, and that expressive arts therapy practices could be treatments for this "Colonialvirus."

Ecological identifying: Relational nourishment as diet

Sociological and psychological literature has long held that identity is fluid and negotiable, depending on interpersonal social interaction (Swann, 1987; Weinstein & Deutschberger, 1964). I suggest that the same applies to ecological identifying and re-membering.

Re-membering our human ecological identity is a process of rekin-dling our relationship with the living Earth. As in marriage, a marriage certificate identifying a married couple's legal status does not promise an intimate and vital relationship. Claiming our ecological identity intellectually also does not guarantee a deep sense of belonging to and a genuine connection with the more-than-human world. To develop an ecological identity, we need to engage in transpersonal ecological interaction, listening to and interacting with the more-than-human beings in a deep felt sense.

In expressive arts-based inquiry, the de-centering process creates a waking-dream state through play and imagination. During the process described in this chapter, I was able to encounter and "listen" more deeply to the nature beings that "showed up" in the art-making experiences. The deep listening intuitively guided me to uncover prehistorical stories of the living landscape where I reside. When the Anishinaabe woman told me that water was "my helper," it was a statement of intellect rather than of experience, but the arts-based exploration has deepened my relational experience with Lake Ontario on a transpersonal level. In this expressive arts-induced waking-dream state, our human "autism towards the world" finds healing, and our interrelating capacity to have a "great conversation with the more-than-human world" can be restored.

Living ecopoietically: Metabolizing imagination as medicine

Because of its art-oriented nature, the de-centering process is also about creating and shaping. In the "studio," I have worked with emerging images (such as "water creature," "womb," "new-born," "wake them up," "learn your song") through movement and poetry. This "alternative world experience" has also continuously informed my creating and shaping in the "habitual world experience" before and after de-centering processes, resulting in me leading a variety of online groups as my unforeseen and spontaneous (aesthetic) response to the pandemic.

The intersecting structural relationship between the habitual world and the alternative world has blurred the distinction between realities and unrealities. In the phenomenological experience of shaping and creating, whether in poetry, movement or creating online groups, I have been able to play with imagination from a deep sense of listening and a wider sense of wellness for all beings, as if the everyday world is also the "studio" in which I can expand the act of poiesis into everyday experience. Stay-at-home orders and social distancing have become situational restrictions, limiting the range of play in my shaping, inviting me to create imaginative resilience and beauty.

This poietic approach to the pandemic sheds light on human participation in partnership with the living Earth. As mentioned, poiesis in expressive arts therapy is the human innate creative response to shape what has been given to us and that equally shapes us. Widening the concept of poiesis to that of "ecopoiesis," expressive arts theorists have proposed that the human capacity for a poietic act is "embedded within the ongoing creative process of the living Earth" (Aktins & Snyder, 2018, p.118). The concept of "aesthetic response-ability" is then expanded by questioning: What does the Earth need? What does a poietic approach to ecology look like? (Levine, 2019).

The act of ecopoietic shaping, in and in between the habitual and alternative world experiences, could metabolize in the embodiment of our participation in the world. Can we hear the sound of the E(art)h crying and rejoicing inside us? Can we not know about the Earth but know the E(art)h? Can we carry ourselves in the everyday life-world as artists shaping and nurturing the relationship between the E(art)h materials and our creation? Can we grow ourselves out of a separated self, into a maturing aesthetic human shaping, one being shaped within the living shaping E(art)h? By living "ecopoietically," we mature our ecological selves in transpersonal evolving relationships with the more-than-human world that continuously defines who we are as a species. We listen deeply to the creative process of life, and shape and play with what is given to us respectfully.

Pandemic narrative: Are we *corona-ing*?

One of the concerns in this inquiry is the pandemic narrative which frames the virus-human relationship as the enemy in us-versus-them terms, aligned with the colonial mindset of separation. After the de-centering process described in this chapter, I realized that the pandemic itself is indeed a collective de-centering experience, and we were all put in a global liminal space to encounter our limitations as a species.

The coronavirus causes us to leave the habitual world experience and enter an alternative world experience—one of seemingly unimaginable realities. In my de-centering process, the images of the water of a mother's womb, and a new-born have shown up repeatedly. Serendipitously, in a community resilience training webinar with Earth Deeds founder Daniel Greenberg, I learned that corona means crown; and that "crowning" is part of a birthing process referring to the baby's head becoming visible in the birth canal after the mother's cervix is fully dilated. "Crowning" is often known as "the ring of fire," because the mother experiences intense burning sensations as the baby stretches the cervical opening. It is the stage when the midwife will ask the mother to stop pushing, to allow the baby's head to work at its own pace. The midwife then guides the baby's head through the birth canal, followed by one shoulder and then the other.

This image casts light on a different narrative: as a species, are we the mother "corona-ing" to give birth to a new world? Are we the midwife witnessing the burning pain of climate disruption, worldwide socio-political and ecological collapse, while guiding the emerging life-sustaining societies? Are we baby Gaia coming into "human-ing"? Or, are we the mother, the midwife, and the baby, "midwiving" ourselves to our own birthing?

Coronavirus is a rough initiation and a painful birth indeed. We have lost many lives to this pandemic, and we are still facing unprecedented challenges and injustice globally. Whether this "wounded" opening will be a breakthrough or breakdown is up to our imaginative shaping, together with Gaia.

Conclusion

In keeping with the tenets of EABR, the final form of presenting the research results is still a creative act (Calderon, 2020). This chapter has documented the research process and findings in a written academic format, although in some ways creatively challenging and playing with the traditional academic writing standard. But the creative act does not feel complete to me. In the spirit of living ecopoietically, I wonder if the ecopoietic act is birthing another group, perhaps prescribing the expressive arts to treat "Colonialvirus"?

One of the aforementioned opportunities I had to facilitate a group experience was to serve young adult activists in Hong Kong who were dealing with socio-political trauma. The creative challenges lay in their tremendous distrust and suspicion of others and of online security. In an expressive arts session, my supervisor and I explored the possibility of facilitating expressive arts from a distance and in darkness. In an improvised movement-based mixed imaginative role play, the images of a mycelium network in the dark and a multicoloured boulder emerged, absorbing my laptop as part of them. The mycelium then turned into a web of landline telephone coil cords. The ancestors holding the handsets were dialing. Nobody had picked up the call. Everybody was busy with other things. My supervisor asked, "Can you answer the phone?" I did, and this is what I heard:

Thank you for answering the call.
We have been calling 24/7 trying to talk to some of you.
Listen, help them to remember who they are.
There is more to who they are than who they think they are, more than their passport identity.
Who they are is in their blood memories.
Help them to remember the minerals in their own earth.
Their tears and blood are the ocean in them.
Their anger and passion is their fire
also burning in the Amazons, burning underneath volcanoes...
We the ancestors have been there, we understand.

Tell them that they are suffering together with the Earth.

Tell them it is the season of Winter now, the time when things go deep into darkness and die,

so they can be born into something new in the Spring.

And once we cross the threshold, there will be no going back.

References

Atkins, S. & Snyder, M. (2018). *Nature-Based Expressive Arts Therapy: Integrating the Expressive Arts and Ecotherapy*. London and Philadelphia, PA: Jessica Kingsley Publishers.

Berry, T. (1999). *The Great Work: Our Way into the Future*. New York, NY: Bell Tower.

Berry, W. (2002). The Gift of Good Land. In N. Wirzba (ed.), *The Art of the Commonplace: The Agrarian Essays of Wendell Berry*. (pp.76 -85) Berkeley, CA: Counter Point Press.

Buzzell, L. & Chalquist, C. (2009). *Ecotherapy: Healing with Nature in Mind*. San Francisco, CA: Sierra Club Books.

Calderon, J.M. (2020). Expressive arts-based research. *Poiesis: A Journal of the Arts and Communication*, 17, 34–35.

Eisenstein, C. (2020). *The Coronation*. https://charleseisenstein.org/essays/the-coronation.

Fiddes, J. (2014). *Lake Ontario*. FirstStoryTO. https://firststoryblog.wordpress.com/2014/04/29/lake-ontario

Gebara, l. (1999). *Longing for Running Water: Ecofeminism and Liberation*. Minneapolis, MN: Fortress Press.

Kennedy, C.C. (1977). *Whales Bones Found*. Special to The Chronicle, Canadian Museum of History. www.historymuseum.ca/cmc/exhibitions/archeo/kichisibi/k300c-clydeswhale.html.

Knill, P., Levine, E., & Levine, S.K. (2005). *Principles and Practice of Expressive Arts Therapy*. London and Philadelphia, PA: Jessica Kingsley Publishers.

Lal, R. (2017). *Encyclopedia of Soil Science*. Boca Raton, FL: CRC Press.

Levine, S.K. (1992). *Poiesis: The Language of Psychology and the Speech of the Soul*. Toronto: Palmerston Press/Jessica Kingsley Publishers.

Levine, S.K. (2019). Ecopoiesis: Towards a poietic ecology. *Ecopoiesis: Eco-Human Theory and Practice*, 1(1). [open access internet journal].

Louv, R. (2005). *Lost Child in the Woods*. New York, NY: Algonquin Books of Chapel Hill.

Macy, J. (2007). *World as Lover, World as Self*. Berkeley, CA: Parallax Press.

Macy, J. & Brown, M. (1998). *Coming Back to Life*. Gabiola Island, BC: New Society Publishers.

McFague, S. (1993). *The Body of God: An Ecological Theology*. Minneapolis, MN: Fortress Press.

Ruether, R.R. (1992). *Gaia & God: An Ecofeminist Theology of Earth Healing*. San Francisco, CA: HarperSanFrancisco.

Swann, W.B., Jr. (1987). Identity negotiation: Where two roads meet. *Journal of Personality and Social Psychology*, 53, 1038–1051.

Swimme, B. & Berry, T. (1992). *The Universe Story*. San Francisco, CA: HarperSanFrancisco.

Tuck, E. & Yang, K.W. (2012). Decolonization is not a metaphor. *Decolonization: Indigeneity, Education & Society*, 1(1), 1–40.

Weinstein, E.A. & Deutschberger, P. (1964). Tasks, bargains, and identities in social interaction. *Social Forces*, 42, 451–455.

Chapter 12

A Process-Oriented Approach to Nature in the Context of Ecological Art Therapy

RUTH HAMPE

The most beautiful experience we can have is the mysterious. It is the fundamental emotion that stands at the cradle of true art and true science. Whoever does not know it and can no longer wonder, no longer marvel, is as good as dead, and his eyes are dimmed.

Einstein, 1953

Introduction

The need for a new attitude to nature is becoming increasingly more obvious in view of the acceleration of climate change and the increase in emergency situations in the world, such as famine, war scenarios, pandemics, and so on. In this context, art therapeutic interventions can become a bridge that supports the transformation of individual and collective consciousness in regard to the natural world. Nature itself can act as a key resource in this process. Creative design is a process of making which follows one's own intuition and inspiration, as well as being determined by the challenges presented by the materials, and takes place with the assistance of the therapist. In a process-oriented design, the end result is not solely about the aesthetic object; rather, it includes all phases of transformation. Pausing and recognizing this process of change can lead to a special significance for participants, and each phase can be captured using digital media, so that afterwards the participants can explore various possible meanings in more depth. In this chapter, this process is viewed from different perspectives, such as the use of "digital storytelling," and further explored through the discussion of several practical examples. In addition, contact with the natural environment can support feelings of confidence in nature, awareness of its beauty, and the sense of being in resonance with the principles of life; these can be supported, as well as a capacity for resilience.

Process-orientated art therapy in dialogical interaction with nature

Transformation during the design process can be traced back in art, for example through the filmed documentation of the creation of an artwork. Artists such as William Kentridge, Andy Goldsworthy, Joan Miró, Pablo Picasso, Jackson Pollock and Gerhard Richter have already worked in front of the camera, documenting playful, spontaneous sequences of action in their creative processes. The changes that occurred while making the work are not immediately visible or perceivable in the finished aesthetic object. The possibility of witnessing this moving transformation conveys a liveliness and a tensile arc, starting from the mostly empty initial space to the resulting work. In comparison, growth processes in nature, such as the life cycle of the seed from germination to growth, blooming, bearing fruit and passing away, have been documented in slow motion on film.

The physiology of visual perception shows that we usually perceive moving objects before static ones. The neuronal stimulus is primarily triggered by movement, which can be overridden by emotionally charged scenes. In this context, eye movement also has a special function in that objects are scanned with the eyes. This has a feedback effect on the processing of experiences; that is, on whether the eye movement slows down, as in deep sleep in contrast to rapid eye-movement (REM) sleep, or is in the state of a dynamic scanning back and forth perception. In the procedure of eye movement desensitization and reprocessing (EMDR) therapy (Shapiro, 2007), specifically targeted eye movement is activated as a therapeutic method to support the stabilization and processing of experiences. This bilateral stimulation of the brain can help people to calm down, to process and integrate stressful experiences. The combination of perception and movement also supports the creative process. For example, in expressive painting (Stern, 1998), the artist works with proximity and distance to the painted picture by painting directly standing in front of the wall and then stepping back to take colors from a table placed away from the artwork, thus perceiving the image from a distance. In moving forward and backward, a form of processing takes place in which the painted image, in its process-related change, is experienced as an inner-psychic resonance.

An ongoing process of change also takes place in dialogical processes of image-making, such as in dialogical or interactive painting (Hanus, 2014), the squiggle game (Winnicott, 1973), and the progressive mirror image (Damman, 2012; Peciccia & Benedetti, 1994), among others. These processes mostly take place without phases of documentation, but the image itself serves as a witness to the process and is saved as a memory trail. By integrating photographic documentation using digital recording, the changing process can be examined independently, meaning that the initial image can remain as a visual or tactile stimulus for ongoing creation. This means that the image and the creator are engaged in a constant dialogic process of change where both inform the other's ongoing development. Incompleteness and change are the main features of this process. Change and transformation occur in the participant/client, therapist and the art object in an interactive time and space. In the triangle or square situation, with the additional stimulus of the materials, resources can be activated in the continuous modification of the dialogical process. Stuck things are transformed into a dissolving and creating process, whereby verbalization only follows after the image has been completed. Each new, final change is documented photographically and is thereby also appreciated. The change is integrated into a playful flow, similar to a rhythmic cycle, where one is the creator and the other the viewer, the observer, and vice versa.

This supports empathic participation with regard to what is emerging in the aesthetic object. The dialogical element of the creative process also stimulates empathic understanding (Bauer, 2004) and contributes to a respectful perception of nature. The creative process stimulates resonance relationships with elementary natural phenomena, as they can also be revealed on a small scale; for example, the client can participate in natural growth processes in the perception of the unfolding of a leaf. Such an experience may lead to the perception of the vital force in nature and resonate with inner-psychic processes. The movement of nature, in the process of becoming, maturing, and decaying, is immediately understandable as analogous to one's own life phases. Change is inherent in all these natural forms and thus creates a vivid counterpart to personal experience.

Sensual and symbolic experience when working with natural materials

Design processes are subject to sensory modalities, which are affected by the materials used. The inclusion of natural materials or creating images in nature can go hand in hand with sensory stimulation including auditory (hearing), gustatory (tasting), kinesthetic (feeling and touching), olfactory (smelling) and visual (seeing) senses as an exteroception. It can be the experience of silence or the rustling of branches or leaves, the activation of taste experience in the smell of grasses, herbs, flowers, fruits, the visual perception of their colorful design and the tactile experience of their surface structure. In addition, other sensory modalities are included as interoception in the design process, such as the vestibular (sense of balance), proprioceptive (depth sensitivity) and also tactile (surface sensitivity), through which a holistic stimulation of physical experience is possible. With every movement of the body, there is a so-called incorporation of the image, in that it becomes part of the inner experience. This process goes hand in hand with biographical traces of memory and inner images (Hüther, 2004), which are activated in the natural environment and can create new possibilities for experiencing nature. Natural materials in their organic or inorganic substance offer different levels of resistance when working with them; for example, stone, metal and wood mostly evoke a stronger process in contrast to soil, sand, clay and wax or liquid materials. In addition, objects can be created that, like recycled objects, undergo an aesthetic transformation. In this case, the process concerns editing, re-arranging, deconstruction, and reconstruction of references to nature.

If natural materials are used to create mandalas outdoors, and small-scale arrangements such as flower arrangements or natural elements are integrated into an artistic context, then nature is always used as a reference and a changed approach to the creative process is stimulated. There is a tension between cliché-determined, sign-like images and symbolic or proto-symbolic forms of implementation (Hampe, 1999, p.202), as far as the inner-psychological response is concerned. Nevertheless, using natural materials conveys an experience of perception that can give meaning to what is done. In the social interaction and integration of natural materials, a relationship to nature and its phenomena can be established. In the art therapeutic process, mirroring and staging of actions leads to changed processes of perception. What has already been exemplified by artists working with natural materials can, depending on the client, provide examples for work in the art therapeutic setting.

For instance, the artist Andy Goldsworthy (Riedelsheimer, 2001) works exclusively with natural materials and incorporates their transience into his creative process. He uses materials that he finds on site, such as stones, petals, wood, and ice. He works without artificially designed tools, using leaves and branches, thorns, sticks, or grass fibers to hold materials together; he sprinkles petals directly into a river or dissolves powdered colored rocks in the flow of water. In addition, he documents the process of transformation through the forces of nature, for instance the processes of melting and dissolving, using photography to track these changes. He plays with the hidden mysticism of the landscape, making the experience of nature into a work of art. This also applies to other land art practitioners, such as Richard Long or James Turrell, who leave traces of artistic images made mostly with natural materials in specific locations (Lailach, 2007). For example, Wolfgang Laib (Sorace, 2009) works with the beauty of pollen by arranging color fields with pollen collected from dandelions, hazelnuts, or pines. He also creates artistic arrangements using milk, beeswax, marble, rice, and sealing wax. His work is about another dimension of perception, about contemplation as well as time and transience. All of these artistic works with natural materials activate a deep experience of nature as well as space and time. The familiar becomes strange, special, and unique in the transformation of what already exists in nature and its respectful reception by the artist. This artistic activity differs from purpose-orientated creative design by working with the aspect of beauty in nature which is already present.

In art therapeutic practice, there are special forms of communication that involve dialogical interaction between therapist and client. Photographing the artwork during the creation process can mark each end of a design phase, allowing it to be appreciated indirectly and to be understood during its different phases of dialogic change. If Werner Hoffmann (2014) assumes that beauty is a line, this also includes reference to the elementary forms of beauty in nature. For example, the curved line shape can be found in the form of a snake's movement or in the river as it meanders. The beach sand rippled by the sea or the dune crest shaped by the wind in the desert landscape also reveal the spiral lines that can be seen in archaeological formations and in various forms of art. They refer to the rhythmic as a principle of life, and to the cyclical change that occurs in nature. These natural rhythms also determine the creative process and its resonating effect on physiological and psychological experience. Correspondingly, harmonious proportions in nature (Doczi, 2005), such as growth patterns according to the golden ratio and also in a spiral structure formation, can stimulate a positive resonance effect on the psyche. Observing the uniqueness of a seed, its germination and growth as a plant, its flowering, fertility, and withering, can also help us understand the principles of life in nature. The following practical examples relate to these effects. In this respect, the application is not necessarily specifically for use with different clients, but depends on motivational aspects and available resources.

Art therapeutic examples of process-orientated practices

The process of creating can take place both inside and outside, depending on the possibilities and limitations of the circumstances of the therapy. Natural materials are familiar to clients and can be selected, compiled, and used in a playful manner. One possible application is "laying a picture," in which, for example, a face (Figures 12.1a–b), a mandala, or a plant pillow, can arise by placing single elements in dialogical alternation, one at a time and one after the other. With the laying of natural materials, narrative stories can be developed associatively in the process of alternating addition and change (Figures 12.2a–b). This is a scenic interaction practice in a two-person or group situation. In this case, it is not the result that is decisive, but the mutual interaction during the process. This interaction creates a playful component that is familiar from childhood and activates resources of a game played in common. As Johan Huizinga (2004) notes, the origins of culture are to be found in the game.

Collages with images of people, natural and cultural objects (Figure 12.3) also offer easy access to narrative exchange during creation without the need for artistic skills. When creating an overall picture, individual, small, laminated pictures, with a Velcro strip underneath, can be attached to a felt pad as a base. For people with disabilities or senior people, this scenic interaction practice is well suited to finding one's own symbolic expression. It also can be used to enrich or process what is experienced in narrative dialogue.

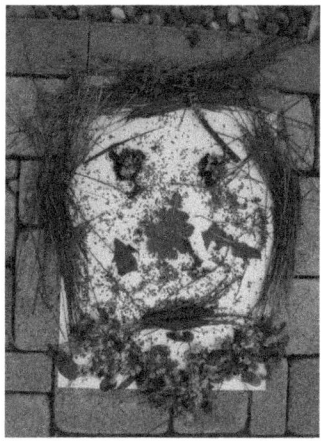
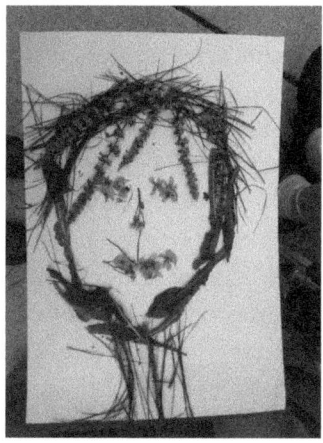

Figures 12.1a–b: Faces made of natural materials together with people with disabilities and students (photos from a course run by Ruth Hampe)

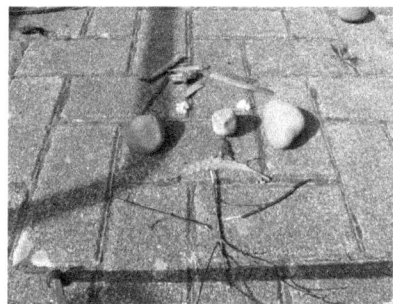
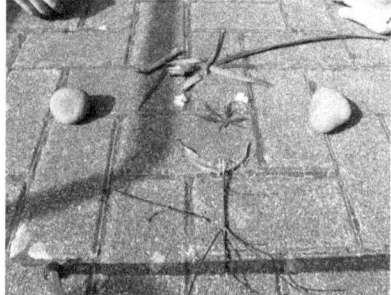

Figures 12.2a–b: Laying game with natural materials, student work (photos from a course run by Ruth Hampe)

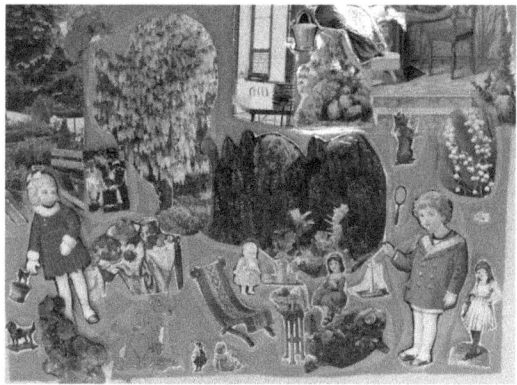

Figure 12.3: Laying picture with laminated felt-based collage elements, student work (photos from a course run by Ruth Hampe)

The situation is different with materials such as sand, clay and soil, that provide a haptic and tactile experience. When using dry sand—for example, in a frame—play on the surface with exposure of the ground can occur using the fingers, one hand, or both hands. Each finished picture brings an element of challenge for the next maker to engage in the continuing process. The dry sand can mobilize intuitive, playful action, without claiming to be a completed picture. Changes in the sand game can be made with the hands and fingers, which triggers a dynamic haptic stimulation (Figures 12.4a–b). Process-based interactive design can easily lead to the experience of a flow, as emphasized by Mihaly Csíkszentmihályi (2000, 2014).

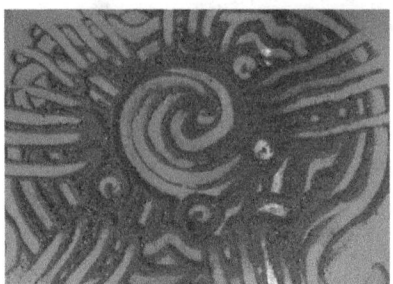 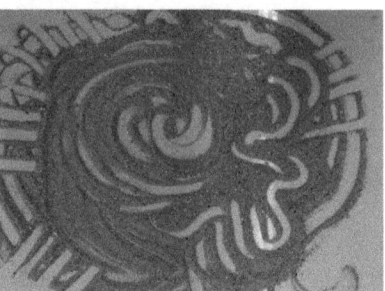

Figures 12.4a–b: Sand play alternating between two people on a white surface, student work (photos from a course run by Ruth Hampe)

When using clay, other proprioceptive sensory modalities can be activated in the process of molding and kneading. The changing additions of formal elements can result in a scenic narrative which can be captured on film in its individual phases so that it can be observed later and lead to a new approach in talking about it and in exchanging memories. The co-creation of the accompanying person provides a supportive function in the enrichment of the design process and can activate resources and encourage the continuity of the process.

To understand art processes in nature, it is also possible to work with charcoal drawing. William Kentridge (Rosenthal, 2010) uses his charcoal drawings to create animated films. The trace of the previous charcoal drawing, which is wiped off in some places, remains partially visible and overlays the new image. These drafts on paper, which are captured in photographs over time, form a narrative sequence. The process may allow the maker to sense the resilience of natural processes and to perceive this as a resource. The charcoal drawing becomes a matrix of an inner perspective, which follows a spontaneous creative flow (Figures 12.5a–b).

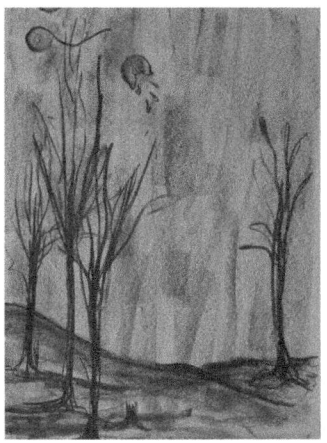 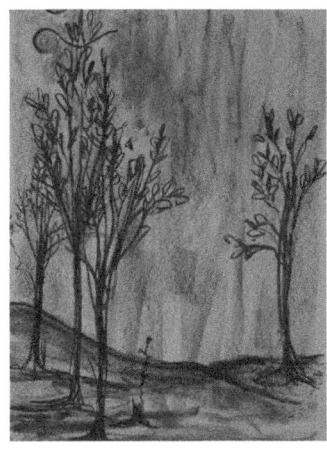

Figures 12.5a–b: Change processes related to forms of growth in nature by wiping away and overpainting charcoal drawings on paper, student work (photos from a course of Ruth Hampe)

A similar process-oriented artwork can be achieved using chalk on the blackboard. A basic picture can be developed by wiping away the dry chalk and drawing over it, producing a layered image that can be traced through photographic documentation. This work on the board can eliminate the need for perfection in a picture and mobilize the creative process, for example in a dialogue between two people without speaking. In addition, when drawing at the blackboard, the person stands—similar to a painting board—and has to get up from their seat to draw. This gives the opportunity to gain distance and to get a different view of the image alternating from near and far (Figures 12.6a–b).

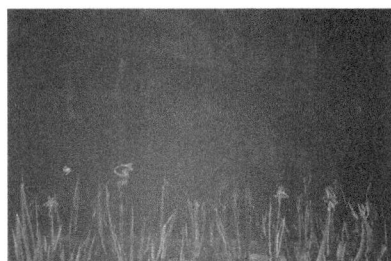 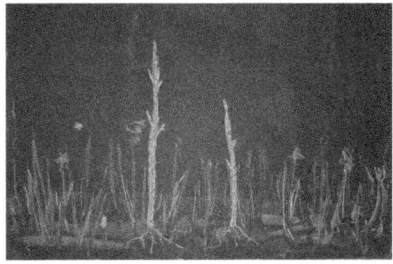

Figures 12.6a–b: Change processes related to forms of growth in nature by wiping away and painting over chalk drawings on the blackboard, student work (photos from a course run by Ruth Hampe)

Digital photographic documentation corresponds to "digital storytelling"

(Mathews-DeNatale, 2008; Meadows, 2003; Sadik, 2008), which is understood as a form of social practice using the support of technical media such as the camera and the computer. Individual images are put together like an animated film, for example using the program *MovieMaker*, and are thus transformed into a digital story. The animation can be saved as a video on the computer or a mobile phone. Digital storytelling enables multimedia editing with spoken word, text, and music inserts, as well as special image transitions and color changes or focus adjustments. This application of digital media is often used in educational and cultural fields, but it can also be implemented in the art therapeutic field, as it has already been shown in art therapeutic work in psychiatric care, where it has been used with disabled people and in therapy with children and adolescents, as well as adults or older people. Working with the digital medium is particularly challenging, and capturing single design phases using digital photography can lead to positive perception of self-efficacy and self-esteem. It can be used in two-person and group settings and requires the technical support and assistance of the accompanying therapist in the implementation of a digital narrative storytelling sequence. When Aaron Antonovsky (1997) speaks of understanding, manageability and meaningfulness in relation to the sense of coherence, this can also be applied to the creative process with digital storytelling. This can lead to an imaginary transformation of one's own life themes as well as experiences. In this way, a change of perspective and new interpretations are mobilized in a playful process.

The medium of image sequencing in the creation of digital films creates a perception of movement that can activate multi-layered sensory modalities in the visual processing of what has been experienced. It requires eye movement in the visual perception of the image sequences, which can cause a different form of processing from what has been experienced, similar to changing the gaze using EMDR. The use of the digital medium depends on the situation, and the participation of clients is always tied to their self-determined influence on the process as directors of the storytelling process. Experiencing and documenting nature in this way differs from other cultural examples, such as those that can be seen on television or in film. What is experienced is anchored in the digital processing and, at the same time, becomes a medium for psychological stabilization, similar to presenting oneself in a social group.

In line with this, the photographic image can also be used to present oneself in an imaginary space, and one's own portrait can be integrated with natural materials. The relationship to self-portrait has been explored in modern art in terms of deformation of the body or as a form of self-awareness (Hampe, 1999, p.257ff.). The exploration of the self in relation to natural phenomena, for example in designing with natural materials or in experiencing natural processes, can provoke a discussion, and nature can be perceived as a reference to one's own self in the sequence of the images presented via the digital medium. At the same time, this process-like design is connected to a realization of what has been experienced in the digital editing stage, by receiving it again and discussing it associatively. In this regard, the images go through different phases of exploration and are subject to enrichment and processing in the sensual-symbolic experience.

It is the play in an art therapeutic setting (Winnicott, 1973) that can lead to an enrichment of what has been designed. A transformation of the design afterwards into a narrative dialogue like a fairy tale as "Once upon a time..." supports an intuitive animation of the designed picture and creates another level of mentalization. This applies, for example, to working within the framework of a sand play using natural materials. It is also possible as a dialogical design by two persons in silence, as the following examples show (Figures 12.7a–b). Creating an environment can lead to a transformation of consciousness about it, as Alexandrova (2020, p.10) has pointed out.

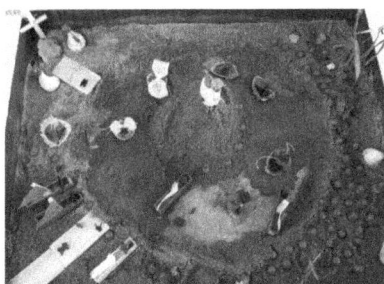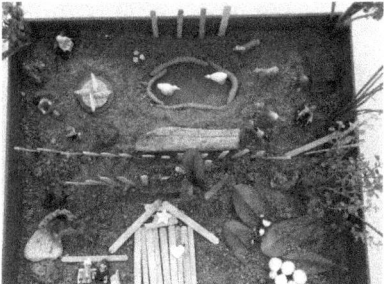

Figures 12.7a–b: Designing an environment with natural materials and figures in a sand tray by two people, without speaking and with a narrative dialogue afterwards (photos from a course run by Ruth Hampe)

In addition, experiencing nature is related to a safe place as an inner resource. Quite often, clients perceive the symbolization of nature as a stimulation for feeling well (Figure 12.8). As a three-dimensional space—like a corner, a box, or something similar as a basic structure—it becomes a field, a small world into which emotions can be projected. In the process of creation, it is the haptic experience in which natural elements are referred to in the construction of a scene. The possibility of holding it in one's own hands and thus making it manageable also has a salutogenic effect.

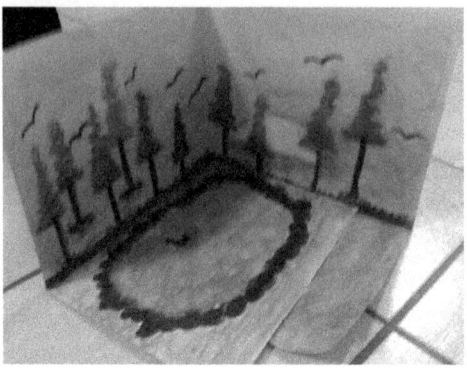

Figure 12.8: Creation of a safe place in symbolizing different environmental aspects of nature. Paper work with natural materials and painting (photos from a course run by Ruth Hampe)

The symbolization of a tree, a plant or a flower as representatives for nature in the art therapeutic process has a particular meaning. For example, inner strength can be symbolized in an animal or another object, mostly in relation to an environment with nature-related elements as a protective space—or natural elements themselves become a symbol of inner strength. In combination with the animal, an environment is often formed in which a tree or plant is added. In creating a tree of life for inner strength, the tree can show the fruition and can be covered with glitter to make it into something extraordinary (Figures 12.9a–b). It is unconsciously perceived as a substitute for one's own growth. For comparison, an American art therapist advised a depressive client to view a tree in the different seasons and to draw it. Over time, this practice helped the client to overcome his depression. In this way, nature can resonate with our inner feelings, and life principles can be understood more vividly.

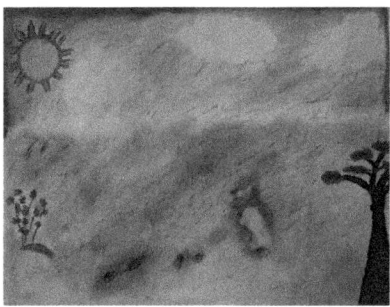 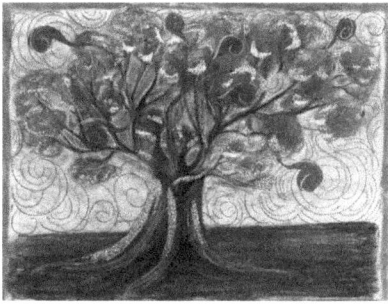

*Figures 12.9a–b. Creating inner strength using natural symbols
as resources (photos from a course run by Ruth Hampe)*

Conclusion

Process-oriented creative activities allow a person to experience their inner self, as well as nature, in a multi-layered way. Such activities are affected by situational and personal circumstances, as well as the particular moment in time and the materials used as a stimulating factor. In addition, they enable interaction in the therapeutic pair or in a group, during which photographic documentation of the process can become significant in enhancing the dialogical element of the constantly changing form. This applies both to the pause after creating each phase of the design and the compilation of images into a digital story, similar to an animated film. Moreover, the stimulation of an empathic connection between therapist and client is expressed in the artistic process. The activation of sensory modalities through the use of natural materials, as well as in the exploration of self-representation in relation to nature, can mobilize changes in the relationship to oneself, others, and the natural world. The phenomenon of nature, in references to inorganic and organic materials, the micro and macro level and self-experience, is an effective therapeutic component in terms of activating sensory perception. In this context, it is not the duration of the interaction that is decisive, but rather the inner attitude in relation to the experience of the process. Artists who are working in nature and with natural materials can inspire therapists to incorporate access to nature in art therapy as well. This kind of work is possible with all age groups and can include people with disabilities. What is special about working with natural phenomena and materials is that they are accessible to everyone due to diversity of perception and biographical anchoring, and can therefore form a fundamental constant in the creative process. In addition, the use of some kind of frame in the creative activity—such as the size of a piece of paper or a box, a given limited space—can support a feeling of security and support.

Nature thus becomes a field of learning in which life principles can be recognized and natural processes can be appreciated in their particularity. The feeling of being a part of nature helps one to overcome loneliness and to display compassion for the natural environment. It supports a change of consciousness by helping individuals to realize the principles in the life cycle, like the principle of the circulation of everything, of vibration as a wave, or the principle of holism and of balance, of cause and effect. As we observe in the cycles of gathering and spreading, separating and uniting, blooming and withering, transmigration and reincarnation, imperfection in perfection and perfection in imperfection, everything is in process. The coincidence or accidental in the creative process creates an inner mobilization and stimulates a new understanding of transitions that appear as constant challenges. This can be thought of as the emergence of the perception of one's own nature, externally and internally. In this context, a process-based design is helpful and brings about a narrative transformation of the experience as a kind of mentalization. Thus, it is a form of ecopoiesis, which supports the development of a changed relationship to oneself in relation to nature and natural processes.

References

Alexandrova, N. (2020). Priorities of the development of ecological education in an art university. *Ecopoesis: Eco-Human Theory and Practice*, 1(1), 6–16.

Antonovsky, A. (1997). *Salutogenesis: To Demystify Health* (in German). Tübingen: DGVT.

Bauer, J. (2004). *Why I Feel What You Feel* (in German). Munich: Heyne.

Csíkszentmihályi, M. (2000). *Flow: The Psychology of Optimal Experience*. New York, NY: Harper and Row.

Csíkszentmihályi, M. (2014). *Creativity: Flow and the Psychology of Discovery and Invention*. New York, NY: Harper Perennial.

Damman, G. (2012). Effective Factors of the Progressive Therapeutic Mirror Image in the Light of New Psychodynamic Process Theories. In G. Damman & T. Meng (eds), *Mirror Processes in Psychotherapy and Art Therapy* (pp.69–85) (in German). Göttingen: Vandenhoeck & Ruprecht.

Doczi, G. (2005). *The Power of Borders: Harmonious Proportions in Nature, Art and Architecture* (6th edition) (in German). Stuttgart: Engel & Co.

Einstein, A. (1953). *Mein Weltbild*. Zurich: Europa Verlag.

Einstein, A. (1954). The World as I See It. In C. Seeling (ed.), *Ideas and Opinions*, based on *Mein Weltbild* (pp. 8–11). New York, NY: Bonzana Books.

Hampe, R. (1999). *Metamorphoses of the Figurative*. Bremen: Universitätsbuchhandlung.

Hanus, O. (2014). *Color Interaction. The Group Dynamics and the Social Image* (in German). Aachen: Shaker Media.

Hoffmann, W. (2014). *The Beauty of the Line* (in German). Munich: Beck.

Huizinga, J. (2004). *Homo Ludens: A Study of the Play-Element of Culture*. London: Routledge and Kegan Paul.

Hüther, G. (2004). *The Power of Inner Images* (in German). Göttingen: Vandenhoeck & Ruprecht.

Lailach, M. (2007). *Land Art*. Cologne: Taschen.

Meadows, D. (2003). Digital storytelling: Research-based practice in new media. *Visual Communication*, (2)2, 189–193.

Peciccia, M. & Benedetti, G. (1994). The Progressive Therapeutic Game Picture. In G. Schottenloher (ed.), *When Words Are Missing, Pictures Speak* (pp.91–94) (in German). Munich: Kösel.

Riedelsheimer, T. (2001). *Rivers and Tides—Andy Goldsworthy Working with Time* [DVD]. Berlin: Absolut Medien. Co-Produktion MetropolisFilm und Fernsehproduktion GmbH und Skyline Productions.

Rosenthal, M. (Hrsg.). (2010). *William Kentridge: .Five Themes*. Ostfildern: Hatje.

Sadik, A. (2008). Digital Storytelling: A meaningful technology-integrated approach for engaged student learning. *Education Tech Research Development*, 56(4), 487–506.

Shapiro, F. (2007). *EMDR in Action: The Treatment of Traumatized People* (in German). Paderborn: Junfermann.

Sorace, M.A. (2009). The intensity can be so strong that there is no separation: On the relationship between art and meditation. *Journal for Christian Spirituality and Lifestyle*, 35(1), 1–34.

Stern, A. (1998). *The Place of Painting* (in German). Eltmann: Daimon.

Winnicott, D.W. (1973). *From Play to Creativity* (in German). Stuttgart: Klett-Cotta.

Chapter 13

Natural and Artistic Aspects of Art Therapy

MONIKA WIGGER

Introduction

For the artist Josef Beuys, nature in its entirety was spiritual and spiritually animated. This included plants and animals as well as crystalline forms such as stone and sand. His art consisted of the need to research an in-depth, multi-dimensional awareness of the relationships between nature and human beings and to repeatedly bring this into a social discourse. His drawings of rabbits and deer created analogies with prehistoric cave paintings. As a result, he repeatedly made references to the origins of human history and to Indigenous peoples. Installations and performances always play a major role in the forces of nature and animals. In his performance in 1983, "How to explain pictures to a dead hare," Beuys can be seen walking through the rooms of a Dusseldorf gallery with a dead hare in his arms. For Beuys, the hare functioned as an ancient Celtic symbol for fertility. He had applied honey and gold leaf to his face and hair and his shoes were weighted down with iron soles that gave him traction.

The art historian Volker Harlan commented:

> When he explains the pictures to the hare, when he describes the deer, swan and other animals, not only when he sees animals, but also plants, soil, planets, the supernatural, etc. as the perimeter of human observation, it is the task of every human being to learn to understand this environment in order to learn to understand oneself, that is, to practice self-recognition by recognizing the world around us. (Harlan, 1986, p.108)

Beuys is serious, he wants to provoke, wants to generate something and even goes so far with his conception that he categorizes the contemplation and understanding of his conceptualization of art as an expanded concept of art "...even if it is only a sound wave that reaches another ear" (Harlan, 1986, p.81). Even as an adolescent, he was interested in many things, including understanding what it is to be human, and the philosophy of Rudolf Steiner. Characteristic of Steiner's natural philosophical view is his reference to the four elementary qualities: solid, liquid, gaseous, and heat, as well as to the levels of nature: mineral, plant, animal, and human. Steiner found equivalence in nature and art for certain physical, psychological, spiritual, and social aspects of humans (Teichler, 1996, pp.86–89). Steiner's anthroposophical perspective has been established in specific educational and therapeutic concepts to this day. Waldorf education and anthroposophic medicine and therapy should be mentioned here as examples. Art and natural interventions have a firm place here, just as nature and art are inseparable for Beuys in the sense of an expanded concept of art.

Contradictions between nature and art

A nature-oriented, therapeutic approach extended specifically to art therapy is not yet in sight. Perhaps it is the contradiction between the two terms "nature" and "art" that makes it difficult to coalesce into a definitive natural art therapy.

> Artistic appropriation of the natural world itself follows a structure of contradictions: on one hand, it removes an object from us by transforming it into a distant image, on the other, its state of imagery grants us the ability to experience it in the first place... It is the nature of art to not be able to understand it. (Berg, 2009, p.5)

The categorical separation of nature and art described in this way allows a distance from the two components in order to see which aspects from the respective areas can be used for one's own approach. The term "nature" in this context could be a reference to material and location—art using natural materials in a natural environment. Instead of working inside a studio, art would be created in meadows, forests, mountains, and along waterfronts using materials and conditions found on site. However, this is by no means an invention of art. Even in primeval times, humans unconsciously and consciously worked and shaped natural objects by stacking, layering, piling, trampling, lying, laying, scratching, gnawing, digging. Natural art or specifically *land art* uses, among other things, this original "processing" of nature within nature. The works created in this way, however, are still subject to change; they are subject to wind and weather, thereby changed and in the end, they fade away. From the artist's point of view, this aspect is inherent to the work.

Belonging to and interacting with nature

One of the best-known representations of the natural art genre, a variation on land art, is by the Scottish artist Andy Goldsworthy.

> I am a part of nature, I don't see myself as being in opposition, and I think it's a strange idea to see us as separate from nature. Our lives and what we do affect nature so closely that we cannot be separate from it. (Goldsworthy in Ilschner, 2004, p.105)

His artistic works are a consequence of site conditions, time of day, weather and weather-dependent energy, as well as the abundant possibilities of the materials that he finds. In addition, most of his artistic works are site-specific and are abandoned on completion.

> A rock is not independent of its surroundings. The way it sits tells how it came to be there. The energy and space around a rock are as important as the energy and space within. The weather—rain, sun, snow, hail, mist, calm—is that external space made visible. When I touch a rock, I am touching and working the space around it. In an effort to understand why that rock is there and where it is going, I do not take it away from the area in which I found it. (Goldsworthy in Ilschner, 2004, p.41)

Goldsworthy has no intention to possess the work of art that he creates within nature. The artist captures the coalescence of the moment and seizes its essence by taking a photo snapshot.

Conservation, preservation, collection, and storage, much like the processing of natural materials, are cultural achievements—skills and resources that are crucial for body and soul. Stored natural foods initially ensure the availability of basic food, but also enable access to emotional preserves. A glimpse at a shell from last summer's vacation can be exhilarating on cloudy days, or a snowball from winter, preserved in the freezer, can be disillusioning in its un-snow-like state. The objects, shell or snowball, have a representative function here—they are objects that resonate a feeling of longing. "We cannot grasp the snow, cannot possess it; if we try, it slips through our fingers, if we bring it into the house, it melts, and if we put it in the freezer, it ceases to be snow" (Rosa, 2019, p.7). Sociologist Hartmut Rosa's idea that one could experience resonance if only one could finally get the world or nature under control proves to be a fallacy. Nature enables us to recognize that not everything is available at all times.

> Nature is the basis of our existence. The ways in which we perceive nature are also part of its reality. In being perceived, nature materializes in different ways, whereby this perception neither coincides with nor is independent of its reality. In this way, the boundaries between "nature" and "culture" are, in effect, a product of culture. Nonetheless, every culture must recognize that it only exists because nature exists, and so, we as natural creatures understand the reality of nature. (Seel, 2009, p.55)

Experiencing nature *live* has its own specific qualities. In everyday urban life, for example, we associate a walk in the forest, in the mountains, or by the sea with *unwinding*. Engaging with the natural world allows us a psychological, physical, and sensory reset. By experiencing phenomena such as distance, proximity, cold, heat, day and night, colors, surfaces, and elements, we are able to leave our daily routine behind in order to find a sensory, cognitive baseline. Abandoning the four walls of indoor space opens up new possibilities; we get moving, to the outdoors.

> We step outside; however, this necessary step is not alone sufficient to truly experience the outdoors. ...it is only when we enter the real outdoors and simultaneously the metaphorical outdoors; when we loosen the ties to pragmatic orientation that determine our normal behavior in indoor space; when we no longer move within this outdoor space with fixed goals; rather, we remain open to the irregular presence of the larger space itself. (Berg, 2009, p.177)

In this situation, new, sensory, emotional, and physical experiences can be made. Every form imaginable to us is present in nature and has its unique properties. Experiences with nature can be varied and extremely contradicting: pleasant, uncomfortable, or frightening. Nevertheless, we continually allow ourselves to be inspired by the diversity and abundance of nature.

Nature as an evolving practical laboratory

According to Huppertz & Schatanek (2015, p.123), "We can experience a strong bond with nature. This experience is the basis of many spiritual interpretations and speculations about the alliance between man and nature, the interconnectivity of all things or an essence that is the source all existence." One aspect of the "primordial source" can be interpreted as analogous to *maternal* qualities. Accordingly, nature also allows regression and interaction with the primordial, and satisfies basic human needs, such as feeling connected and held, to touch and to be touched. "Sometimes everything intertwines so well that we cannot distinguish between what nature contributes and what we contribute (for example when breathing or swimming)" (Huppertz & Schatanek, 2015, p.287).

In this way, experiences of nature enable psychological and physical "development" to compensate for a deficit. Such experiences can be an important countermeasure. Of course, the natural world is not without contradictions and resistance. Existential borderline experiences through natural disasters are threatening and can profoundly shake our confidence in nature. Creating art within nature is not always harmonious. The unpredictability of wind, weather, tides, and the strain and unpleasantness experienced are uncomfortable. As a result, one's mental and physical limits are challenged, sometimes destroying ideas. We, at times, question the basic principle of cooperation. *Mother Nature* does have a disagreeable side—and that can make perfect sense.

When we observe nature, we must not overlook that fact that she is a patient herself. Deterioration of flora and fauna, marine pollution, global warming—nature is beleaguered and needs our empathy and care. We inform ourselves, try to be mindful, and are righteously indignant about exiting agreements that aim to protect our environment. Despite this, we still look to the natural world to fulfill our need for peace, relaxation, recreation, spirituality, inspiration, pleasure, joy, desire, humility, and gratitude. In this instance, art facilitates access to the cultural manageability and availability of nature's endowment. Pictorial representations (including plastic arts) offer the opportunity to approach the beauty, unpredictability, harshness, and destruction that the natural world endures and creates. Art enables us to examine nature, including our own, human nature.

> Within the visual space of art, the natural world appears in such a way that every overwhelming emotional impact is always simultaneously controlled and distanced through the knowledge of the artistically created situation and aesthetic discernment. (Adolphs, 2009, p.55)

A work of art *grounds* nature, confines it, gives it a defined context, lends access to it, and simultaneously provides a definitive perspective. At the moment of viewing, we are in a protected space; we have choices, we are not simply *exposed* to nature. This enables the recipient to *get acquainted, to warm up, to move in closer*; it also offers the opportunity to distance oneself if things get *too hot* or *too stormy*. Self-awareness within a natural landscape is always multidimensional. Unlike using paper, the outdoors has no formal boundaries, yet it refuses "to see the big picture," demands the use of the body and the senses, "so that even the greatest foresight becomes blurry" (ibid., p.179). We can never commandeer the natural world, or functionalize it as a backdrop. Being in the outdoors always implies being involved, whether by the sea, in the forest, in the mountains, or at home in your own garden.

Visualization of nature and one's own well-being—the painter Claude Monet

The painter Claude Monet (1840–1926) was being coy by claiming that "he could do nothing but garden and paint" (Gockel, 2015, p.260). Unlike Goldsworthy, who works with nature, Monet dealt with particular intensity in *observing* nature, viewing it as a subject of research independent of a representation of reality, symbolization, or abstraction. Monet was fully engaged with daily studies in his "natural laboratory." He conducted dozens of studies from a haystack alone. The motif probably had a particular charm in its simplicity, offering Monet a welcoming surface on which light and color could play and project.

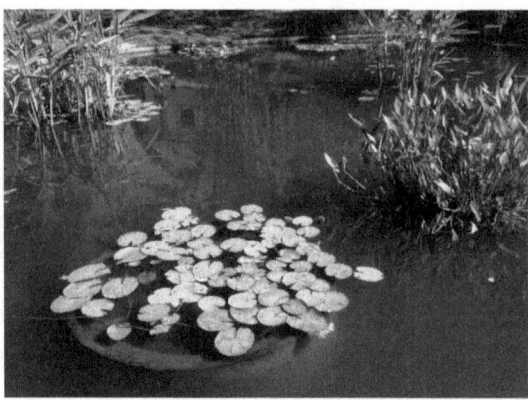

Figure 13.1: Water lily pond in the Freiburg Botanical Garden (photo by Wigger)

His renowned, large-format oil paintings of evanescent subjects such as clouds, water, plants, and reflections completely engage the viewer, demanding absolute attention, analogous with the visually receptive demands of perceiving these subjects in the natural world. Despite the permanence of painting, when stepping forward and backward while viewing Monet's works, we find that visual phenomena of constant change can also be perceived, much like those that occur in the natural world through light and shadow, day and night or seasonal conditions. "To experience sight by recognizing oneself within the view" is how Gockel describes the essence of Monet's endeavors (Gockel, 2015, p.262). As Monet aged, his eyesight deteriorated due to cataracts. The resulting alterations in his eyesight and associated depression were presumably terribly stressful and a huge sensory challenge for the painter.

> "The distortions and exaggerations of the colors that I now experience are frightening. If I were condemned to only see nature in this way, I would prefer to remain blind and remember its beauty." (Monet around 1926, quoted in Kutschbach, 2006, p.64)

During the time of Monet's acute illness, the natural world can be seen as an equivalent of the bizarre, threatening, and frightening, not only for individual physical, psychological, and social changes and the suffering of the resulting discrepancies, but also for the painter's irrepressible energy, and the way he faced and dealt with *visual distortions*. Monet experienced his own physical and psychological limitations while he was ill. In 1922, he was almost blind, but his painting did not stagnate.

He became inventive, pushing himself beyond limits; shapes became almost abstract and seemed to dissolve, and he found himself and his perception of nature anew.

The principle of plastic arts and sculpture in nature

Principles of nature and life can also be transferred to multi-dimensional forms of art. For example, let's examine plastic arts and sculpture. In a narrower sense, a sculpture describes the addition of plastic media, such as clay, wax, or paper, to form an object. The development of a bone, a tree trunk, a stalactite through the deposits of calcite follows exactly the same principle.

A sculpture is created by reducing, removing, grinding, sawing, or carving. Equivalent processes can also be found in the natural world. The artist Josef Beuys speaks of a natural work of art. Every pebble is afforded its shape through the grinding process and thus becomes a naturally formed plastic work of art. "One can of course imitate something similar, there are sculptors who try to imitate this, to imitate a naturally produced sculpture" (Beuys in Harlan, 1986, p.83). Understanding nature through shapes, thereby learning about oneself within them could apply to plastic arts and sculpture. The sensory experiences with and within nature, the individual, sensory-related state of being *impressed*, as well as the interest in and the desire for perception itself facilitate experience and development.

Images of longing within nature— photography as a window

Permanent—that is, non-changing—representations of nature in the form of painting, drawing, and photography can evoke sensory experiences and effect emotions in much the same way as when we experience the natural world. Let us remember the aforementioned paintings by Monet. In 2005, as part of the redesign of a closed ward for acute psychiatric patients, several large-format landscape photos by the Münster artist and photographer Thomas Wrede were installed in the corridors and common rooms of the Clinic for Psychiatry and Psychotherapy at the University Hospital Münster. The decision was accompanied by an artistic design concept for the entire psychiatric clinic (Borgmann & Wigger, 2006)

Wrede's works from the 2004 series "Seascapes" feature images of the sea, the sky, and the horizon, as well as beach tents and people playing or swimming. As the works were being installed, conversations about the sea were spontaneously prompted: "I've been there before." Memories were awakened; at some point, most people had been to the sea. The topic lent a feeling of belonging, and conversations arose. The horizon of the protected ward expanded through the images captured from nature.

One older gentleman was so excited by the sight of the sea motif that he began singing the song "My Bonnie Lies Over the Ocean" and attracted astonished listeners. The photographs have been an integral part of the ward ever since. It must be noted that the viewers were not left to fend for themselves in front of the works. The positionings chosen by Wrede, the perspectives, the precision of captured moments, the size and color of the photographs provide the viewer with a calculated composition that guides the perception process.

The photographer is effectively on site as the works are viewed. For patients experiencing acute psychological crises, this can harbor an important *auxiliary ego state* function. Visual art can, in this way, serve as a controlled perception test in a titrated and filtered manner, effectively avoiding overstimulation. Acute patients, whose activity radius is limited to the dimensions of a psychiatric ward, are enabled to have an interaction with nature receptively through the presence of images of oceans and beaches.

Existential experiences with inner and outer nature

Water and sky are primeval. Walking on water is a biblical motif and, in essence, all life originates from water. With solid ground under our feet, we revert to this basic natural principle.

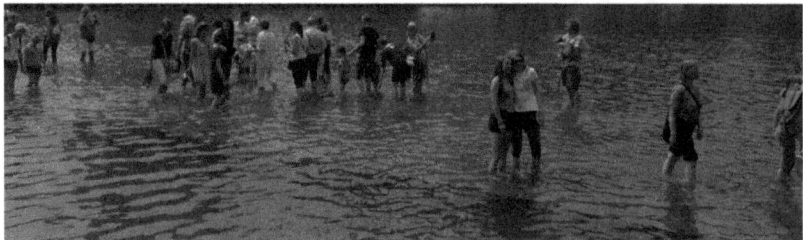

Figure 13.2: Sensory and magical—the installation On Water by the artist Ayse Erkmen during The Sculpture Project, Münster in 2017 (photo by Wigger)

With her current work *On Water* in Münster's harbor, Erkmen offers an active, sensory space of experience in and above the water. A biblical, magical image of being able to walk on water reveals enjoyment, excitement, and fright. It opens up the possibility to ignore the laws of nature. A collective, unifying feeling of *it'll be alright* arises among those who actively wade.

> I want to create a trustworthy space in the water... Water is difficult to handle, which makes it very attractive to me. I created an easy way to become acquainted with water: above it, in it, and yet, everyone is safe. It's a way of dealing with the element at its best. (Erkmen, 2017)

Life sometimes requires symbolic solutions, such as those offered by Erkmen when walking across her safely submerged footbridge. Confronting a life-threatening illness can be such a moment.

A tumor diagnosis triggers feelings of helplessness, existential threat, and deep despair in those affected. In addition, related treatments, such as surgery, radiation, and chemotherapy, are often cause for concern. Whether the tumor is benign or malignant, accompanying symptoms such as physical complaints, anxiety, and depression ensue and impact the quality of life of those affected.

The overall situation is complex, inscrutable, often difficult to grasp, and frightening. Those affected are faced with the task of accepting the vulnerability and dysfunctionality of their inner nature. They can't rely on anything anymore or take anything for granted. The rug has been pulled out from under them.

To trust that *everything will be alright* is essential in this situation; this is not naive, but rather courageous in a positive sense. Much like the way Erkmen uses wading to cross the expanse of water in order to reach the other bank, patients allow themselves the positive energy to look to the future.

Since 2012, patients with brain tumors have had access to art therapy in the neurosurgical ward of the University Hospital Münster in Germany. In addition to access to museums and the outdoors, the standard materials for therapeutic interventions in the form of active artistic work include natural materials such as sand, water, clay, wood, objects found in the natural environment, and plant material. In this context, dealing with nature with all your senses is of particular importance. The materials transform into a sensory exercise. A branch becomes a tree, a pile of sand becomes an island, a stone becomes a mountain—arranged in a defined space, designed and structured. The colors of an autumn leaf are scrutinized and enlarged as a painting, the structure of an orange is explored, the lines on the palm of a hand are drawn and transformed into a landscape. Sometimes a brain is modeled, which is not necessarily part of everyday perception but within these circumstances, is somehow inherent in nature. The invisible and the incomprehensible are expressed with the help of natural media. The artistic materials create a mental and physical balance that allows patients to take something into their hands and control it. In this way, patients are not just passively receiving treatment, they are proactively exercising control.

An excursion

May 25, 2012: A group of five young brain tumor patients, an intern, and I are sitting on the terrace of the painter's workshop. The conversation revolves around complicated organizational procedures in hospitals. We discuss communication problems with treating physicians and everyday bureaucratic hurdles. In the end, tumor surgery is the focus of the conversation. Patients describe their individual experiences. They question which physician and professional advice can be trusted to make important decisions demanded over the course of their exceptional disease situation. The surgery itself is usually classified as stressful or traumatic. The same applies to the entire in-patient phase. Patients exchange ideas regarding subsequent rehabilitation. The individual, altered relationship to their own body represents a plethora of issues.

S. decides to paint the view from the terrace onto the field as a landscape and chooses Indian ink for her medium. While the other patients are working on their spatula paintings in the workshop, S. positions herself at the communal table on the terrace. She asks how she can transfer the composition onto the picture surface, and I refer back to our drawing exercises. We measure our field of vision with a pencil, recognize gaps, overlaps, and proportions. I also take a watercolor paper to transport the view into the landscape. S. delineates her picture area onto the paper with an individual format. At the edge of the picture, she creates color samples...

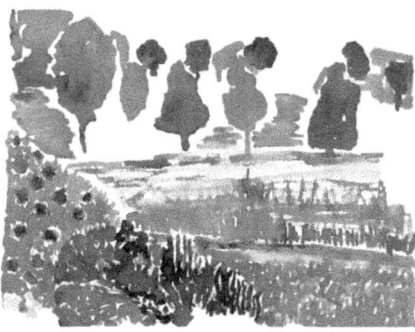

Figure 13.3: Watercolor from May 25, 2012

In this young woman's watercolor, not only the visual, but also the emotional reaction to the tranquility of the landscape can be felt within the individual lines. The activity of painting not only reveals the image of a landscape, it also opens the possibility for intensive self-awareness: *I paint; therefore, I still am.*

In this instance, it is the view of a landscape, at others, the inspection of the intricacies of one's own hand, the peel of an orange, an autumn leaf, your life partner's feet—in the here and now. Through active art therapy, patients remain connected with nature and life itself.

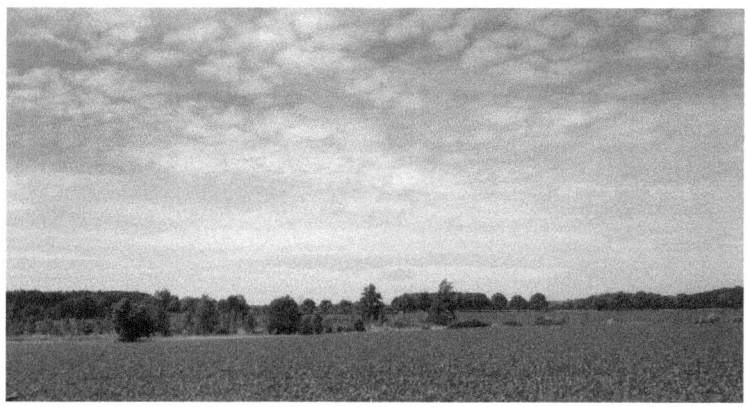

Figure 13.4: View from the painter's workshop in Münster (photo by Wigger)

References

Adolphs, V. (2009). The Own and the Other: The Construction of Nature in Art. In V. Adolphs (ed.), *Nature in Contemporary Art* (pp.49–135) (in German). Cologne: Wienand.

Berg, S. (2009). Longing and Distance. In V. Adolphs (ed.), *Nature in Contemporary Art* (pp.5–15) (in German). Cologne: Wienand.

Borgmann, P. & Wigger, M. (2006). Development and realization of an artistic design concept for the Clinic for Psychiatry and Psychotherapy at the University Hospital in Münster. Unpublished paper (in German).

Erkmen, A. (2017, 8 July). It is not good to have wet feet. *Berliner Zeitung.*

Freyberger, H.J. (2018). *Psychrembel Online.* www.pschyrembel.de/Hilfs-Ich/P04FT.

Gockel, B. (2015). Equivalents: Monet's Painting and his Garden in Giverny. In A. Lutz & H. von Trotha (eds), *Gardens of the World: Places of Longing and Inspiration* (pp.256–264) (in German). Cologne: Wienand.

Harlan, V. (1986). *What Is Art?* Workshop talk with Beuys. (4th edition 1992) (in German). Stuttgart: Verlag Urachhaus.

Huppertz, M. & Schatanek, V. (2015). *Mindfulness in Nature: 84 Nature-Related Mindfulness Exercises and Theoretical Basics* (in German). Paderborn: Jungfermann Verlag.

Ilschner, F. (2004). Embodied Periods of Time: An Examination of Land Art in the Works of Andy Goldsworthy, Richard Long and Walter De Maria (in German). Dissertation for Doctor of Philosophy in the Institute for Foreign Language Philologies (English/American Studies) of the Faculty of Humanities at the University of Duisburg-Essen (Campus Duisburg).

Kutschbach, D. (2006). *Monet and His Gardens: His Art, His Life* (in German). Munich: Prestel Verlag.

Rosa, H. (2019). *Unavailability* (in German). Wien, Salzburg: Residenz Verlag.

Seel, M. (2009). The Own and the Other: The Construction of Nature in Art. In V. Adolphs (ed.), *Nature in Contemporary Art* (pp.49–181) (in German). Cologne: Wienand.

Teichler, U. (1999). Internationalisation as a challenge for higher education in Europe. *Tertiary Education and Management,* 5, 5–23.

Chapter 14

From Ikebana to Botanical Arranging: Artistic, Therapeutic, and Spiritual Alignment with Nature[1]

ALEXANDER KOPYTIN AND TONY YU ZHOU

Ikebana: Reflection of Japanese and East Asian worldview

Ikebana is one of the important traditional Japanese arts and has been in existence for 600 years. The word Ikebana, which is composed of *ikeru* (生 け る, *keep alive*) and *hana* (花, *flower*), means "giving life to flowers." It is also called *kadō* (華 道 or 花道), which means the way of the flowers. Ikebana originated from China, derived from the Buddhist tradition of offering beautiful objects to the dead, mainly in the temples. In the 7th century, Ono-no-Imoko, an official envoy, brought the practice of this Buddhist flower arrangement on an altar from China to Japan. While Ikebana continued to be part of Buddhism in China, it became a real art in Japan. It was an early sign of the Buddhist integration into Japanese religious and social practices. Contrary to the art of flower arrangement in the western world, where the quantity of flowers seems to have a high priority, Ikebana reaches far beyond the philosophical ideas of beauty and forms a cultural worldview, centered around ideas of living in harmony with nature. In Japan, nature has always been the

---

1   Reprinted with permission from the journal *CAET, Creative Arts in Education and Therapy: Eastern and Western Perspectives*, (2019), 5(2), 96–105. http://caet.inspirees.com/caetojsjournals/index.php/caet/article/view/192.

highest manifestation of truth and beauty. Japanese poetic attitude to nature remains a strong feature of Japanese culture (Danylova, 2014).

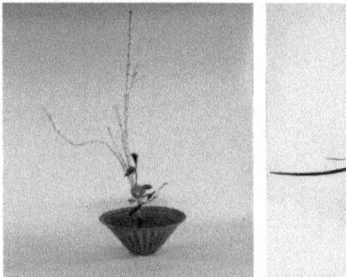 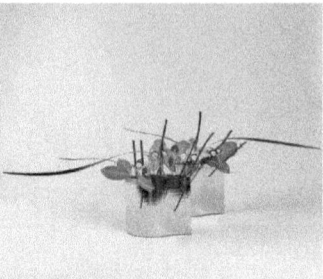

Figure 14.1: Ikebana, Ikenobo School (courtesy of Reginaldo Bockhorni)

In Ikebana, attention is focused on the lines, asymmetry, space, contrast, and harmony (Figure 14.1). Nowadays, it is considered as a disciplined art form in which nature and human creativity are brought together. Ikebana requires technical skills and is backed by solid theory. This form of art remains a vital medium for creative expression. Similar to the other practices in Japan like calligraphy, tea ceremony, and Haiku, which have been valued in Zen Buddhism as a means of self-cultivation, Ikebana is seen as one way of body-mind training. Immersion in the physical practice of this art can lead to both psychological and spiritual emptiness (no-self), which is thought to be the source of skillful action and the basis for empathetic and ethical behavior. Self-transformation is the result of such diligent practice. The reduced role of the humble artist allows objects to reveal their inner essences (Hovane, 2017). The health benefits of Ikebana practice in enhancing the well-being of both patients and the general population are supported by some empirical and evidence-based research (Hannemann, 2006; Homma, Oizumi, & Masaoka, 2015; Sasaki *et al.*, 2011; Watters *et al.*, 2013). In modern society, where abundance, wealth, and egoism are mostly valued, Ikebana brings the notion of simplicity, modesty, and gentleness to the foreground and reminds us that the power of nature and human beings does not necessarily come from the *yang* or the "condensing" quality (i.e., strong, direct, free, and quick). Interestingly, until the 18th century, Ikebana practice was only for men. Such appreciation toward similar quality of arts and practice can also be found in the Four Arts (四藝, *siyi*): *qin* (the guqin, a stringed instrument. 琴), *qi* (the strategy game of Go, 棋), *shu* (Chinese calligraphy, 書), and *hua* (Chinese painting, 畫), which were the four main academic and artistic accomplishments required of the aristocratic ancient Eastern Asian scholar-gentleman.

Unlike other art forms, Ikebana directly employs materials from nature, which thus builds up an explicit connection to nature and embodiment experience for Ikebana practitioners. The traditional structure of Ikebana arrangements has three main stems emerging from a central point and often forms the shape of a harmonious triad, symbolizing unity among the heavenly realm, humans, and the earth. The human body is thus very much present in the composition that forms the basic entity to interact with the Universe. Different body organizations such as radial symmetry, head/tail, upper/lower, homo-lateral, and cross-lateral are the patterns visualized in Ikebana. Grounding and center of gravity/levity can be felt on the plant as well as on our own body. Dynamic alignment and body phrasing can be projected onto the flowers and plants. Ikebana masters usually integrate the breath, spatial intent, and different body movement quality when creating Ikebana. This sensing and embodiment form the basics of the practice. During this ritual, which requires strong personal presence, the rhythm and pattern of breathing is adjusted and aligned with flowers and nature. Our breath is strongly associated with Ch'i, which is interpreted as the vital energy, moving power, and psychophysical energy in East Asia (McNiff, 2016). Apparently, through this alignment process, human beings get empowered via this Ch'i from nature. The Ch'i further enhances our creativity and artistic expression. On the feeling level, where the energy and dynamics are the main parameters, the inner drive toward weight (strong/light), space (direct/indirect), time (quick/sustained), and flow (bound/free) is manifested by the construction and composition of the flowers, and even by the cutting of the plants themselves. The indulging and condensing energy can be used as a strategy to create Ikebana as well as a way to exert and recuperate during this creative process. Although Ikebana presents a still form at the end, the whole process of creating is an interactive and dynamic "dance" between human beings and flowers, and with nature at the physical, mental, and spiritual level. The wider the spectrum of the movement and the clearer the intention of the "dancer," the richer the interaction will become. The art of balance is essential: structure/freedom, symmetric/asymmetric, stability/mobility, outer/inner, self/other, part/whole, all implemented in the Ch'i (flow) of an Ikebana master who has the eye for detail and the appreciation for creativity and spontaneity.

In Ikebana, emphasis is placed on accentuating the lines and individual shapes of each flower, leaf, and branch. The surrounding empty space is just as important as the materials themselves. The Japanese ma (or Mao, 冇, in Chinese), for the concept of interval or void in both time and space, is full of energy and feeling instead of "negative space," which is highly valued in Zen meditation. Ma creates rhythm and flow, engaging the viewer with the composition. Ma allows us to understand that less is indeed more. The space element of Ikebana triggers our thinking regarding the general space, our inner space, as well as our kinesphere (personal space) in terms of different spatial zones, reach space, and pathways (central, peripheral, and transverse). Different points in the space as well as the dimensions (vertical, horizontal, and sagittal) are taken into account.

Besides space, the Ikebana practitioner is consistently creating relationships with the flowers before eventually reaching out to the environment. That requires the intuition of a person. How do we see the still shape form of ourselves and the flowers to give a clear self-image that will be brought to the flowers? How strongly do we focus on ourselves with our physical sensations before we open ourselves to the flowers? How do we interact with the flowers and the environment? Is it a spoke-like direct reaching or more art-like indirect reaching? How capable and comfortable are we to accommodate ourselves to the other (flowers, space, environment), which sometimes requires more three-dimensional shaping from us? What kind of rhythm or pattern do we decide to make this relationship?

The motif becomes one of the characteristic symbols of Ikebana and a tool to remind us to project our worldview to the flowers. With its simplistic concept and presentation, Ikebana requires the concentration and mindfulness of practitioners to create the clear motif of the flower arrangement. This is usually the single-task action that is nowadays not often and easily practiced in our daily life and work. Thus, Ikebana helps us to experience the other deficient polarity of the duality that is essential in keeping ourselves in balance with others and with nature.

Ikebana involves "human interventions" with the cutting and arranging of flowers and spaces. But eventually we realize it is not a human intervention but an interaction with nature, and a process for us to learn to realign humanity with the laws of nature. This process can be interpreted as the practice of wu-wei (无为), widely described as "non-action" in Taoism tradition, which is a person's innate and authentic virtue (te/de, 德) action/expression in accordance with the movements of nature—an approach that carries within itself a timeless guide to well-being (McNiff, 2016).

Ikebana and ecological art therapy

Although Ikebana remains one of the symbols of the Eastern cultural traditions of China and Japan based on their philosophy and artistic, ritualized daily practices, it assumes a new meaning and role in the context of the contemporary globalized environmental, ecological movement. This movement, together with many other effects, has brought new significant implications for contemporary psychology and therapy, in particular creative/expressive arts therapies. Throughout the last two decades, such new scientific disciplines as environmental psychology, ecopsychology, and ecotherapy, with their concepts and practices, have been brought to fruition and helped us understand Ikebana from a new, environmental perspective.

Nowadays, a significant increase in the use of various ecotherapeutic, nature-assisted environmental therapies applied on different clinical and non-clinical populations with therapeutic, rehabilitation, and preventive purposes is observable. As global culture becomes more urbanized, clinicians are increasingly looking for strategies to optimize the beneficial aspects of nature in a client's life. Findings from numerous studies support the premise that contact with nature is beneficial for human health and well-being (Burls, 2007; Heerwagen, 2009) and supports human growth and development in cognitive, emotional, spiritual, and aesthetic domains. Here, one of the techniques of ecological art therapy, the technique of botanical arranging, which has some connection to the philosophy and practice of Ikebana, will be presented.

Botanical arranging, an ecotherapeutic activity, has certain connections to Ikebana on the conceptual and practical levels. Botanical arranging draws its theoretical model from the literature and research of art therapy, ecopsychology, and horticultural therapy, and is focused on the use of cut flowers, greenery, and other botanical ephemera as a metaphorical and artistic modality. It implies a helping practitioner, such as an art therapist, a horticulturist, an occupational therapist, or other therapist, facilitating the creation of simple arrangements of botanic materials as an art product on the part of a client and then studying it for embedded meaning with the client. Botanical arranging establishes an affiliation with horticultural therapy and ecopsychology/ecotherapy by integrating organic materials into an art therapy approach.

In the process of botanical arranging and interacting with compositions, the phenomenon of subjectification of natural objects can manifest itself, which supports the subjective-ethical mode of attitude towards nature. According to Deryabo (2002), the process of subjectification of natural objects has the following basic functions: a) to provide people with an experience of their own personal dynamics, b) to act as an intermediary in a person's relationship with the world, and c) to act as a subject of joint activity and communication.

Although botanical arranging can be a form of creative leisure, it will be described here as part of the art therapy process, implying the interaction with a helping specialist, an art therapist, horticultural therapist, occupational therapist, and so on. A specialist supports a meaningful interaction of people with their creations, subjectification of natural objects and, thus, the subjective-ethical mode of attitude towards nature.

Montgomery and Courtney (2016) emphasized that when botanical materials are utilized in art therapy, the client and the therapist may engage in another dimension of feeling and association not present with non-organic materials. Botanical products are evocative in ways that may be personal, ancestral, experiential, or archetypal in different layers of conscious and unconscious awareness. Plants enter a spectrum of experience through color, symmetry, scale, texture, scent, and shape, whose attributes merge with an individual's own history. These are primary sensory impressions that belong to a pre-verbal, pre-narrative world—the biophilic (Kellert, 1993; Wilson, 1984, 1993) component of human experience. Simply touching, smelling, and arranging botanical ephemera into pleasing symmetries can bring pleasure, alertness, and a sense of accomplishment. Formulated by Wilson in 1984 and then elaborated by Kellert and Wilson (Kellert, 1993), the biophilia hypothesis is described as the "innately emotional affiliation of human beings to other living organisms" (Kellert, 1993, p.31). Kellert (1993) presumed that it is a "human dependence on nature that extends far beyond the simple issues of material and physical sustenance to encompass as well the human craving for aesthetic, intellectual, cognitive, and even spiritual meaning and satisfaction" (p.18).

Montgomery and Courtney (2016) believe that an increase in the varieties, structures, and types of materials, including vines, leaves, fruits, flowering branches, and seed pods, as well as flowers, yields a richer, more complex visual and psychic field for the client's exploration in art therapy sessions.

> Culturally, flowers for adornment in wedding celebrations, liturgical practices, and memorial traditions, among others, all indicate that there is an emotional content to flowers whose presence often signifies personal transformation. Thus, botanicals acquire metaphorical vitality that individuals may experience at conscious and unconscious levels of experience. Within this interwoven relationship, it is unsurprising that botanicals become signifiers of specific human events as a part of the common language. (Montgomery & Courtney, 2016, p.19)

According to Diehl (2009), flowers can release neurochemicals that help "eliminate pain, induce sleep, and create a sense of well-being" (p.170).

Botanical arranging as a form of ecological, nature-based art therapy can be a viable expression of the art of biophilia (Kopytin, 2016, 2017), defined as a form of creative activity in and with natural environments (green spaces), supported by biophilic reactions. Creative acts as perceived from the art of biophilia or ecopoiesis perspective (Kopytin, 2020) are rooted not so much in the need for individual creative self-expression in the traditional sense of the word, but in the motivation to support and serve nature and life and achieve non-duality, a balance between natural and cultural milieu by embracing the transpersonal realm of being (Davis, 2011).

The process of botanical arranging occurs in three phases: preparation, experience, and debriefing of the experience. The first phase introduces clients to botanical arranging as an ecological art therapeutic activity and to the materials needed for a session. Then there are some warming-up indoor or outdoor exercises aimed at awakening sensory awareness—through touch, taste, smell, and so on—of natural spaces, objects, and materials and providing change in the modes of environmental perception. Setting a focus related to the topic of the session, choosing a question or situation that could be most relevant for the day, can be also included in this part of the session.

The second phase is the actual working session wherein clients create an art product using botanical ephemera and interact with it or through it with themselves and the environment, installing their creations in the landscape or using action-based creative activities such as performance, dance and movement, personal or group rituals, or multimedia events.

More concentrated forms of reflexive and creative activity such as journaling and creating narratives can also be implemented in the session. In the third phase, clients step back from their creations and observe and discuss their work for insight.

Assignments related to botanical arranging can be open ended or based on certain themes. Open-ended assignments encourage participants to walk outdoors in the environment or explore natural materials indoors and pay attention to scenery or objects they find most interesting or appealing for them, and then to select materials. Mindful interaction with the natural environment and botanical materials is considered the significant component of sessions.

Case example 1: Botanical arranging as a result of a meditative journey in the institutional green area, accompanied with selection of natural materials

A mixed group of helping professionals took part in a brief wellness-focused supportive art therapy program with the goal of learning ways to develop self-regulating stress management skills and mindfulness based on their creative interaction with the natural environment. The three-hour weekly sessions included art-making with the use of environmental botanical ephemera as a mindfulness practice.

In the beginning of one session, the therapist offered the group the possibility to spend one hour outdoors in order to explore the institutional environment of the community center where sessions took place: an enclosed field with sports ground and some wild plants and apple, pear, and birch trees. The therapist explained that the participants were allowed to select and use any type of organic materials available on the institutional ground, including vines, leaves, fruit, branches, seed pods, wild flowers, and other botanical ephemera as well as stones, soil, sand, and water, but not to destroy any life.

Participants were encouraged to take a meditative journey through the environment and find some natural materials and objects in order to do a small botanical arrangement. The therapist recommended participants to use small ceramic containers, plates, or cups up to 12cm in diameter as a holding space for their creations. The therapist also encouraged the participants to find some place in the environment to install their artwork and arrange the surrounding area, if needed. Later, they were invited to present a brief performance, a ritual in the environment, and somehow interact with their creations as meaningful objects. This part of the session was followed with participants sharing their experience and the meaning of their performances and creations.

While presenting his artwork, a 62-year-old man, a university teacher, sat on the bench below the birch tree, holding his botanical arranging in his right hand and an apple in his left hand (Figure. 14.2). He explained his performance in the following way:

> "The apple is a symbol of ecological learning and the birch tree is a symbol of my connection with nature. I also created a composition by putting water and the burning candle in the vessel. I meditated for a while sitting on this bench under the birch tree and holding the vessel in the right hand and the apple in my left hand. I felt tranquil and I was inviting great powers of nature in the form of water, fire, earth, and air to be with me and around me. I was absorbed in the peaceful state of mind. I felt being grounded in the mystery of life."

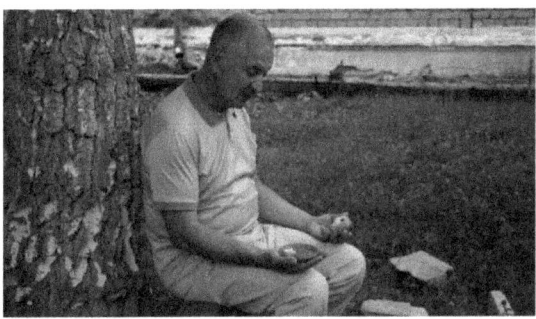

Figure 14.2: A group participant performing his ceremony

While sharing their experience and effects at the end of this session, the participants mentioned their improved affective state of decreased stress and energetic restoration. Some of them emphasized that by exploring the environment in their meditative walk, creating their artworks, finding and arranging a place to install them, and interacting with their creations in the environment through rituals and other activities, they felt physically, emotionally, and spiritually connected to the natural environment.

Case example 2: Botanical arranging as a form of environmental art expression with substance abuse clients

Art therapy was carried out with substance abuse clients taking a course at the specialized rehabilitation center in St. Petersburg. The course was attended by people aged 30–60 years who had problems with the use of psychoactive substances. The majority were alcohol-dependent (70%); the rest were drug addicts in remission. Approximately ten percent of the clients used the so-called new drugs (salts, acids, hallucinogens). Men made up about 80 percent, whereas women comprised 20 percent of the rehabilitated clients.

Some sessions involved creating botanical arranging from natural materials, mostly from botanical ephemera found in the environment, with the goals of relieving emotional tension, multisensory and emotional stimulation, supporting mindful interaction with the environment, cultivating a sense of beauty, raising environmental consciousness, and improving self-perception and self-understanding.

Botanical arranging and other forms of environmental art activities using natural materials and found objects took place regularly during the course. In some cases, participants were invited to go outside for a period and, while walking in the park, especially in autumn, collect natural materials they like. Returning then to the studio, they were asked to create a composition from them, for example in the form a botanical arranging ("green mandalas"), using cardboard plates as the basis for the construction.

One of these sessions was held in the second half of September 2018. Having created simple botanical arrangement from natural materials found and discussing the work and their impressions of the lesson, the participants noted that they could see the beauty of simple things, how surprisingly diverse and harmonious were the shades and shapes created by nature itself. The beauty of natural ephemera had become more apparent due to the organization of the found materials into simple compositions (Figures. 14.3 and 14.4). The participants also noted that as a result of a relatively short walk outdoors (15–20 minutes), their emotional state improved and a feeling of joy and satisfaction from the activity was experienced.

Describing his botanical arrangement made of leaves in the form of a mandala, Valery (name changed) (alcoholism, 57 years old) said that it resembled his life, in which different colors were mixed. He associated the left side of his "green mandala" with his childhood, while the middle part of his artwork, made of leaves with different shadows, was associated with the present period of his life, and the right part, with its yellow and reddish hues, was associated with the future. Valery considered an acorn located at the top of the composition as the symbol of rebirth (Figure 14.3).

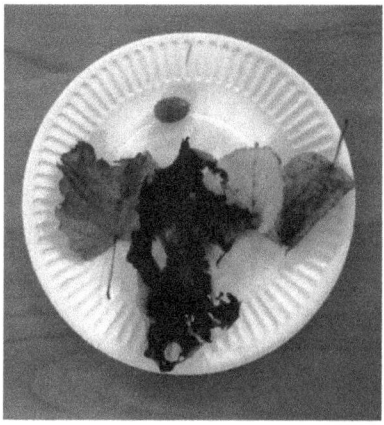

Figure 14.3: Botanical arranging made by Valery

Rooslan (name changed) (alcoholism, 48 years old) realized that his arrangement reflected running in a circle, but with a stronger intention to come out of the circle and to bring his talents associated with acorns into fruition.

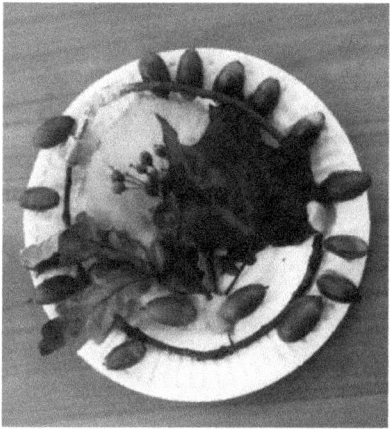

Figure 14.4: Botanical arranging made by Rooslan

Conclusion

The ancient art of Ikebana is a vivid example of the creative collaboration of humans and nature, allowing us to see and create beauty as a manifestation of natural and cultural forms and, at the same time, to support self-transformation and spiritual enrichment of a person.

The art of Ikebana takes on a new meaning and role in the context of the modern environmental movement. This movement, along with other effects, supports the development of innovative approaches in modern psychology and therapy, in particular in art therapy and creative/expressive arts therapies in general.

The chapter has presented one of the techniques of ecological art therapy—the technique of botanical arranging, which has a certain connection with the philosophy and practice of Ikebana. Botanical arranging is a kind of creative artistic activity that gets its rationale from the standpoint of art therapy, ecopsychology, and horticultural therapy. It is not only a means of healing, but also of harmonizing relations between human beings and the more-than-human world, and the development of environmental awareness.

The conceptualization of botanical arranging from the ecopsychology perspective was presented, as well as examples of its use as an art therapy tool in the training of helping professions and as part of a rehabilitation program for drug and substance abuse clients.

References

Burls, A. (2007). People and green spaces: Promoting public health and mental well-being through eco-therapy. *Journal of Public Mental Health*, 6(3), 24–39.

Danylova, T. (2014). Approaching the East: Briefly on Japanese value orientations. *International Journal of Social Science and Management*, 2(8), 4–7.

Davis, J.V. (2011). Ecopsychology, transpersonal psychology, and non-duality. *International Journal of Transpersonal Studies*, 20(11), 137–147.

Deryabo, S.D. (2002). The Phenomenon of Subjectification of Natural Objects. Post-doctorate degree thesis. Moscow State Psychological-Pedagogical University.

Diehl, E.R.M. (2009). Gardens that Heal. In L. Buzzell & C. Chalquist (eds), *Ecotherapy: Healing with Nature in Mind* (pp.166–174). San Francisco, CA: Sierra Club Books.

Hannemann, B. T. (2006). Creativity with dementia patients. *Gerontology*, 52, 59–65.

Heerwagen, J. (2009). Biophilia, Health and Wellbeing. In L. Campbell & A. Wiesen (eds), *Restorative Commons: Creating Health and Wellbeing through Urban Landscapes* (pp.39–57). Washington, DC: USDA Forest Service.

Homma, I., Oizumi, R., & Masaoka, Y. (2015). Effects of practicing ikebana on anxiety and respiration. *Journal of Depression and Anxiety*, 4(3), 187–190.

Hovane, M. (2017). *Ikebana: The Japanese "Way of the Flower."* www.zenvita.com/blog/ikebana-the-japanese-way-of-the-flower.html.

Kellert, S.R. (1993). Introduction. In S.R. Kellert & E.O. Wilson (eds), *The Biophilia Hypothesis* (pp.18–25). Washington, DC: Shearwater Books/Island Press.

Kopytin, A. (2016). Green Studio: Eco-Perspective on the Therapeutic Setting in Art Therapy. In A. Kopytin & M. Rugh (eds), *Green Studio: Nature and the Arts in Therapy* (pp.3–26). New York, NY: Nova Science Publishers.

Kopytin, A. (2017). Environmental and Ecological Expressive Therapies: The Emerging Conceptual Framework for Practice. In A. Kopytin & M. Rugh (eds), *Environmental Expressive Therapies: Nature-Based Theory and Practice* (pp.23–47). New York, NY: Routledge/Taylor and Francis.

Kopytin A. (2020). Archetypal psychology in the context of the eco-human approach. *Ecopoiesis: Eco-Human Theory and Practice*, 1(2), 6–16.

McNiff, S. (2016). Ch'i and artistic expression: An East Asian worldview that fits the creative process everywhere. *Creative Arts in Education and Therapy*, 2(2), 12–20.

Montgomery, C.S. & Courtney, J.A. (2015). The theoretical and therapeutic paradigm of botanical arranging. *Journal of Therapeutic Horticulture*, 25(1), 16–26.

Sasaki, M., Oizumi, R., Homma, A., Masaoka, Y., Iijima, M., & Homma, I. (2011). Effects of viewing ikebana on breathing in humans. *The Showa University Journal of Medical Sciences*, 23(1), 59–65.

Watters, A.M., Pearce, C., Backman, C.L., & Suto, M.J. (2013). Occupational engagement and meaning: The experience of ikebana practice. *Journal of Occupational Science*, 20(3), 262–277.

Wilson, E. (1984). *Biophilia*. Cambridge, MA: Harvard University Press.

Wilson, E. (1993). Biophilia and the Conservation Ethic. In S.R. Kellert & E.O. Wilson (eds), *The Biophilia Hypothesis* (pp.31–40). Washington, DC: Shearwater Books/Island Press.

PART 3

Sustainable Development and Eco-Human Perspectives in the Contemporary Arts

Chapter 15

Interview with Newton Harrison

THE INTERVIEWERS: ALEXANDER
KOPYTIN AND STEPHEN K. LEVINE

Brief note about the interviewee

Newton Harrrison is Research Professor and Director of the Center
for the Study of the Force Majeure at the University of California at
Santa Cruz, Director of Harrisons Studio, and Professor Emeritus at the
University of California at San Diego. He was among the pioneers of the
eco-art movement, a member of the collaborative team of Newton and
Helen Mayer Harrison (who died in 2018) that worked for over 40 years
with biologists, ecologists, architects, urban planners and other artists
to initiate collaborative dialogues to uncover ideas and solutions which
support biodiversity and community development.

The Harrisons' concept of art embraces a breathtaking range of
disciplines. They are historians, diplomats, ecologists, investigators,
emissaries, and art activists. Their work involves proposing solutions and
involves not only public discussion, but also community involvement
and extensive mapping and documentation of these proposals in an
art context. Past projects have focused on watershed restoration, urban
renewal, agriculture and forestry issues, and urban ecologies. The Harrisons' visionary projects have, on occasion, led to changes in government
policy and have expanded dialogue around previously unexplored issues,
leading to practical implementations variously in the United States and
Europe. There is a large body of literature on their work. They have
exhibited extensively in the United States and Europe, and been awarded

grants from the National Endowment for the Arts, the European Union, and the German, Dutch, French and English governments.

Alexander Kopytin (AK): You and Helen were pioneers of environmental art and were involved in your influential joint career together that lasted nearly half a century. You made a serious impact on the contemporary policy and practice of environmental art. You were among the first artists in the 1960s to address the issues of environmental protection, including the issues of climate change, the extinction of biological species, pollution, and renewable natural resources, and you emphasized that they can no longer be perceived as secondary and should instead become central in everyday politics: in the economy, in everyday life, in education, and so on. The field of environmental art has developed alongside an increasing awareness of ecological issues and the rise of the environmental movement since the 1960s. Once an area of interest for a relatively small group of people, art that addresses environmental issues has in the last years to become part of the powerful artistic mainstream, its forms and methods. How has the Harrisons' art evolved since the 1960s? How would you characterize the current situation in the environmental artistic milieu and your recent projects aimed at building a new and more continuous future?

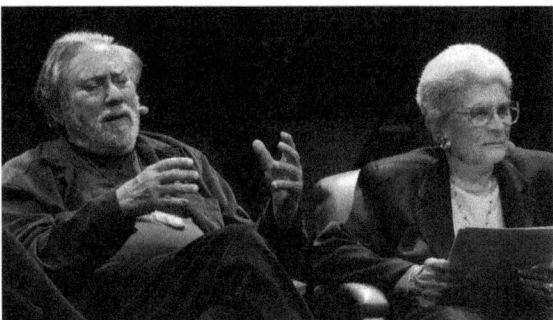

Figure 15.1: A Counterforce on the Horizon. Helen Mayer and Newton Harrison. TEDxSantaCruz, April, 2015

Newton Harrison (NH): First to clarify timing, in Helen's and my first work together, where we didn't actually know we were collaborating, she was an intelligent wife and academic helping a husband academic. The work was a world map of endangered and extinct species done for an exhibition entitled "Fur and Feathers" by the Contemporary Crafts

Museum. It took four months of research and the assistance of two graduate students. We were chosen to supply content and overview, since we were known to have looked at the ecosystems from which all the fur and feathers emerged.

We began thinking and doing this work together in 1969 and so we continued and never changed. My foundational work separate from Helen was the question, how does a cell grow, since I either began with the largest or the smallest in seeking understanding. My very first work was *The Birth and Death of a Lily Cell* and was first exhibited in Howard Weise Gallery in, I believe, 1968. Our *Fur and Feathers* piece was done in 1969. Helen and I agreed to make a joint career, combining our diverse talents to do no work that did not benefit the ecosystem that year. Our first few years working together were about finding out exactly what ecosystems were. Now, 50 years later, looking at environmental art, most of the work looks to me as if many artists are taking on local ecological problems and raising the issues at community levels. It is my opinion that our field needs to be trained in how to read the life web itself. After all, it continually speaks to us. And in reading this life web, we need to become obedient to its wishes. Its principle wish, from my perspective or my understanding, is that the human race would do best to seek ways to join the web, stop consuming it, but rather become niches in the life web which would then reinforce its evolution, but above all its ability to continue. The consciousness in our small group is that continuing becomes more difficult and dubious with our present civilization, in which the leadership or the elite have committed to, on the one hand, growth and, on the other, consuming the life web itself. This shockingly negative outcome is taken up by critics like T.J. Demos, but the larger issues are avoided as, in my judgment, over-attention and the majority of resources, at least in our country, move toward social justice funding and away from funding systems breakdown.

So, my characterization of the current situation in the environmental artistic milieu is that we are too little and too late in coming to the kind of understanding and behavior that would let all of life continue in an amiable, convivial, nurturant manner. Most disturbing is the increasing ice melt and ocean rise, reduction of oxygen in the atmosphere, disappearance of the world forest down to about 30 percent, topsoil distress due to industrial agriculture (quite a few million miles of this), deep oceanic stress, and accelerating extinctions. So much denial! All our work in the last decade can be seen as counter-extinction work.

You have a number of the works. They begin with *Greenhouse Britain*. We are attaching one of the most recent, *Apologia Mediterraneo*. In this work done last year, I ask and answer the question: Can I stretch my empathy to include a small ocean? The answer is, maybe. Then, when you look at the other work, *Sensorium*, if you blow the image up big enough to read it, you will see that I'm now closer to being able to stretch my empathy to deal with the whole ocean. Would an oceanographer ask such a question?

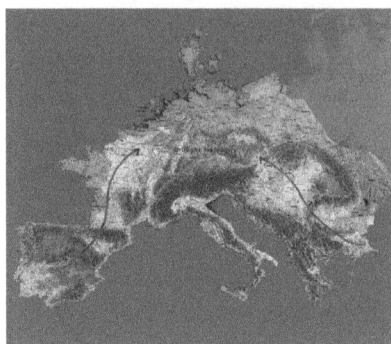 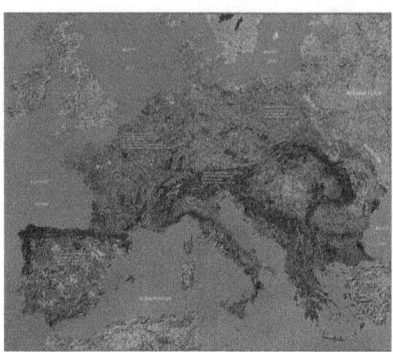

Figure 15.2a and 2b: Artworks from Peninsula Europe: Part II and IV (2007–2008)

To quote the text accompanying the artworks:

> To a very different world than we now inhabit
> The greatest difficulty in this new beginning
> Is not so much the research required
> Or the science or the experimental design
> In which concept and design can be tested in small patches
> Rather it is overcoming the inertial properties
> Embedded in the major cultural forces that define
> Most human behavior toward our life-support systems
> They are
> Democracy and capitalism
> Technocracy and some religions
> For this level of experimentation to succeed
> All must yield agency enforceable by law
> To the lives that are not ourselves

AK: Art possesses its own means of responding to the problems facing the planet. How can art impact the environmental crisis? Does it need a seat at the table where decisions are made? One of your most recent works, *The Force Majeure*, is about that. You and Helen used the exhibition format in several ways, often in the sense of a town meeting, always with the intention of seeing your proposals move off the walls, land in planning processes, and ultimately result in interventions aimed towards social and environmental justice. So, you were mingling with policy-makers through being artists. Is it possible to artistically engage with policy-makers and make them more sensitive to environmental issues through the use of art? What is the difference between problem approaches taken by the artist and most other disciplines?

NH: Yes, I'd like to talk about the dramatic difference between problem approaches taken by the artist and most other disciplines. The best way to get at this in my and Helen's work is opening our book and engaging with the work entitled *Green Heart Vision*, which began in 1994 and concluded successfully in 2002. We were brought in by the cultural council of South Holland, the Dutch art government group, to see if we could save the 1000 square kilometer center of the country from a $230 billion development. This center of Holland was known as the Green Heart—it's all in the account we wrote in our book. The important thing for the non-artist, the scientist and social scientist, the planner and the politician to grasp is the artist's way. This differs from artist to artist, but has in common freedom of expression, freedom of research, and freedom with improvisation. In fact, my career is not about research, it is about search and discovery and taking immediate responsibility for that which is discovered. The Dutch example suits well. For instance, in the first couple pages you will read our public warning. It was published far and wide. In it, we were able to condense it into a two- to three-minute read on the *Urgency of the Moment* (it works best read aloud). The danger the country was facing, which above all was the extraction of its whole history, its early history, is the story of the formation of a primitive kind of democracy where all had to work together and agree to work to keep waters pumping from the land to maintain itself below sea level. To do this, a large number of communities had to find agreement and act out this agreement collectively.

After presenting the text warning of the "urgency of the moment," we then made a map of the country printed backwards with 300,000 of the 600,000 houses proposed penciled in. It quickly became clear that the green heart of Holland would disappear from development, into a

600,000-house city, which endangered the city of Rotterdam. Actually, the whole history of Dutch culture would disappear: windmills, the ecology, farming, 13 villages, and for what? Creating a city that does not need to be built in the first place. It was proposed in the wrong-headed belief that the best lands in the country have to be sacrificed in order to handle population growth. We showed that the perception was wrong and that this kind of development could easily and fruitfully be accommodated within the open spaces around all the cities that surround the green heart. We subscribe to the notion that if you want to criticize a big plan, come up with a better one, which we did, exhibited it, and finally our plan was accepted by Dutch parliament. Can you imagine your local planner presenting a map of a region to be planned printed backwards and explaining to the planning community that the concept itself is based on wrong-headed beliefs? Moreover, pointing out that resolution is easily at hand if you change how you perceive your environment. This Green Heart of Holland work is about a sharp change in perception and accepting the limitations this brings on, as well as the opportunities. So, this is what I as an artist come to the table with. These are the improvisational skills and vision designing skills, so to speak, that I see often in sharp contrast to the belief structures around me—but always done to the advantage of the life web.

Put most simply, I as an artist am unafraid to offend. I as an artist feel compelled to improvise in much the way my other companion species do. I improvise my existence as best I can with the material at hand. The intention is to improve that which is around me. The materials at hand in Holland were based on their planning group's misperception of their countryside and the stresses that it faced. So, the image sequence can be understood as follows. We sent a warning in a text entitled, On the *Urgency of the Moment*. We printed the Dutch map backwards. Everybody then can see the Green Heart broken up into parts, Rotterdam endangered, and the history of the country lost. We were then asked if our map was backwards by the Dutch, who were quite blunt and annoyed with us for embarrassing them. What then is forward? Another image explained what we meant by *forward*. This image made clear how to save the green heart, how to save the country's history, how to increase the biodiversity, save the farming, and 13 villages which collectively are the deep expression of Dutch life. A later image drawn by our landscape architect student showed how you can disburse 600,000 houses easily, fruitfully, even to the benefit of immigrants, and at the same time preserve the integrity of Holland's green heart. Ultimately, our intention was to create and secure in the culture a new nurturant narrative that would permit and indeed encourage the green heart of Holland to continue to be itself.

Moreover, we believe that our thinking and seeing approaches are both revolutionary and revelatory. We find that our work over time tends to bring to pass unintended consequences. For instance, in Holland, rather than making a biodiversity ring, the Dutch accepted our general principles then redesigned our work in part. They discovered that biodiversity would be more advantaged if their major rivers were widened. Then flood control would be improved, and biodiversity at the edges would be do far better work than our biodiversity ring. But designing the ring encouraged the Dutch to do it more effectively with their concept, which was much more open and improvisatory than ours. I must say, it was a pleasure to see the Dutch improve our plan in this way, while at the same time making our original boundary around the green heart the law of the land. This meant you couldn't develop beyond our line unless it was for small, intimate family reasons. I go into all this detail because so much of the sciences deny passion, and seek to minimize risk-taking, therefore shrinking their capacity to deal with the scale of the problems we face. Actually, the positions we took in text and image could as easily have been used by the Dutch to dismiss us.

I conclude with some comments on science itself. I find in most of my work a need to refer to scientific discovery as subject matter—much of which I agree with and some of which I do not agree with. I get my confidence to do this from an attitude I developed in the early 1970s where the sciences were concerned: if the science I needed did not exist, I could and would do it myself. Hence, if you look at the seventh piece in *Survival Series*, it is about how we decoded the mating behavior of a Southeast Asian crab. We did so in open competition—we were told—with 60 other scientists, some of whom objected to non-scientists getting such a grant. To give you an example, John Isaacs, one of the sub-directors of the Scripps Institute of Oceanography, and I were friends. He literally commanded us to go for a sea grant because he explained that the $17K we used to decode the mating behavior of our crab was like six or seven percent of the $300K they spent trying to decode the mating behavior of the lobster, and we were successful and they were not. Their standard scientific behavior was to begin by dismembering the lobster to see how it worked. I remember thinking to myself, "Well, how about asking them to put it back together so we too could see how it worked?" Instead, I asked an entirely different question which had nothing to do with how a crab worked physically, but much to do with its environment. Helen and I set out to make an environment that crabs would be happy to mate in. We had no notion that we would cut up some poor crab to see how it might go about the business of mating. Of course, I had some specialized information. I understood that crabs mated in small ponds four paces by five paces and waist-high, therefore we felt comfortable in this knowledge. The other thing we artists do is question differently. I remember one of the great Bauhaus problems, I taught it many times. It was in two parts. Make a light thing look heavy. Make a heavy thing look light. My position on that, and many artists do the same, is to turn their work upside down to continually give ourselves new perspectives on what we were doing. I did not notice the other lobster folks turning their lobsters upside down or making a lobster feel comfortable enough to mate. Please note that the crab finally turns up to be a central figure in a major work of art titled, *Lagoon Cycle*. Thus, the scientific experiment leads to a complex narrative that turns out to be a 160-foot long mural, now in the possession of the Centre Pompidou as part of the French National collection.

AK: My perception is that you have a long-standing and extraordinary grasp of strategies of multidisciplinary collaboration, that your work together with Helen was driven by a deep understanding and respect for ecological systems and fueled by great empathy for the Earth. Works such as *The Serpentine Lattice* or *The Force Majeure* posit that unless artists, scientists, industry, and government begin creating working environmental projects together which actively acknowledge our future needs in light of our current environmental issues, habitable environments that can sustain future generations of life may not exist. Do you believe that artists must have a firm grasp of a number of disciplines in order to intelligently and effectively engage large-scale projects that can make a difference in artistic, environmental, economic, and other social systems that determine the fate of the many living creatures on which our existence depends?

NH: Such a nice question. So easy to answer. My answer to your question is: Yes! My earlier responses may make clear why I say this. At the end of your elaborate question, it is true that we introduced the idea of sustainability. It is also true, however, that by the 1980s we were in disagreement with sustainability. To sustain something in a particular state, given the laws of indeterminacy, is a physical impossibility. And the term "sustainability" has been hijacked by the growth of good people saying that to grow itself is sustainable. I consider this a form of madness. Our real discourse has to be about continuing and what we are doing to permit ourselves to continue. And what must we discontinue in order for life to continue? Could we be talking about leaving all the fossil fuels in the ground? Could we be talking about our new energy abundance being the sun? And the careful nurturing of photosynthesis? Don't you think the physicists should be biologically educated? Don't you think politicians should understand the fundamental laws of the conservation of energy, particularly since our systems of consumption are producing entropy in big systems? Many of these are—to use MIT talk—entering perturbation in preparation for collapse.

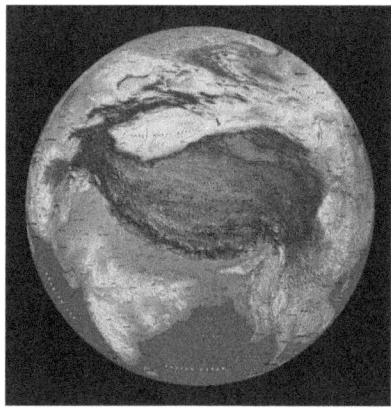 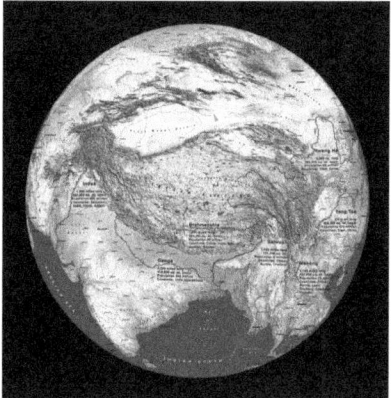

Figure 15.3a and 15.3b: Works from the book, Tibet is the High Ground (2008–2012)

As quoted in the text accompanying the artworks:

The research of Chinese glaciologists
As well as those from India appears to be right
And more than 80 percent of the glaciers in Tibet
And surrounding areas
Will disappear in the next 35 years
As the temperatures rise
Six degrees Celsius or more

Thus, producing conditions of
Flood and drought negatively affecting
The Salween, Mekong, Hwang Ho
Brahmaputra, Yangtze, Ganges
And Indus River systems
That nourish both the ecosystems
And the well-being of those living within them
The Force Majeure
Will work to the disadvantage
Of about one-sixth of the earth's population
All those who live in these seven drain basins
That constitute so much of continental Asia
The countries of China, Burma, Laos, Cambodia,
South Vietnam, India, Bangladesh, and Pakistan
Will need to put aside
Differences of culture, governance
Race, religion, and legal systems
In order to create a counterforce
At virtually continental scale

AK: I know that you often use poetic language in your environmental art projects. What do you think about the power of poetic gesture in your work? Can a very simple poetic gesture have an effect on policy? You once said that poetry avoids planning language, science language, all those kinds of languages, so that if somebody reads our work carefully, they can understand.

NH: The answer to your question is: Yes. The examples exist in the Sava River work, in the Pacific Northwest text, and the Holland work. You might read the *Urgency of the Moment*, which affected the planners considerably in Holland.

AK: Why is the act of artistic/poetic expression important? Do you think that poetic expression is written not only to be understood, but also to be read out loud, so that it's not just the written word but also the spoken word that is very important? Why do you think so?

NH: I am influenced—and Helen was, too—by the work of the ancient bards, particularly in Ireland and Scotland. In those times, nothing was written down, everything was an oral tradition. The poets in their poetry were policy-makers and were listened to by the leadership and policy-makers of those countries. So, we took lessons from them as well as Heraclitus, Socrates, and the Noble Eight-Fold Path of the Buddha, with a little help from Gandhi. Our work is meant to be read but often does best as a performance where Helen and I did alternate reading. If you go to our book and review *Lagoon Cycle* you will find much of it is written by both of us and you can understand this by looking at the difference in our handwriting—mine being a little bit awkward and Helen's being elegant. When others read the work, we tell them, let the male voice speak the words that are written awkwardly, let the female voice read the words that are written elegantly. Where influencing policy-makers is concerned, the last works in our poem "The Urgency of the Moment" did the work for us and affected the planners considerably. You might quote this.

AK: Your book, *The Time of the Force Majeure: After 45 Years Counterforce is on the Horizon,* actually does offers a 21st-century manifesto. Could you please comment on the key points of this manifesto?

NH: I choose not to comment on the key points. The manifesto is meant to be read and thought about and acted on. It is literally a call to action. Without this call and many others like it, we appear to be traveling the road to our own destruction. I actually believe our most recent works on the Mediterranean, the *Sensorium*, and the work on Peninsula Europe are all about what we mean by the term "counterforce." However, the counterforces that we have put on the table are weak forces.

Stephen K. Levine (SKL): Can you say a little about *Helen's Town*?

NH: It started with the Swedes—a Swedish art group invited us to Stockholm to help them add something to the greening of the harbor. So, we said, well, that's a big notion, let's go look. We spend a week there and found out that in the main they were building as many apartments as they could and going a little green, but it's green-washing. We wrote them a letter and said no, we've met your planners, we've seen it and this is not enough, you need to begin again. *Helen's Town* is our beginning again. We wrote a brief thing on why we wouldn't do it and then wrote *Helen's Town* and said we want to do this. It didn't work out there, our presentation maybe wasn't clear enough. It's gone through re-writings to become simpler, clearer and more humble.

I took our rejection and difficulties as useful criticism, once I got past my exasperation and recreated it. Sometimes criticism that comes at you is not what it appears to be—it's about what they are not saying, and you need to pay attention to what is not being said. *Helen's Town* says what they are—when the heat rises, the trees die and maybe new trees come. What you can grow for your food changes. What grasses and flowers grow in the meadows that would nourish cattle and the like. We proposed that *Helen's Town* began with a series of botanists living in a small community and starting to grow the future of farming, herding, the overstory in a forest, the understory in a forest, and as such you have six or seven simultaneous experiments that collectively take a look at what your environment can grow and produce and enhance biodiversity, on the one hand, and human development, on the other, and utterly defeat capitalism.

What does that mean? Capitalism is very skilled and it will utterly defeat itself. Not because of some Marxist theory where the proletariat rise—we've got rid of the proletariat, there is only the very rich, the rich, and the starving. The laws of conservation of energy are being turned upside down, and they don't work when they are turned upside down.

We can keep business as usual, doing what all us Americans are trying to do. The best of us, who I find boring, are trying to make the environment a little belter, do a little less damage, so that we can continue making money. They don't want to hurt the environment as much as we are. But I believe we are done for. We need a whole new discipline, a belief analysis. How much does a belief cost? The cost of the belief...

SKL: What does the new form of belief require?

NH: It's too simple to believe for most people... All species overproduce for survival reasons. Produce a million eggs, only a hundred will develop—it's a natural phenomenon that causes growth. If we harvest redundancy appropriately, we will assist in the health of ecosystems. For instance, if I have 1000 hectares of forest and I harvest on a 200-year basis. I only cut 20 hectares of trees any given year, so I harvest from different places, then biodiversity happens,

As a human being, I can take that redundancy for my own benefit—I'll take only the redundancy and only take it in such a way that the forest improves. Otherwise I do not pull out the tree. And that's the rule. That's the wealth of our future: in nurturing the web of life and harvesting the excess to our benefit for trade and making sure that the harvest improves or at least sustains the systems. Right now, our harvest eats up the system. That's my answer to capitalism. My second answer is if we don't do it, we're dead.

Thanks for these questions.

AK: It was our pleasure to talk to you.

Chapter 16

Sensorium: The Voice of the World Ocean—The Thinking

An Immersive Global Classroom and Interactive System for Civilization Recovery

NEWTON HARRISON

The World Ocean is the mother of us all and its well-being is our well-being.

Introduction

Sensorium is a physically beautiful, immersive, interactive space (approximately 30 x 50 feet) with total surround visuals. It invites the audience to "walk the world ocean," interact with it, ask it questions, listen to its voiced response, hear its challenges and discover fresh new insights for ocean recovery solutions to the stresses placed on it, particularly those stresses that exponentially increased during the last hundred years.

It is designed as a deeply felt experience, a classroom, and a systems solution tool that is valuable to students, general audiences and scientists alike. Its LED-lit interactive floor and walls are powered by sophisticated artificial intelligence tools. The construction and aesthetic presence generated by Sensorium are performative in nature and evocative of the kind of revelatory feelings that can emerge as it expresses cathedral-like properties. In fact, Sensorium blends research work with the aesthetic experience. It is the latest in scientific, ecological, biological, economic thinking and precise measurements. This makes the Sensorium a powerful communications tool and instrument to create with. Enhanced by the surrounding poetic and artistic expressions, the intention is to evoke creative imagination.

Thus, the world ocean becomes a teacher when the Sensorium, acting as a new kind of classroom, manifests stunningly informative properties. It is informative even to the point that there will be questions asked of it for which there are no answers. The voice of the world ocean is then empowered to visualize an array of answers from which a synthesis can be derived. Sensorium functions in the conceptual space that everyday humanity functions in. It is a space that operates between the far seeing of the telescope and the micro-visualizations available in a microscope.

In addition, Sensorium is a unique poly-disciplinary communication system. For instance, we envisage Russian oceanographers from the Baltic Sea, people from Scripps Institute of Oceanography, and Woods Hole in the United States all talking to each other about a common problem—and the voice of the ocean then answering in response as well as acting as interpreter, information source, and conversational participant.

In conclusion, we believe that Sensorium is the first poly-cultural, poly-aesthetic, poly-scientific global classroom. The profound hope is for Sensorium to answer a multitude of questions of great variety. By this we mean the questions the scientists would ask, the social scientists, the humanists, by everyday people, even children. The long-term intention of this work is to generate the possibility and avenues of approach for human communities large and small to become niches in the web of life itself.

Sensorium: The thinking

Sensorium is a work both of art and of science that sets out to synthesize the survival problems that the world ocean faces in our emerging heat-shocked future. The work is designed by me, and emerges from the Center for the Study of the Force Majeure, located at the University of California, Santa Cruz. Personally, I am grounded in the arts, the sciences, and have been working for the past 50 years on systemic environmental problems such as topsoil degeneration, planetary warming, atmospheric imbalance, forest and oceanic degeneration. Sensorium is our most recent effort in addressing the ongoing degeneration of our world ocean's life web. Attached to this written proposal/explanation is our book entitled *The Time of the Force Majeure: After 45 Years Counterforce is on the Horizon*, written by myself and my life partner Helen Mayer

Harrison, now deceased. By way of history, our work is acknowledged as foundational to the rapidly growing eco-art movement, with our first global warming work done in 1974. Sensorium is an example of what we mean by counterforce. Through Sensorium, I am proposing a form of expression that references the whole systems knowing that our ancestors practiced as part of their everyday survival mechanisms, and which has now faded to a whisper in modern western life.

I begin this commentary not in the present but imagining myself as living a tribal life, one hundred thousand years ago, standing in the high grasses not far from the open canopy forest from which I emerge. The grasses are tall, but I can see above them. A hundred yards away the tall grasses wave in a manner that signals a large animal is present (a classic example of figure ground perception). A tail is then seen and instantly the image of a tiger comes to mind—as one of my human visual talents is to create a whole from seeing or hearing only a part. If the wind is blowing away from me, then I need not flee. If the wind is blowing from me towards the tiger, then flight takes over as the tiger would smell me. At the same time, my personal sensorium is picking up sound, wind and subtle changes taking place in many different forms, while registering places to escape and hide, all at once and all together. I am having a whole-systems fight or flight response to a clear and present danger. The survival principle at work is scanning, which led to this nearly instantaneous, un-rationalized and holistic response. I believe that the potential for this kind of perception and survival response from the human sensorium has been so reduced by modern life that large-system scanning and improvisational response has ceased being an environmental survival strategy in contributing to safety in everyday life.

Instead, this talent has devolved (with some notable exceptions) to what can be derived from the computer screen experience. I believe that this human loss is catastrophic for the life web of the planet. This is because decision-making, still mainly Cartesian in nature, is now made part by part, in a fragmented, environmentally disassociated manner, which requires the world to be viewed as a mechanism rather than a living, changing system. This is typical for much present-day research and most modern people, who no longer see and act on what is happening all over and all at once, like our ancestors once did. Even though the ancients' historic perception was local and ours in this very complex modern world must become global, I believe our original capacity for whole-systems scanning and response is vital to our continued survival.

In the brain, cognitive science reveals that neurons devoted to visual processing number in the hundreds of millions and take up almost 50 percent of the cortex, as compared with eight percent for touch and just three percent for hearing. This indicates that retrieving and evolving our original scanning skills is necessary if we are to successfully respond to the problems operating in all systems all at once due in good part to planetary heat shock.

In response, we at the Force Majeure Center propose the Sensorium intervention as a digital expression of how we, in modern world terms, can go about re-establishing whole-systems seeing, decision-making and, above all, action. The intention is to bring whole-systems scanning back as a part of everyday experience, and to use this once common and natural practice both in scientific research and everyday life.

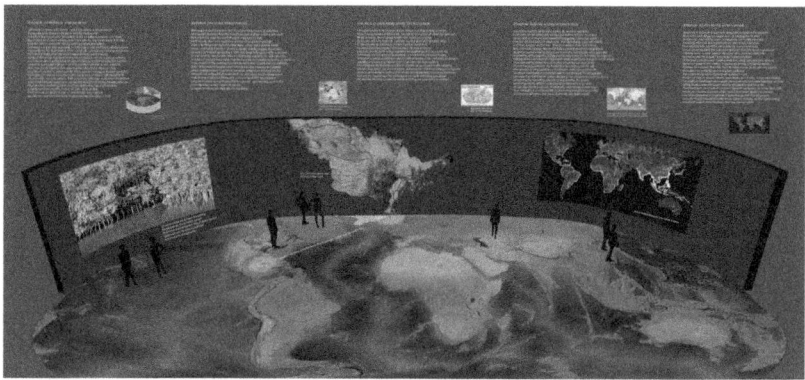

Figure 16.1: The Sensorium general layout (please, see the section towards the end of the chapter titled 'Sensorium footnotes')

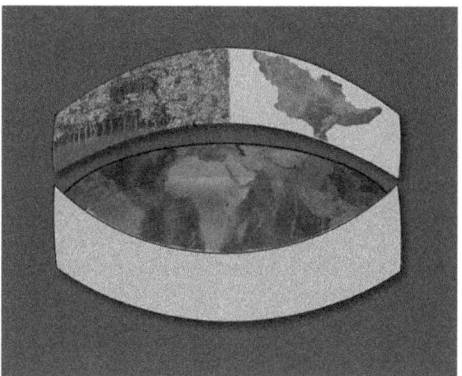

Figure 16.2: The Sensorium complete is in the round

To this end, we are in the process of designing a new kind of instrument that takes up the middle ground between the telescope, which sees far, and the microscope, which sees near. The instrument—the Sensorium—sees in the now and is supported by scientific research which demonstrates the large proportion of our brain that is committed to processing visual information.

We note that a great deal of restorative oceanic work takes place in a one at a time, problem-solving, reflexive manner—whether we are looking at the loss of coral reefs, dead spots, heat pollution, fish farming pollution, acidification, rising oceans or plastics removal (obviously, the total list of problems is much longer).

In contrast, the immersive work we propose, by combining art and science, opens up space of mind for a new, useful-for-all kind of oceanic narrative to emerge. We start with the concept of creating a fully interactive three-dimensional human centered interface, where the floors, walls and even the ceiling all act as "live" surfaces, connected to real-time data, information and modeling/simulation tools. Building on and incorporating elements of two dimensional, three dimensional, virtual reality and sophisticated audio tools, the goal is to create an experience for the user that brings visual, audio and haptic experiences together in real time.

In this chapter, we won't describe the technology in depth but focus on the experience of the user. The experience begins with an interactive, programmable floor, which is on a raised platform. Sensorium requires a large space, an area of at least 1500–2000-square feet. On the floor is a potentially ever-evolving world map with all the world's oceans delineated. Emerging from this digitally expressive surface, the walker encounters the ever-changing locations of the principle ocean stressors. For instance, if one is walking the ocean close to Chile, one of the principle stressors would be fish farming, particularly shrimp, the pollution from which has a negative impact on normal oceanic ecosystems. In this case, a local solution would be taking the polluted waters and pumping them on land to a swamp-type wetland. This action would purify the polluted water sufficiently so that when it returned to the ocean it would be oxygenated and function as nourishment, rather than generating hypoxic conditions.

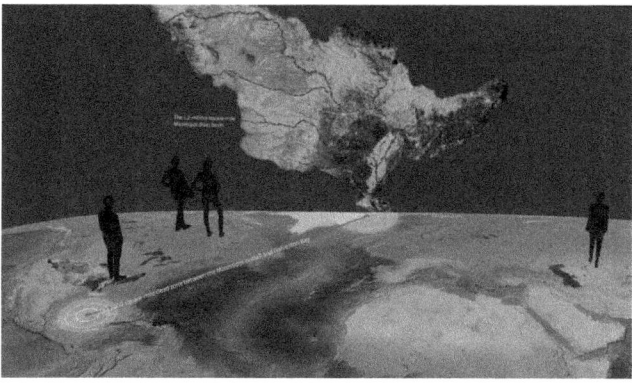

Figure 16.3: Mississippi river basin

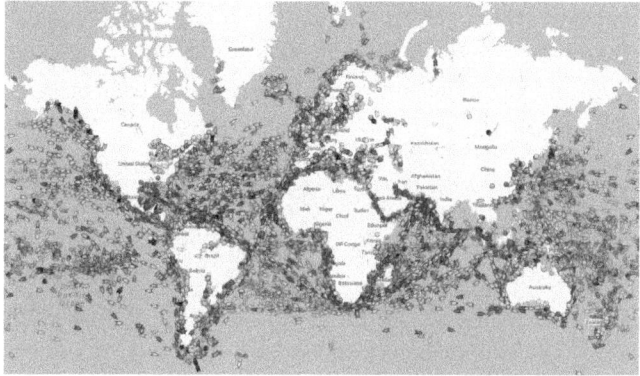

Figure 16.4: Sensorium reveals a transoceanic pattern for wetland restoration where every ship on the whole ocean is marked

In addition to presenting solutions to such local problems, part of Sensorium's purpose is to dramatically express the need for global ocean governance that could enforce a whole-system rule of law. This global system of governance would need to have the power to penalize polluters on a global scale and demand drastic changes, such as the invention of biodegradable plastics. Sensorium also holistically demonstrates the profound benefits that will arise from a regenerated ocean and, in the long-term, exceed the costs required to bring about such changes. Moreover, visualizations that come out of Sensorium will illustrate what might be done about ecological problems facing the world's oceans, what it might cost, and also what would be the cost of not taking action.

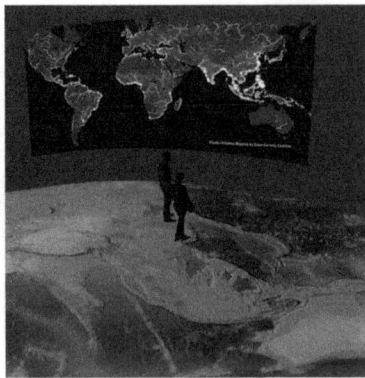

Figure 16.5: Mapping plastics pollution

In response to a certain question, a tsunami might be projected onto the walls for a minute or two, followed by another environmental catastrophe and then another. Such emotive imagery might be projected repeatedly on different walls at different times—but only as requested and within the context of a large, oval, cathedral-like space. Questions asked of Sensorium will be responded to visually, auditorily and with printed text. Sensorium is designed to present information comparatively. For instance, those who engage Sensorium might choose to examine the overall death risk facing the world ocean. Sensorium might suggest six factors which are destroying ocean life simultaneously:

- Increase in atmospheric carbon.
- Increase in oceanic acidity.
- Decrease in the ocean's ability to sequester carbon, its capacity reduced mainly by increased acidity.
- Decrease in production of oxygen both in the atmosphere and oceanic waters.
- Perturbations from extractions in virtually all life support systems.
- Dramatic cross-oceanic ecosystem disruption through pollution, particularly plastics.

What I am describing here is a first sketch for perhaps one of the most complex immersive systems ever put in place. It has multiple functions—first, it educates and allows people to engage personally with the ocean. More significantly, Sensorium can function as a generalized pre-emptive planning environment, where oceanographic problems, mostly of human creation, can be seen and acted on because their interconnectivity is understood all at once and all together. Of particular interest is how oceanic stressors interact with one another, and where solutions can be sought out that are not models or bits and pieces of larger problems, but real-world, large-systems solutions.

Furthermore, Sensorium can give details of the local place of each oceanic problem, with poetry in the language of the visual arts in tandem or interacting with the language of science, always with the life web as the instructional source. Sensorium may use poetic language, including metaphors, such as only a fool picks a fight with the ocean or every place is the story of its own becoming, to communicate more deeply and holistically.

Accompanying this narrative is a 42" by 98" sketch presenting how Sensorium works visually (Figure 16.1). This image makes clear why we believe Sensorium is of great potential importance. For instance, the sketch image demonstrates a potential resolution for dead zones, which involves the recreation of land-based wetland purification systems. What becomes visible, through Sensorium's unique way of presenting such ecological problems, is the multifaceted ecological value such wetlands have worldwide, as they also function as sanctuaries for birds and other, often endangered species. Sensorium is then asked, perhaps by a different group, a question such as: how can diverse types of pollution generated as waste from ocean vessels be managed? The answer, stimulated by the newly visualized wetland pattern, is to mandate wastewater from all shipping to be introduced to these newly created wetlands. The new wetlands work thus integrates the process of purifying highly polluted water from ships, which can then return to the ocean.

Sensorium is actually a form designed in consultation with the life web. Properly used, the oceanic Sensorium can become the voice of the world ocean. Sensorium works to make visible what is happening in transoceanic waters at any place and any time, always assuming programming is up to date. Finally, in the attached Sensorium sketches we reflect on the oceanic voice, speaking truth about its nurseries, its sanctuaries, its dead zones and the endless infusion of plastics from large to tiny. Acting on these four voices all at once, from our position as artists, generates deep empathy for the ocean, literally the mother of life itself, which is endangered by our own actions. The cathedral-like structure and presentation of the images and information add emotive power to Sensorium's expressive and pre-emptive planning capacities.

The intention of Sensorium is for the scientific, governmental, cultural and industrial communities to be able to visualize the ocean as a whole and to do so in each other's presence. Sensorium encourages holistic decision-making about how to connect disparate parts of the bigger picture and ensure total oceanic well-being. Sensorium is a whole-systems visualization digital structure that automatically generates transdisciplinary outcomes. It tunes itself to whole-systems seeing, thinking and being, in this case with the world ocean as beneficiary. Finally see the addendum at the end of the chapter, where the value of Sensorium can be projected onto the Plains of Russia, even as far as the North Pole.

Sensorium footnotes
Text 1: Sensorium: The beginning. A partial sketch
Sensorium is a space cathedral-like sensibility created to enable anyone to generate and experience discourse with the world ocean

Sensorium presents visually in scientific detail complex oceanic life web threats by revealing dead zones' endless plastic input with the distributed waste from ships from fish farming and ocean netting creating bottom dead spaces

Sensorium can give voice and image to both oceanic and land-based pollution sources responsible for the degeneration of the oceanic life web now experiencing extinctions

Sensorium permits multisystem scanning and seeing simultaneously similar to the envisioning developed by our ancestors to survive in their ecosystems and become niches setting tribal life support patterns in place for long-term survival

Sensorium is speculative design work that manifests complex oceanic problems all at once and all together often requiring transdisciplinary efforts by many

Sensorium's visualizing system permits direct work on multisystem problem resolution

For instance sensorium envisions oceanic nurseries as a network that can call forth a transoceanic sanctuary pattern, then envisioning revitalized dead zones transformed simultaneously revealing an unexpected resolution to global shipping pollution simultaneously visualizing plastics and their elimination from the food chain as fundamental to a healthy oceanic life web, as imperative

Sensorium has the power to express relationships not previously seeable therefore knowable thereby opening new space of mind

Text 2: Sensorium: Dead zones transformation

Well-mapped dead zones over 450 in number have formed at coastlines with oxygen depletion from the overproduction of algae as the death cause

Sensorium first maps the worst of places making clear that most oceanic dead areas happen as a result of land-based pollution often river inflow from agro-industrial waste urban and industrial waste

Worst is the outfall from the 1.2-million square-mile Mississippi drain basin pouring into the Gulf generating a 1000-mile-long 7000-square-mile dead zone

Soon to be 8000-square-miles from the Mississippi outfall to the Galveston Bay

Sensorium's visualizations make clear the need for land-based purification systems to be created on the coastline between the Mississippi outfall and Galveston Bay

Short-term solutions happen when saltwater wetland swamps are created with pumping systems invented to exchange newly clean waters from the Wetlands and polluted Gulf waters from the dead zone newly reoxygenated

First become productive living zone or even a candidate for sanctuary

Long-term solutions require all pollution sources, agro-farming in particular need resolution at their source of creation

Complex in solving but imperative in the doing

Text 3: Sensorium: Ocean nurseries and pattern recognition

Sensorium's pattern visualization process makes clear that oceanic nurseries these diverse mothers of oceanic life are mostly local places all calling for sanctuary

When nurseries, the mangrove forests, the mouths of estuaries, coral reefs, estuarine wetlands, swamps, nursery slicks and upwelling areas in their entirety are conjoined and developed as sanctuaries

Sensorium can then visualize a transoceanic life support system with protected nurseries acting to protect the beginnings of most oceanic life

Collectively protecting nurseries makes for a valuable new pattern discovery

Sensorium envisions conjoining a nursery sanctuary pattern with revitalized dead zones revealing a complex eco-regenerative transoceanic sanctuary pattern

This envisioning further indicates that an oceanic sanctuary pattern this complex

Wherein dead zones the worst of places and nurseries the most endangered of places conjoins in an ongoing foundational source for oceanic life webs, continuing evolution

And with the beginning of life protected and oceanic well-being guaranteed

The invisible beneficiary is land-based life including our own ability to continue

Text 4: Sensorium: Expresses a global wetland pattern
Sensorium reveals a transoceanic pattern for wetland restoration

If saltwater and brackish water wetland purification systems are created whose work is to receive and transform deoxygenated eutrophic waters from the 450 land-adjacent dead zones, then exchanging them with healthy nutritious reoxygenated waters, with dead zone waters can be transformed into the healthy biotope that existed before extreme extraction and pollution

Sensorium seeing a new global pattern of wetlands reveals alternative outcomes responding with a mapping of daily oceanic vessel presence in a shocking snapshot making clear a necessity that ships transfer waste to wetlands at nearest port of arrival

Thus relieving the ocean from yet another intractable pollution assault all costs borne by polluters, the beneficiary the world ocean's life web with recovering fish populations and extinction reduction as outcomes

Sensorium continuing in transaction with multidisciplinary human explorers can make clear that only the overproduction of fish populations can be the harvested envisioning the harvesting redundancy as preserving the system protecting oceanic systems' biota population balance to stay intact and become the life web's way of continuing while serving human need

Then criminality is associated with overharvesting and pollution creation as are human behaviors that cause oceanic life web degeneration

Text 5: Sensorium: Plastics and the ocean's life web

Sensorium in the beginning of its development responds to the question
What is the most dangerous single element infecting the life web?

Its response, now held by many, is that plastic particularly micro bits
negatively affects life that ingests it first in the oceanic food chain then
infecting land-based life particularly the human food chain

So, sensorium visualizes this vast plastic infection from land-based
manufacture infecting rivers, oceans, oceanic life and all who consume
oceanic life

Sensorium sees the Benioff Clean Ocean Currents Coalition as the
most comprehensive viable approach to whole-systems plastic removal

Sensorium presents the coalition mapping oceanwide as force full
evidence coalition then choose 9 of 1000 rivers to install massive plastic
recovery systems

Their discovery is that 80 percent of plastic pollution into oceans
world-wide is transported by these 9 rivers

Plastic river capture removes plastic waste before ocean entry, a
short-term solution

This coalition simultaneously engages in eco-politically land-based
long-term solutions calling for recyclable alternatives dealing with plastic
pollution on site

The beneficiaries are all oceanic and land-based life particularly the
human food chain

Sensorium visualizes the value of the reduction of plastic production
possible only when agreement is developed to leave coal gas and oil in
the ground

Sensorium's search found no better whole-systems thinking and
work safeguarding virtually all oceanic life in the doing than this coalition's work

Sensorium addendum: The Vastlands

We think the Sensorium concept is repeatable at scales large and
small—the differences being in the main the energies available, the
lands available, the waters available, including the lives, ourselves and
our companionate species. For instance, a vast new northern landscape
becomes visible as haven for the life web especially when looking northward from Moscow past the Urals into the Siberian Plateau and even
the East Highlands. For instance, the four-million square kilometer

Russian Plain joined with the vast Siberian sub-plains forms a unique body of land, serving a unique grouping of species, endangered and not, within what I call the Vastlands. The creation of a Sensorium for the whole of these lands, although smaller than the world ocean, enables the workings of a complex new future that would allow the life web's survival with human populations functioning as a niche within it. This would ensure the continuing of the human race, which at present seems uncertain. We use the term *continuing* since we consider it important to emphasize the non-static continuous changing that is inherent in all life forms. The more common word *sustainable* does not convey the nature of the indeterminacy principle and we consider it misleading. This new envisioning of a Sensorium for this whole region would then produce a survival-based eco-human collaboration. The outcome from this collaboration we envision is a bi-continental biodiversity continuum. This can be evolved where species from both Asia and Europe—driven northward by the heat—would be then able to create a niche in the heat-transformed biota of this vast terrain. At the same time, if syntropic farming, topsoil regenerating, biodiversity technologies are introduced in the food-producing sector of this vast terrain then finally food production and biodiversity can be conjoined. If this course of action is developed, we would have a bi-continental drought compensatory system at work. Where food is no longer sufficiently produced in drought-ridden Europe and drought-ridden Asia it can be produced in a re-considered Russian Vastland. We see this effort as of equivalent value to the World Ocean Sensorium. We also see great benefit from creating a scattering of regenerative Helen's Towns across the Siberian steppes and reaching back into the Russian Plain.

A Vastland Sensorium coupled with Helen's Town settlements answers a multitude of questions that are scientific in nature and also human and fundamentally ecological as well. The total formation, the concept of human community becoming a self-made niche in a large environment of their own creation, is a profound life web acknowledgement, even apology collectively ecopoietic in its visualizations as well as autopoietic in its structure.

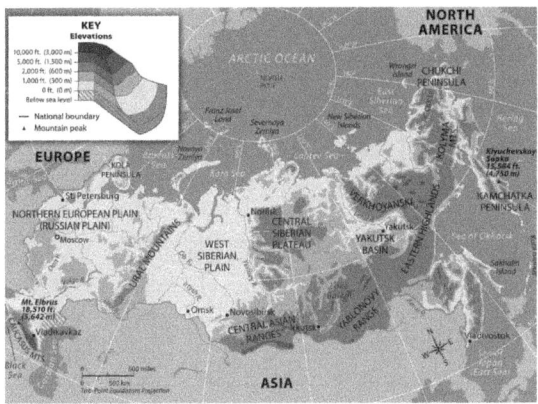

Figure 16.6: Diversity of altitude acts in support of diversity of species, farming and human cultures

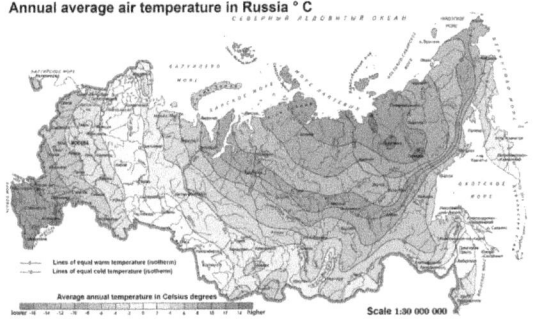

Figure 16.7: The temperature gradients for the whole region move from warm to very cold. This mapping suggests the complexity of change that must be adapted to across the whole region

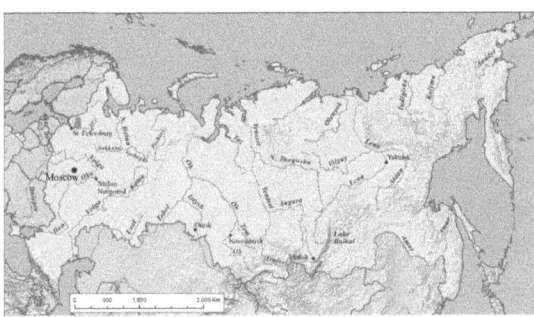

Figure 16.8: Twenty watersheds made visible by major rivers all shape the lives within them, both similar to and different from each other watershed, adding its own biota and productivity to the whole

Chapter 17

Interview with Teagan White

THE INTERVIEWER: ALEXANDRA DVORNIKOVA

Brief note about the artist

Teagan White is an artist living in Portland, Oregon. Teagan received a BFA in Illustration from the Minneapolis College of Art & Design in 2012 and is a member of the VACVVM illustration collective. Their paintings have been exhibited in dozens of solo and group shows across the United States, and they have worked with *Nature Conservancy Magazine*, *Smithsonian Magazine*, Pangeaseed Foundation, Patagonia, Mondo, Nike, Target, American Greetings, Penguin Random House, and many other magazines and journals. In addition to their nature-related art, Teagan makes picture books and other products for children under the name Tiny Moth Studios, with six books published to date.

During their time in Minneapolis, Teagan was a volunteer in the Avian Nursery at the Wildlife Rehabilitation Center of Minnesota. They are currently a member of the University of Washington's Coastal Observation and Seabird Survey Team (COASST) and Oregon Shores' Coast-Watch, two citizen science projects dedicated to monitoring ecosystem health and public land use and collecting baseline data to help assess patterns of seabird mortality due to natural and human-induced events.

Alexandra Dvornikova (AD): Please tell us a bit about yourself and your approach in art.

Teagan White (TW): I'm a 29-year-old artist and illustrator. I grew up in the Midwestern United States (born and raised in Chicago and lived most of my adult life in Minneapolis), and relocated to the Pacific Northwest in 2019. I make detailed, allegorical gouache and watercolor paintings based on my experiences with nature, usually depicting animals that appear dead or struggling for survival.

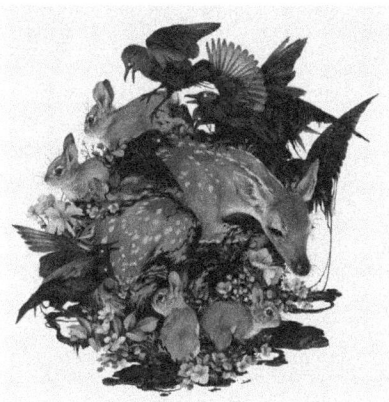

Figure 17.1: Last Concern (24" x 24"), gouache and watercolor on paper

AD: Let's talk about your relationship with nature. How did it begin and evolve? How would you describe your connection with your land?

TW: I can't pinpoint the exact origins of my affinity with nature, but for as long as I can remember I've felt out of place in modern society. As a kid, I was less interested in making friends than in reading books about heroic mice and bats, or staring out the window trying to identify the birds I'd memorized from a field guide.

But I grew up within a huge sprawling city, so my relationship with nature was definitely stunted until I moved to Minneapolis. There I began exploring urban forests, riverbanks and wetlands, and taking trips north to Lake Superior and the Boundary Waters Wilderness. Finally discovering the private immensity of nature felt like finding a missing piece of myself, or like my soul opening up and pulling everything in so it could all become a permanent part of me: small brittle bones scattered in the dry grass, the shrill shriek of a fox nearby when the moon is high, the ceaseless lap of frigid lake water against a smooth slab of sun-warmed rock, the sagging weight of road kill in my hands, bits of floating ice that clink together like wind chimes until they melt to nothing at the river's edge.

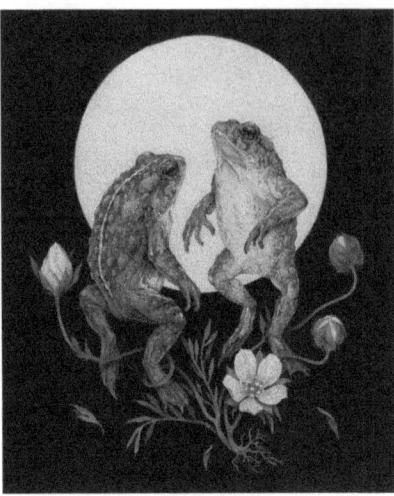

Figure 17.2: Moondance (8" x 10"), gouache, watercolor and colored pencil on paper

I get around by bicycle only, which dictates what types of places I have access to, so I primarily experience nature at the fringes of human life. I find beauty in railroad tracks overrun with invasive plants. I internalize the sadness of shorelines dotted with little pieces of styrofoam. There are all these threads of meaning I'm trying to unravel in the indefinable spaces where human activity ends and nature begins. For years, I buried every animal I found dead in a bike lane; I feel strong kinship with the "pest" animals that live among us, that have adapted to cities or backyards or distressed remnants of habitat. They help me make sense of my own life.

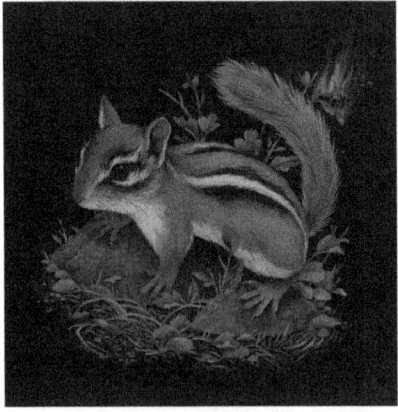

Figure 17.3: Ash (6" x 6"), gouache and watercolor on paper

Moving to Oregon was accompanied by a sense of loss; when the land you live on becomes a part of your identity and the way you understand and heal yourself, being uprooted is a little traumatic. But I quickly realized that even if the specific species or ecosystems around me were unfamiliar, I could still relate to them in the same way I always had. I've never been very interested in traveling to far-off places or seeking out impressive sights, preferring to choose a small number of places to visit frequently and learn about exhaustively. Like any other relationship, your relationship with a place becomes strong when you show up consistently, when you appreciate its beautiful complexity and stand witness while it changes and grows, when you are personally invested in its health and well-being. For me, being in love with a place and the things that live there conjures the same powerfully magical feelings that being in love with a person does, and at times I believe that nature reciprocates that love as well.

AD: Tell us about your experience of co-creating with nature.

TW: I have a hard time separating what is "art" and what is "nature." If I'm being honest, I think that my real art in its purest form is the relationship with nature that I've cultivated over the years. It exists in the space between nature and myself and shouldn't need a physical form to justify itself, so the paintings that I make based on it sometimes feel like a disappointing failure of communication. I paint anyway, a little because I enjoy it, a little because once in a while I believe in art's potential to have a positive effect in the world, and a lot because my pretentious "pure art" has no value under capitalism and won't translate into food or shelter unless I turn it into something marketable or useful.

These days I don't so much decide what to draw, as nature asks it of me. I learned a while back that my best work comes from direct experience, and I avoid subject matter that doesn't emotionally resonate with me. This doesn't necessarily mean that I have to see a certain animal or plant in person to draw it—my work isn't that literal—but it encourages me to put in the time to engage with nature on a regular basis so that I accumulate experiences that can potentially inspire future work. I've found that when I go to a natural place with an open receptiveness towards what that place might have to teach me that day, I'm answered with an avalanche of incredible experiences and the urgent need to share them somehow.

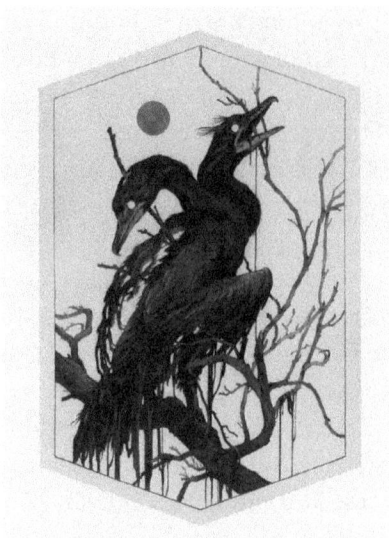

Figure 17.4: Silent Aviary (16" x 20"), gouache,
watercolor and colored pencil on paper

I'm very intentional about allowing nature to be my co-creator, but I'm also cautious about keeping a respectful balance between how much I take and how much I offer back. Besides supporting all our lives, nature has brought me so much joy; it is the foundation of my career, and in many ways the art I make relies on the exploitation of the Earth's resources. I don't think it would be ethical to use plants and animals as my subject matter without recognizing the ways that they are suffering because of us, depicting that with honesty, and using whatever influence or money the art generates to help protect and restore them. Art sometimes seems like an ineffective way to change anything, but when I take on other conservation-related roles—volunteering in songbird rehabilitation, removing invasive species and planting natives, monitoring beaches to collect data on seabird mortality—some part of those experiences inevitably becomes subject matter for my art, as if my work isn't complete until I've processed it by creating something as well.

AD: I can see that the theme of life and death, the cycle of life, inspires you a lot. Can you tell why it is important for you?

TW: Themes emerge in my work when I'm fixated on a concept that is new to me, and need to spend time looking at it from different angles to decide how I feel about it and integrate the conclusions with my larger understanding of the world around me and my place in it.

When I was first becoming more familiar with the natural world I was struck by how often I encountered death all around, and particularly by its unthreatening beauty. Most of us are taught to assign all sorts of negative qualities to death, to see it as ugly and as an end to something, and all of these perspectives betray a total lack understanding of the harmonious cycle of life and death. So for a while I was fixated on depicting my revised understanding of death, as part of an intricate and life-sustaining system that I'm overjoyed to be a part of.

But over time my attention shifted to the deaths that could not be as easily celebrated: road kill, pest animals that are shot or poisoned for our convenience, the ones we treat with cruel indifference because they are only food, the forests we strip for lumber or clear for farmland, the native plants displaced for prettier and more useless species. Here the concept of a cycle is broken, and death is a sentence passed down by the unchecked power of a species that kills based on value judgment rather than need, kills not within sustainable limits but with the goal of extermination or with a heedless gluttony that consumes until there is nothing left; it's a barreling toward doom. As I learn more about the land I live on, I see fewer healthy cycles playing out and more irregularities triggered by collapsing ecosystems, poisoned air and water, human-fueled disasters, and climate breakdown. Each death I stumble across comes with uncertainty—is this one natural or did we cause it in some way? So now when I draw death, I really do connect with the sadness and horror that society told me I should associate with it all along. But the death isn't what's scary. What's scary is seeing the places you love dearly fall apart before your eyes, and to feel complicit in their destruction. Ultimately, death itself isn't really my subject matter anymore, but has become a shorthand visual language that I'm trying to use to portray our entire human relationship with nature, to process my guilt and hold myself accountable, and to focus my mourning on something smaller and less overwhelming.

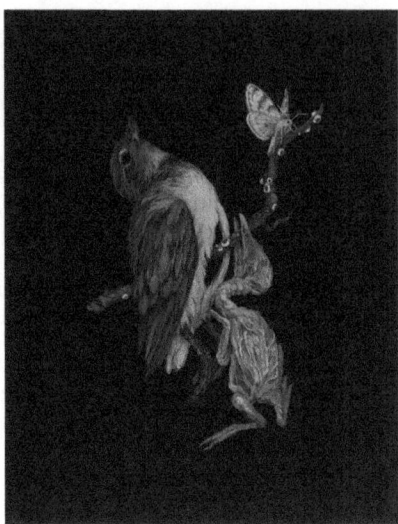

*Figure 17.5: Hollow Bodies (11" x 14"), gouache,
watercolor and colored pencil on paper*

AD: How do you think relations between society and nature/environment should develop in the future? What is the role of creative expression in this development?

TW: We need societies that are aligned with the land they live on, that respect the intrinsic value of nature irrespective of its usefulness to humans, and that understand that a realignment of human activity with nature is not only essential for the survival of our species but also a cure to all sorts of problems we have as individuals and as communities... There are Indigenous cultures that have held onto these truths, but they are met with violent repression instead of looked to for leadership, and I don't know if any progress can be made until we undo the legacy of capitalism, settler colonialism, patriarchy, and anthropocentrism.

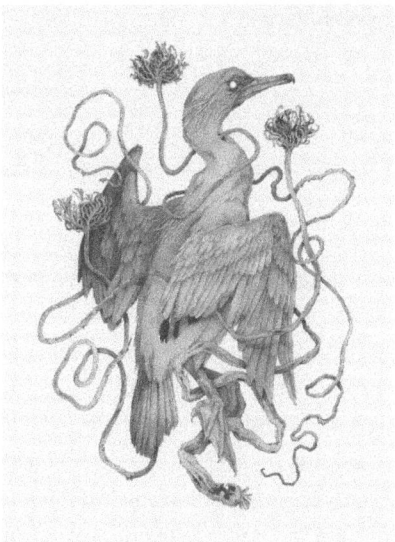

*Figure 17.6: The Restless Sea (16" x 20"), gouache,
watercolor and colored pencil on paper*

My partner and I sometimes laugh about Henry David Thoreau, who complained in the 1800s about fences being built around private property... Wouldn't it be nice if fences were the worst of our worries? What would Thoreau have to say about oil pipelines, or plastic islands in the sea? But really, he was right to fixate on the fences, because the direst problems in the world today are all symptoms of the same worldview that created the concept of property. You can't just tell people not to put up fences; we need cultures of people who have a strong enough relationship with nature to intuitively understand that the very concept of a fence to keep people out or claim ownership over something that can never be yours is evil; people who would never have the desire to build one in the first place.

I do think art can have a role to play in developing this kind of understanding in the world. Big changes of perspective only happen if they originate in a place of subjective truth, which can't be dictated by scientific fact or an authoritative code of ethics. I think art can stir the emotional part of the brain that needs to be activated for you to take personal responsibility for a problem, instead of leaving it for someone else to solve.

AD: Do you see any possible ways to overcome our estrangement from nature?

TW: It's incredibly difficult for anyone living in a developed country or a culture that has lost its grounding in the ecology of their region, because the estrangement is so deeply ingrained and all-encompassing, and we've virtually lost all frames of reference for what a healthy relationship with nature would even look like. For me it comes in waves... Sometimes I feel an intense, blissful sense of understanding of and belonging to nature, and sometimes I feel intensely foolish and embarrassed for thinking I know much of anything or that I'm anything but a burden to the Earth. But I think that's a good combination of things to feel. One gives you purpose, and one wills you to action. Maybe the estrangement is not something we need to overcome, but something we need to exist inside of and allow it to motivate us. If you're even aware that you are estranged from nature that's a good first step, because it means you're listening, and if you listen hard enough I think you'll hear your own sorrow wrapped up in the sorrow of the Earth, and recognize that the only way to heal yourself is by working towards healing the world.

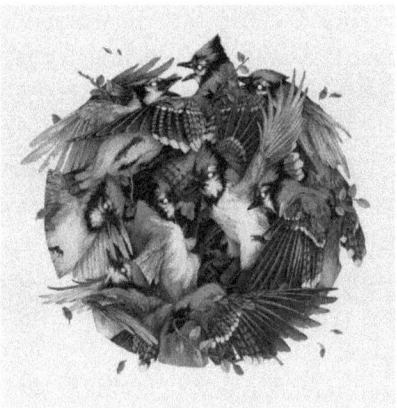

Figure 17. 7: The Cull Racket (14" x 14"), gouache,
watercolor and colored pencil on paper

Note: Teagan White's works can also be seen on their website, www. teaganwhite.com, and on Instagram, www.instagram.com/teaganwh.

Chapter 18

Interview with Diana Sudyka

THE INTERVIEWER: ALEXANDRA DVORNIKOVA

Brief note about the artist

Diana Sudyka (pronounced Soo-dee-kah) is a Chicago-based illustrator. As a child, she was the one always looking under logs for snails and bugs, and not much has changed since. Early in her career, she created screen-printed posters for musicians, and from there moved into the publishing world by illustrating middle grade and children's picture books. She works mainly in gouache, watercolor, and ink, and the subject matter and aesthetic choices for her paintings are inspired by a passion for nature and science, as well as a love for various folk-art traditions. When not working, Diana tries to get outside as much as possible with her family and still sometimes volunteers in the Bird Lab at the Chicago Field Museum.

Alexandra Dvornikova (AD): Please introduce yourself and tell us a bit about your art and inspiration.

Diana Sudyka (DS): I have always been a very visual learner, and have found comfort in drawing and painting from a young age. However, I never really planned to do this full time as I do now. It's been a pretty organic progression over the years, with plenty of odd jobs in between. I do have two fine art degrees, and my focus at university was print-making, specifically intaglio. I spent some of my earlier years working as a printing assistant for a Chicago artist, then gradually moved into making my own work. I spent some years creating screen-printed posters for Chicago's very active indie rock music scene, and that eventually led to my first forays into illustrating books. I now work full time as an illustrator, and almost exclusively for children's picture books. Growing up in the 1980s, I spent a lot of time outside, and many of our family friends lived on farms. As a result, I am still very much an outdoors person, and getting out and connecting to the natural world is critical for my mental well-being. It provides almost all of the inspiration for my personal and commercial work these days. I am also inspired by many traditional folk-art traditions, such as those from my Slavic background and American history.

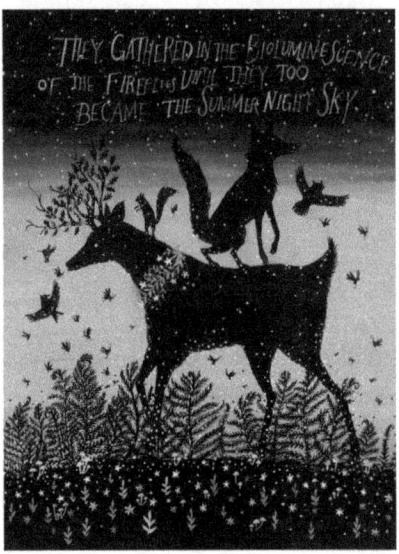

Figure 18.1: Bioluminescense, gouache on clayboard

AD: What do you want people to feel looking at your art?

DS: I don't know that I think about this too much! But, when I do, my hope is that they will feel my respect and connection to all forms of life. And that connection then will maybe spark a memory of their own connections to the natural world and encourage them to seek it out more. I want to normalize a less human-centric way of understanding and valuing of the world, if that makes sense.

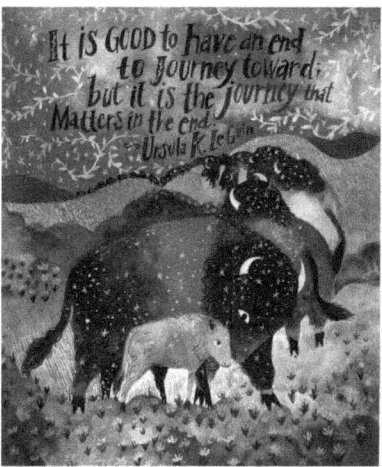

Figure 18.2: Bison, gouache on paper

AD: Please tell us how the imageries of your paintings are born. What is the role of the environment in this process?

DS: When I create an image, and I am really just talking about my personal work and not so much the work I do for children's picture books, I am seeking to create something that has both elements of the spiritual and pagan, but also with elements of the specificness of science. In recent years, my images are very much born out of what I see on my outings to our local forest preserves, and where my focus is at that time, for instance birds, fungi, or these days I am really into native wild plant species and oak trees.

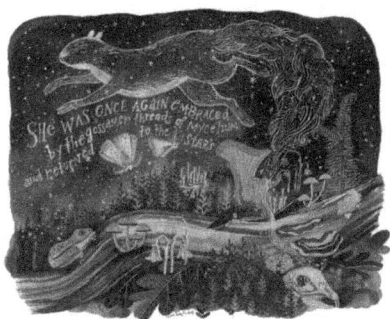

Figure 18.3: Ghost Squirrel, gouache on paper

I live just north of Chicago in an area of the United States called the Great Lakes and Midwestern region. There was a time in my life when I really wanted to move away, but that window has passed as my roots are deep here. I had to find a way to love this area. That's when I started the long learning process over many years of exploring and educating myself about our regional ecosystems, and native flora and fauna. This led to years of volunteering at the Chicago Field Museum of Natural History in their bird lab, and those experiences helped me to find my voice in my art. Living in this area for my entire life did not mean that I knew anything about our native habitats, and the species of plants and animals that exist within. I knew so little! The more I learned, though, the more I wanted to celebrate and share what I was connecting to in our Midwestern environments with others, and the best way for me to do that is through my images.

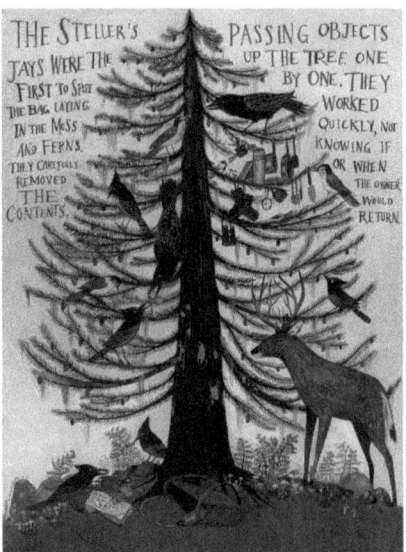

Figure 18.4: The Backpack, gouache on clayboard

AD: You worked a lot with nature as a volunteer and as an artist. Could you describe differences and similarities of both process? What is the connection between ecology and art?

DS: For over ten years I worked in the bird lab at the Chicago Field Museum preparing birds as research specimens using a simplified form of taxidermy. There are many volunteers who do this work. The birds are prepared in such a way that their plumage and body shape are preserved, but they are not posed as in taxidermy mounts. They are laid out so that they will fit into collection drawers. The ornithologist who trained me had started this program of collecting birds that had died by colliding with Chicago's many downtown buildings or confusion from artificial lighting. He and a network of dedicated volunteers collect and bring these birds to the museum to be preserved, especially during the fall and spring migration seasons. These specimens have provided a lot of valuable data and insight into the impact that human-made environments are having on wild bird populations, and it has inspired many cities around the world to seek ways to reduce avian casualties of this sort.

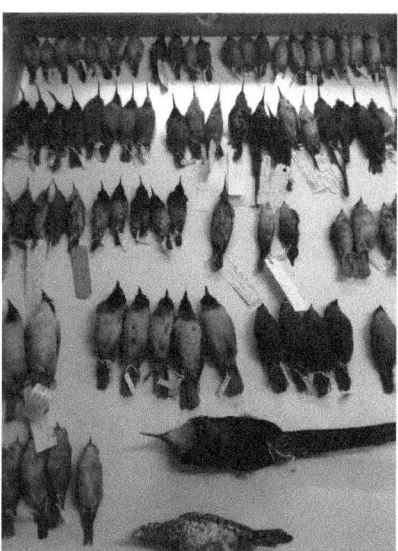

Figure 18.5: Field drawer, bird lab at the Chicago Field Museum

Meeting these extraordinary people who were so generous in sharing their love and knowledge of birds really affected me and my work. I was inspired every time I went in for my shift. I was inspired by what I learned, but also by working so intimately with the beautiful birds. I have always loved working with my hands. There are many aspects of preserving a bird in this manner that engage the same skills of hand-to-eye coordination and aesthetic decision-making that are involved in making art. Also, the powers of observation that you develop as an artist, whether visual or sound, are very much needed for developing a deep sense of ecology. Whether it is bird watching, wild foraging for plants and fungi, or growing a garden, you will thrive more if you have an understanding of the environment, how any given plant or animal has adapted to it, and to do that you must observe and note many details.

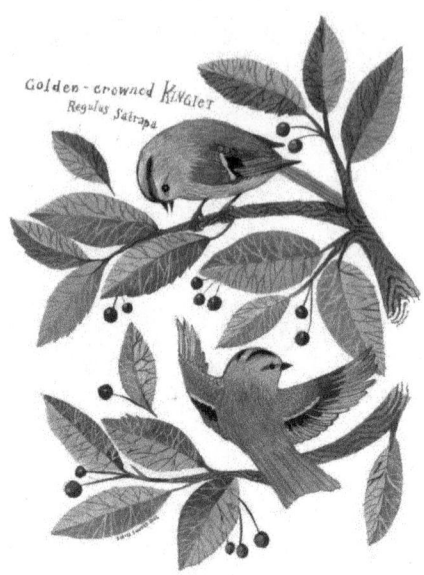

Figure 18.6: Golden-Crowned Kinglet, gouache on paper

AD: You have a daughter and it looks as if you are very close to each other. How did motherhood change your art perspective and the understanding of nature (if it did)? How can we teach children to appreciate nature? What can you highlight as the most important aspects?

DS: Yes, my daughter is nine years old, and we are close. Becoming a parent, especially a mother, turned the intellectual exercise I had with myself over the years of whether or not I should have a child, into an animal experience. When I had my child, all of that intellectualizing went out of the window. In some ways it changed me profoundly, and made me question some of the things I had believed about my life, such as how much agency and choice I really had. Experiencing the bond between myself and my child, and these other very immediate primal needs to take care of her and have her thrive, connected me even more to other life forms on Earth. I do want to say, though, that for all of the change, making artwork is more important to me than ever. It's more challenging in that I have to find that eternal balance between work and family, but I find the rewards to be stronger than before becoming a parent. I am well aware how much of a privilege this all is.

Like so many people, we have been influenced by Richard Louv and his book *The Last Child in the Woods*,[1] which talked about what he calls "nature deficit disorder" and how that is affecting children in particular. My personal experience in parenting and cultivating a connection to nature, is that all children are born with an innate interest in the natural world. It is there, right from the beginning. What happens, I think, is that there are so many opportunities in our culture for children to lose touch with this connection. Many times, I have seen it actively discouraged. People can be very phobic about the outdoors! A lasting connection to nature must be supported by providing regular opportunities for children to be exposed to it in a positive manner, whether at home or at school. It's simply no longer a part of the culture at large, though. We are becoming an "indoor species" in many ways. I have been shocked at how little is taught in schools about biodiversity and local flora and fauna at the elementary levels. It's complicated by other things too, such as race, class, and economics. There have been some really great programs on Chicago's south side in underserved neighborhoods that are working to get black and Latino high school kids out into the preserves to learn about their local biodiversity, as well as helping to remove invasive species. It's so critical for the most underserved young populations to be exposed to experiences that show that nature can be tremendously healing, and can cultivate a sense of ownership and pride over their local ecosystems. For my part, I make sure to get my daughter outside as much as possible. We are lucky to have a yard, as well as some nearby forest preserves. We are hoping, when this virus is no longer a threat over everyday life, to volunteer more in our local preserves with our daughter. We also try to do simple things like raise a few monarch butterflies over the summer, or tadpoles. I try not to push it too much, though, as I am sure she gets tired of me talking about this stuff all of the time!

---

1   Louv, R. (2005) *The Last Child in the Woods*. London: Atlantic Books.

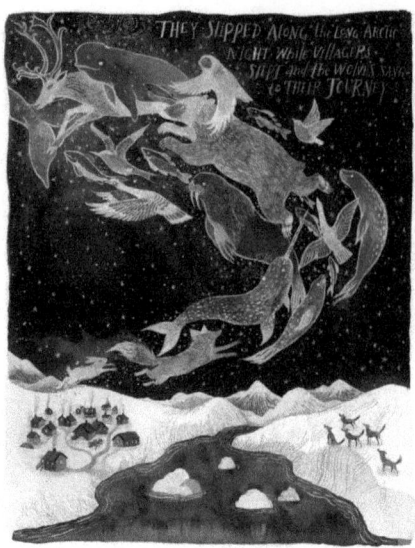

Figure 18.7: The Long Arctic Night, gouache, watercolor on paper

AD: How would you describe the relationship between nature and art/ creativity?

DS: When I was young, people encouraged me when they saw my draw-ings. I was told I was "talented" and had a "gift," and of course I believed this for a while and wanted to do it more. Many artists start this way, by drawing from a young age. As an adult and a parent, I can see that, sure, some of us from a very young age may be more creatively inclined. But what does that mean specifically? Does that mean you are less of a linear thinker? Does that mean you can draw things more accurately than a classmate? I think we are all creative, and that creativity is by no means the exclusive domain of the arts. You can be creative in farming, sports, teaching, medicine, and so on. We need creativity and innovation. Creativity is a survival skill, and is, for me at least, at the root of nature and life. To adapt, one must be creative. My daughter, not surprisingly, is not a very linear thinker...just like her parents. This can be challenging at times, especially when it comes to the way school work is taught here. She is very visual and has a keen eye for observation, though. We sometimes refer to ourselves as having "nature brains," meaning that for better or worse, perhaps we are naturally more sensitive to certain visuals and sounds than our more neuro-normative peers. I am not saying we are special, and certainly many artists are very much this way. These are qualities that can feed the appearance of being an eccentric or outsider. I have given a lot of thought to how these qualities and skills required to make my art, any art of course, may really just be this "misplaced" adaptation that long ago would have helped an ancestor of mine determine what plants and fungi were good to eat (or not!). Paying close attention to subtle differences in color or form could have meant the difference between life and death for that ancestor. Now that I don't have to rely on foraging or hunting for my food, this attention to detail gets applied to other things, such as my art. I still constantly get inspiration, though, from the natural world. These days I seek to find that balance of using these powers of observation for creating work, sharing my feelings of connection to nature through that work, and simply observing the remarkable and beautiful things unfolding in a forest or my backyard.

Note: Diana Sudyka's works can also be seen on her website, www.dianasudyka.com, and on Instagram, www.instagram.com/tinyaviary.

Chapter 19

Interview with Beverley A'Court

THE INTERVIEWER: ALEXANDER KOPYTIN

Brief note about the artist

Beverley A'Court, BSc.Soc.Sci. (Joint hons. Phil. & Psych.), Dip. AT. After a brief research career in architectural psychology, Beverley has been practicing art therapy since 1981, initially employed in acute and long-term psychiatric services, learning disability, special and adult education, then pioneering holistic eco-art therapy via supervision, summer schools, and courses for professionals and students. As a long-term member of the Findhorn Foundation Community, she has contributed to international conferences, festivals, and sustainability education programs, and developed many applications of eco-art therapy. She is an advocate for the recognition of the place of poetic language, the body, ecology, and cultural wisdom traditions in art therapy.

Alexander Kopytin (AK): You have an artistic and art therapy background and were involved in ecological activism for many years. How can you describe the connection between art, therapy, and ecology?

Beverley A'Court (BA): As an artist, art therapist, environmental activist, and member of the Findhorn Foundation Community, I find that the practical and even political question was and still is: How can an ecologically inclusive paradigm be applied in art and clinical art therapy practice? I rely on sensitive attention to the systemic interplay between the human being and the more-than-human environment, attuning to present-moment resonances between the authentic, expressive art-making and the activities of nature and wildlife.

My journey in art and art therapy since the mid-1980s has been to acknowledge, explore and integrate these related streams:

- The body and its role in the creative and art therapeutic process.
- The presence and influence of local and distant ecological and cultural environments.
- The best of psychodynamic, relational wisdom.

The pre-historical, perennial roots of art were very much grounded in the relationship of human beings with the environments which they inhabited. All our perception and cognition arises within our embodied existence. From a bio-cultural, evolutionary view, the arts appear to have been effective instruments for attunement and adaptation to the natural environment, such as developing perceptual and cognitive skills in discernment for survival and for establishing socially bonding rituals. Ancient artworks are often our only or primary window into understanding our ancestors' lives, societies, and beliefs. In addition, ethological perspectives on the arts help us to understand the role of the body as the focus of adaptive activities closely interwoven with "the behavior of art," as Ellen Dissanayake (1988) puts it.

From stone tools, clay figurines, rock reliefs and cave paintings, from bone and horn puppet-toys, to ceremonial body ornament and costumes decorated with shells and stones, animal teeth, horn, fur and feathers, and later, metal jingles, and embroidered patterns of healing plants and dancing "goddesses," what we call "arts and crafts" were a core element of everyday life, where clothing and every implement had to be hand-made, mostly from locally sourced materials, and worked with in a visceral, cooperative process. This suggests a quality of attuned attention, an embodied presence of mind-in-body in relation to materials, "mindfulness," eloquently described by contemporary therapists seeking to integrate into therapy and care non-dual, holistic wisdom from Eastern traditions and discoveries concerning neuroplasticity and global ecological imperatives.

In environmental art and holistic art therapy, introducing natural materials and access to outdoor nature immediately stimulates action, and interactions with nature, in art-making which vividly evokes and echoes the ancient traditional activities of our hunter-gatherer ancestry: selecting, gathering, wrapping, weaving, and binding. The assembly of "fascicles"—bundles of visually or symbolically similar or categorically disparate natural objects, which together have meaning and signify some kind of power—is a frequent initial response to the invitation to make art outside in nature.

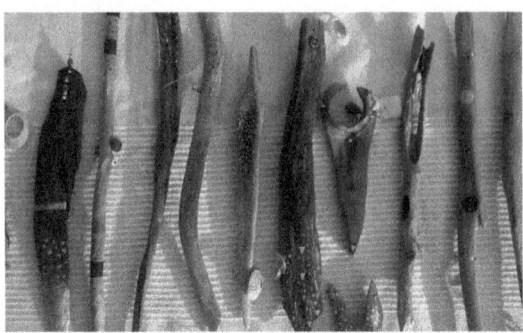

Figure 19.1: Talking Sticks. Beverly A'Court. Painted and decorated natural objects

As an artist and art therapist, through environmental practices I have also come to rely on my own body as a sensitive instrument of resonance to the natural field. I believe that body, mind, and "environment" are always present and interwoven in art-making and art therapy, but the complex dynamics and effects of their interactions have remained largely implicit in our theoretical analyses. The body, its place within the web of life, its structure and movement, though central in making and perceiving art, has not been regarded as such. I believe that the body plays a very important role in environmentally sensitive, earth-based art and therapy.

AK: Could you please explain the role of the body as "an environmental phenomenon" in the art-making process and therapy in more detail?

BA: The following might be regarded as premises of a holistic art and therapy, in particular holistic eco-art therapy, which I practice and have developed over the years:

- Including the body in the art-making process and art therapy leads to including the "environment," because we are spatial beings and all our activity is in relationship to our life-space and those beings who share in it.
- Our body is our closest "wilderness," our own territory of wild nature, most of whose vastly complex processes occur outside our conscious control, without our "thinking" them into happening or directing them.

- Bodies as living systems communicate at gross and subtle levels, locally and at distance, with the field of interdependent living systems. We radiate and transmit ourselves biochemically, electrically, and via empathy, as we also sense and empathize with others' mind-body states, feelings, and motivations, via our mirror neurons and other physiological systems.

"Health" globally increasingly means multifaceted "well-being," a state of body-mind-world in which individual and collective vitality and opportunity are maximized in concordance with other living systems. In therapy, this is typically manifested as awareness, "presence," the ability to remain a fully embodied, connected, compassionate, and attentive witness to self and others, amid disturbance and distress. Images from many cultural traditions of the fulfilled, happy, "enlightened," or holy person often portray them within a complex natural environment, a landscape or garden, where they appear in peaceful harmonious existence with all life forms there, which are also in harmony with one another. The entire field is integrated, harmonized. The blessed person blesses the land. The footsteps of the holy person bless the path.

AK: Could you please give an example of how the body is involved in art-making and holistic art therapy?

BA: The gestural drawing technique I often introduce evolved as a tool to mindfully explore the body's inherent skeletal geometry and the natural gestural marks that emerge from resting in deep attention to this. It has become one among many forms of mindful, somatic preparation for outdoor eco-art therapy work, as it invites authenticity within the micro-environment, the potential space of the large paper. "Drawing" is facilitated to flow from the body as a form of non-doing, without direction and what Feldenkrais calls the "white noise" of effort, contrivance, and striving, while being witnessed as we monitor our felt sense. I also use "breathing drawing'" and the slow tai chi of writing-drawing your name as ways to meet the emergent authentic self with kindness and to recognize its tendency towards harmony, an "emptiness" (of fixed, rigid identity) in a Buddhist sense, and meaning.

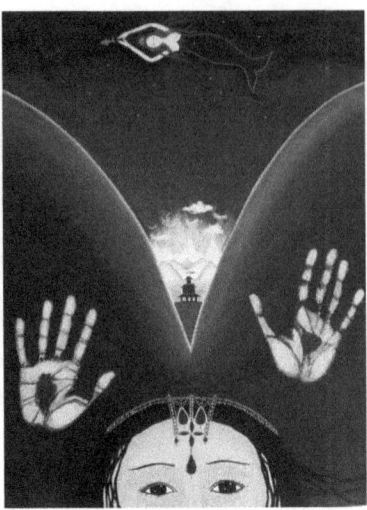

Figure 19.2: Green Tara. Beverly A'Court. Acrylic paint on canvas

Such exercises reveal and relax habitual attitudes of mental grasping at agendas, desires, identity, and outcomes, facilitating a more open, receptive psyche-somatic state in which to experience and listen to both the body-mind and the field of nature. The process of "being drawn" rather than drawing resembles the being "drawn" along, "called" by nature to follow a path toward or into an unfolding landscape. A metaphoric resonance, mirroring how we move through everyday life, is often felt in such moments. The rich discipline of authentic movement has been a long-term inspiration to me in this exploration.

The role of walking in the creative process and in therapy has its own traditions, often overlooked. Walking is associated with the rhythm and movement of mind and can be seen as a metaphor for how we move through the world. The power of walking to bring our body and creative mind into synchrony, to settle and awaken creativity in art, poetry, and music, is testified to by painters, composers, poets, scientists, and inventors. Walking facilitates the loosening of intensely focused attention on the logistics and mechanics of a problem to be fixed, in favor of a roaming awareness that scans the immediate bodily context and synthesizes diverse elements from experience, creating new images, associations, concepts, and insights. Neurologically speaking, in relaxing our default attachment to pre-practiced, familiar verbal concepts, we are providing opportunities to allow new neuronal pathways to develop, entirely new thoughts that let us cognize beyond established boundaries.

As far as therapeutic practice is concerned, in trauma work, for instance, the inclusion of embodiment within therapy can support the journey of recovery, for example in the use of somatic awareness practices to bring clients out of dissociation and post-traumatic flashback, providing short-term "fast aid" and longer term psycho-educational, self-help tools. Mindful body-environment awareness and eco-art exercises can support therapeutic aims by fostering reconnection, returning us to the ground of sensory experience, meeting ourselves and nature in the here and now, as an embodied self-system within a living, physical world-field.

During art therapy, clients spontaneously relate physically to their artworks, or find ways to embody them, extending them into the space and environment via postures and gestures, then into slow movement and occasionally vocalization before, during, and after art-making or by making marks from subtly emergent impulses and expressive gestures. With permission and support, clients can learn to notice the subtle emergence of somatic changes. They may make images of specific body parts, sensations, symptoms, or whole-body experiences and follow urges to somatically express their imagery in facial expression, posture and movement, dance, song, and spontaneous prayer or poetry. Before, during and after art-making, clients can practice, here and now, embodying states unfamiliar or inaccessible to them in their everyday life and seek resonances in the natural world around them.

AK: What particular environments, apart from working in the studio, do you use in your art and holistic art therapy?

BA: We can extend the idea of the relational field around artist, client, and art therapist to include place and its inhabitants as significant contributors to our inner development and life. I use various natural environments, wherever I am working. In Findhorn, I encourage clients to use the studio, surrounding garden, woodland, and beaches, and to notice and include objects and life forms encountered there in their installations and constructions.

Shamanic earth-based traditions, and many contemporary Indigenous societies, have always viewed the health of one person as interdependent with the health of all the systems in which they participate: family, land, animals, ancestors, and god-spirits of place. They respect nature's ability to perceive and involve us and to "talk back." Fairy tales abound with whispering forests, talking animals, and saints and heroes who can converse with more-than-human life forms. Nature and her creatures, including our industrial surroundings, erupt into our awareness via loud sounds or sudden shifts of light/dark and other presences, at moments in therapy instantly recognisable to clients as precisely timed, marking a subtle inner impulse and amplifying its significance, or, during ceremonies, for example as support for healing rituals.

It is a reciprocal relationship: as art therapists we do not simply use nature merely as a passive scenic backdrop, exploitable for inspiration and resources. We attend to the relationship, to what happens between client and nature and to the client-art-nature-therapist field, just as many Indigenous communities use ceremony and ritual to re-establish and harmonize the person-world relationship, often using the arts as the bridging medium.

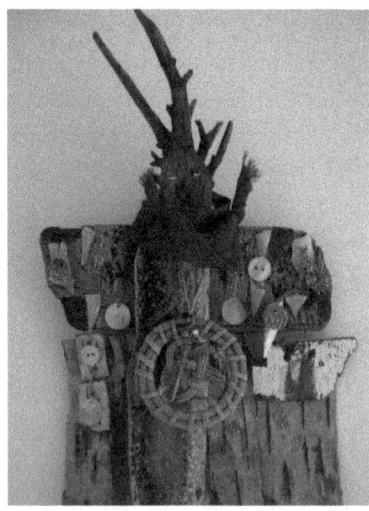

Figure 19.3: Birch Shaman. Beverly A'Court. Natural and non-natural objects.

In open door sessions, I invite the client, if they wish, to loosely include the garden in their awareness and to look and venture outside if, or when, they feel a "call," sometimes initially to go to a place that intuitively feels right for them. Invariably, this place has some supportive or challenging meaning for them, and an encounter occurs which enters and colors their therapeutic process. Therapy itself, at times, becomes a narrative, in which causal and other non-causal, but significant, connections appear. Complex, synchronistic field phenomena occurring during eco-art therapy, especially during the client's art-making, can be observed to have a powerful catalysing and clarifying effect, "speaking" directly to the client's imagination.

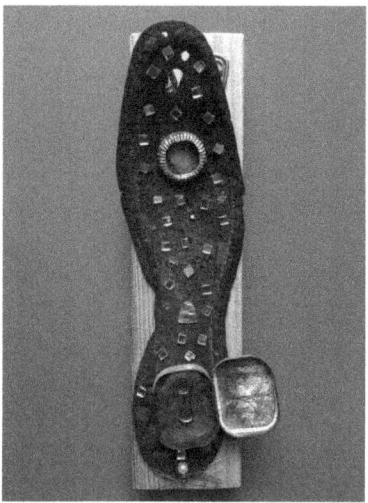

Figure 19.4: Carbon Footprint. Beverly A'Court. Natural and non-natural objects

AK: Is it also possible or relevant for your art and art therapy to use some nature even while working indoors?

BA: Yes, definitely. I advise arts therapists to do this, to include some living nature in the therapy space, even though of course it, we, are all ultimately "nature." Art therapists report that even a single flower or plant becomes a focus for attention and some kind of anchor in the natural world. For example, I keep a basket of driftwood forms, bones, shells, feathers, and stones, on show and available during sessions both for my own art and for clients to choose to handle, to hold onto, especially when speaking of traumatic loss, and to bring some part of their awareness into the present, to awaken and nurture their senses and at the same time to invite subliminal wonder. Where the wood came from, from what tree, brings them ever more present in their bodies and connected to the wider sphere of the natural world. Forest trimmings and driftwood from the seashore embody the natural elements of the area, with their qualities as once-living material sculpted into organic forms by wind, sand, and saltwater. Clients report comfort, warmth, softness, and solidity from these objects, which often appear in the artworks in various ways, symbolically holding physical and emotional experiences and memories. The "talking stick," carved with traditional symbolic forms, and the antler horn-handled Scottish Highland walking stick and hazel or willow wands of Celtic tradition also often feature in clients' art, crafted in distinctive ways expressive of the person's emotional concerns and life needs.

Some objects we find, or which find us (I call these "given" objects and advise clients to choose these rather than take living plants and so on for their creations), seem to be already "art"; others we deconstruct and re-assemble to make art. Archetypal forms emerge from our inter-actions with found media: faces, figures, tiny houses, birds, and ships are common, naturally dynamic shapes found in wind- and water-worn wood and stone. Bird forms often morph into boats and vice versa.

When we make art from found or given materials, there is often a feeling that they belong back in the world, with work to do, and should at some point be returned to nature or placed in another significant location. Often their final destination arrives in the mind as they are being made, and this becomes part of their meaning.

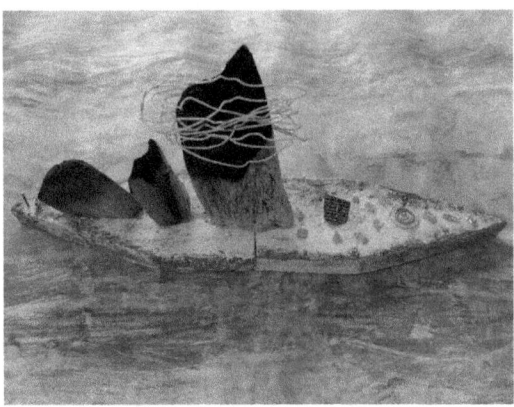

Figure 19.5: Ice Ship. Beverly A'Court. Natural and non-natural objects, gouache on paper

AK: How do you think your approach to art and art therapy is connected to the eco-human paradigm with its emphasis on the unity and co-creation of the human being and nature?

BA: The holistic eco-human paradigm informing art and therapy is an alternative rationality with its own internal logic, requiring appropriate modes of thinking and practice. Buddhist, pre-Buddhist and Taoist meditative, yogic, and western pre-Christian and Christian contemplative traditions have all informed my understanding and therapeutic approaches. We honor the "integrity" of eco-art, valuing it as one of many non-verbal-conceptual forms of knowing, emergent from the communion of subjects, in the process of "making meaning": the intersubjective space, where the impulses of self-directing life forms meet and communicate. Honoring embodied experience and our clients' creativity frequently challenges conventional perceptions and values, but art has historically carried this role and demonstrated great power to energize, liberate, and evolve new perspectives on reality. Environmental art and art therapy offer opportunities to validate, and advocate for, forms of "communion" between sentient subjects—special relationships with the more-than-human world, characterized by recognition of a shared reality and a tenderness and intimacy that many people lack or marginalize in modern life. These experiences have the potential to restore a damaged sense of self, an "eco-identity," and a power to contribute to the multifaceted consciousness and well-being associated with inner and outer sustainability.

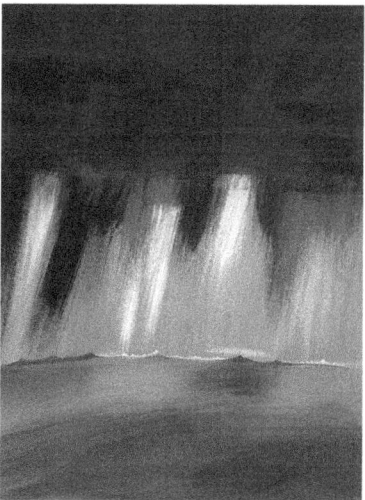

Figure 19.6: Arctic Circle. Beverly A'Court. Acrylic paint on canvas

Holistic eco-art therapy invites and empowers clients to become their own eco-artist healers, to attune deeply to their nature-within-nature for communing with nature's vast field and to listen inwardly and outwardly for its song and find ways to express this. As global medicine increasingly includes eco-bio-psycho-social factors, art and art therapy assume a unique role in revealing the creative, healing self at work within the field of causes and conditions, potentially contributing to the reframing of many areas of care, attending to the root causes of body-mind and planetary conditions.

Note: Beverley's works can also be seen on her website, https://holisticartherapy.wixsite.com/painthorse and her Facebook page, Painthorse holistic eco-art therapy. Some works and workshop images can also be found at https://beverleyacourt.wordpress.com.

References

Dissanayake, E. (1988). *What Is Art For?* Seattle, WA and London: Univerity of Washington Press.

Chapter 20

The Vital Exodus: Éxodo Vital[1]

JUDITH ALALÚ L. AND ODETTE A. VÉLEZ V.

Introduction

Urban life today, particularly in Latin American cities like Lima (Peru), is a little bit like living lost among the dead. De-natured, polluted, and soulless landscapes dominate. Violent scenes, accelerated rhythm, chaos, vertigo, vortex, strident sounds, overcrowding, psychedelia, and fulminating epidemic (like the one we are currently experiencing all over the planet) govern many capitals. In this pandemic scenario (or "desert of modernity," as Hillman (1981, p.41) calls it), we live: human beings, animals, plants, insects, and thousands of unclassifiable beings and objects. There, exposed to infinite difficulties, we try to adapt and find sense in life. Sometimes we make it, but sometimes we don't. So, we get tired, we get sick, we feel stunned and trapped, survivors of terrified cities. We regret, we question what we are doing here, we want another life, we claim another place, we beg for a change, and, finally, we scream at the top of our lungs: "Enough!" It is time to move, to leave, to find a way out. Fed up, we set off for somewhere else; we flee into the cosmic void. It is time to appeal to our resources, ancestral memory, creative capacity, ecopoiesis, hope, and the possibility of resisting. Something begins to crumble, deform, and die as it meets new life. We return to water, to the sea, to connection with the body, nature, and origin. Silence begins to arise. We are alive. We are still swimming.

This is an outline of the pictorial and poetic story that this article discusses. Images that scream as the only possibility to respond aesthetically. They shout to rebel because "Beauty must be raged, or outraged

---

1   First published as Alalú, J. y Velez, O. (2018). *Éxodo Vital*. Lima: Editorial Tae Perú.

into life" (Hillman, 1981, p.42). Beings affected by the contaminated life in the city. Beings who are confused and forced to leave their natural habitats, turned into unlivable places. Beings who initiate an exodus, a migration, looking for other spaces where vitality can resurface. The search for a new planetary, sensory consciousness arrives that nourishes the soul of the world, which has become so technologically hyperconnected and so disconnected from life. Each one of my pores has become an ear and I am deaf; skinless skeleton is my being. These animals are all living beings on the planet that already collapsed long ago due to the irresponsibility of human actions.

This two-handed work (painting and poetry) is an expression of resistance. We make art as a way of being and being-in-the-world, because, as the expressive arts perspective reminds us, the arts allow people to connect with their creative capacity, to reactivate their capacity for poiesis ("making art," "creating" in Greek), and to respond creatively to difficulties and challenges (Levine, 1995). The arts, in the ancient shamanic tradition, are a way of recovering the soul: "When illness is associated with loss of the soul, the arts spontaneously emerge as remedies, medicine of the soul" (McNiff, 1992, p.1); they are a way of soul-making, that is, a way of recovering passion, vitality, and a sense of existence (Hillman, 1975, 1981). *The Vital Exodus* is a book in which, over and over again, the images achieve dialogue through the force of their lively strokes, full of color and play, and also through the voices of their characters, full of pain and despair. The possibility of deforming impotence inhabits the lines, gestures, and poetic words of the paintings. The ability to transform experience, to exaggerate its shapes and take them into fantastic realms, is present in the works, strengthening the potential that we human beings have to shape the situations we face. A tree has been falling...the fish fly, the birds swim.

Fortunately, from an ecopoietic perspective, not even the desert lacks heart because it is inhabited by the lion, and if we want to return to the sensitive heart, we must look for it there, provoke it and make it cry out: "The more our desert the more we must rage, which rage is love" (Hillman, 1981, p.42). Thus, these images roar, howl, bark, shriek, squawk—they call us and ask us to appreciate their presence and will, to recognize their inherent value, to see and hear the world from their own point of view. Listening to them requires abandoning our egocentric vision and developing an ecocentric vision, interested "in the wild, undomesticated side of beauty" (Stoknes, 2017, p.259). Expressive arts invite us to live a more primordial and animistic perception. And it must be remembered that:

Animism is not superstition or worship of nature. It is reverence for the created realm, for all life, it is a feeling of belonging, and of being an integral part of this vast and varied landscape. It is the full recognition that all things have spirit or soul, that all things are alive and aware. (Rugh, 2020, p.56)

Facing the anaesthetic mechanisms of the current times demands roaring to activate our senses and boost our sensory capacity, that is, to put into effect the political implications of our ability to respond aesthetically. That is the desire of this work: to inspire a way of being and being-in-the-world that is in connection with mystery, listening to the voice of the non-human, recognizing the soul of the world, far from our usual instrumental and technological attitude, allowing:

...the body [to] explore again the speech of things and of the land. This brings with it the attitude of wildness: an attentive wonder that draws us into the mystery, the unpredictability, the many voices of the more-than-human world around us that have been silenced for too long. (Stoknes, 2017, p.260)

It is about recovering the enchanted vision of the world, the one we lost with the western predominance of the modern scientific vision and its mathematical understanding of nature, governed by various separations (subject/object, mind/body, self/world, nature/culture). It is time to rescue the sacred vision of the world of the original peoples, the *anima mundi*, where nothing is a different object and apart from us, where everything belongs to an interconnected network. The challenge of re-enchanting the world in the 21st century lies in restoring the lost bond with the cosmos, and recovering the mythical and poetic dimension of existence. It is not a question of condemning modern scientific thought and idealizing the pre-industrial way of life and the animistic worldview of ancestral peoples. We have to rethink our relationship with nature and regenerate a more attentive and sensitive connection with it, in which modern technology and instrumental reason can occupy a generous place, far from hyper-individualism. It is the challenge of recreating a perspective of interdependence, reciprocity, and cooperation, where we treat others and nature in a different way from how we do so today.

It is surprising how the arts are in the vanguard and anticipate the facts. Artistic language is always in communion with the life of the world through the sensuality of its visual, sonorous, kinesthetic, and olfactory images: "Art is not just a universal language for humans—it is the cosmological language of form, the sensory realm from which we construct our very thoughts" (Rugh, 2020, p.58).

The creative project *Vital Exodus* arose several years before the planetary pandemic we are experiencing, and today more than ever its spread makes sense and is aligned with ecopoiesis. Its images not only scream but also speak of the need to hibernate, which is precisely what we have been doing now out of necessity and obligation. Perhaps hibernation is a way to initiate the vital exodus of ecopoiesis. Stop, take perspective, contemplate, and pause to learn to breathe differently. We hibernate and the world seems to rest from us. Hopefully, hibernation will allow us to sharpen our senses and dance again to the rhythm of the universe to which we belong.

In the Andean world each flower, each star, each stone, spider, bee, each drop of dew, each human being... is a Universe—a Pacha—, a perfect totality, which in turn is complemented by another Pacha even bigger and more perfect, and this process never ends. In the way that the rhythm and flow of fluids in a cell embrace the same rhythm and flow of the liquids of the galaxy... generating infinite movements of love and harmony thus...if I touch a flower, I am touching a star. (Vera, 2014)

References

Hillman, J. (1975). *Re-Visioning Psychology*. New York, NY: Harper & Row.

Hillman, J. (1981). *The Thought of the Heart*. Dallas, TX: Spring Publications.

Levine, S. K. (1995). *Poiesis: The Language of Psychology and the Speech of the Soul*. London: Jessica Kingsley Publishers.

McNiff, S. (1992). *Art as Medicine: Creating a Therapy of the Imagination*. Boston, MA: Shambhala.

Rugh, M. M. (2020). Sitting on the edge of wonder: Art and animism in the service of person and planet healing. *Ecopoiesis: Eco-Human Theory and Practice*, 1(1), 56–61

Stoknes, P. (2017). Why Eco-Philosophy and Expressive Arts? In S.K. Levine & E.G. Levine (eds), *New Developments in Expressive Arts Therapy: The Play of Poiesis* (pp.258–260). London: Jessica Kingsley Publishers.

Vera, A. (2014). *Kintu: Offering of Sacred Flowers a la Divinidad, Symbol of Unity*. http://ludoterapiaautocreadoragestalt.blogspot.com/2011/06/kintu-ofrenda-de-flores-sagradas-la.html.

here I am
lost
among the dead

aquí
estoy
perdida
entre los muertos

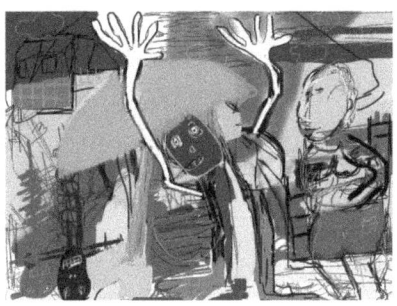

they push me
excuse me, look out, coming
through

me empujan
disculpe, permiso, necesito pasar

I am still
my bones
my hands
in this city psychedelic and
amorphous

todavía soy
mis huesos
mis manos
en esta ciudad psicodélica y amorfa

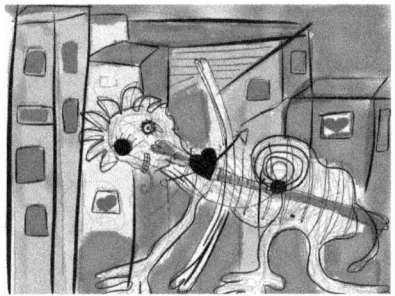

thefishflythebirdsswim
in a fulminating epidemic

vuelanlospecesnadanlasaves
en una epidemia fulminante

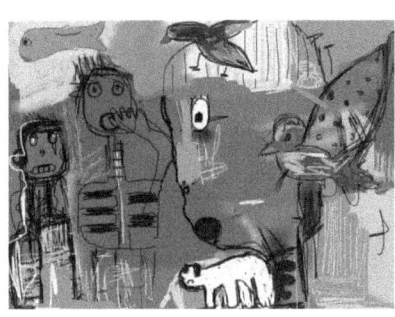

I walk among tangled wires
I dance upon cement

here I play
I draw
I live
between vertigo and vortex

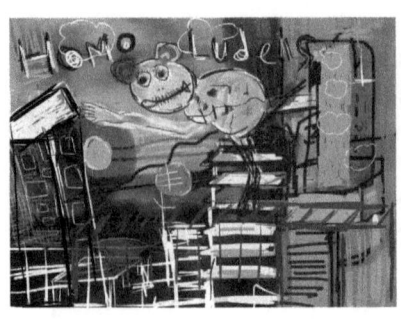

camino entre alambres enredados
bailo sobre cemento

aquí juego
dibujo
vivo
entre vértigo y vorágine

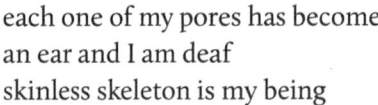

each one of my pores has become
an ear and I am deaf
skinless skeleton is my being

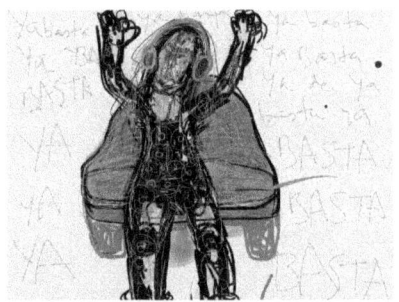

cada uno de mis poros se ha vuelto
oído y estoy sorda
esqueleto sin piel está mi ser

it would be better to go back
try it under the sea

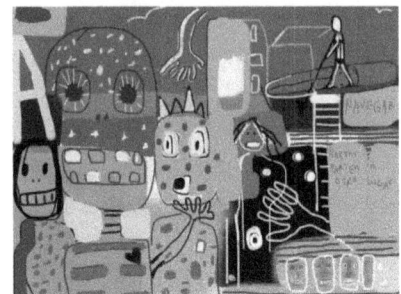

mejor sería volver
intentarlo bajo el mar

myhandsscreamenoughalready
maybe I will have to leave them
behind in this apocalypse

below the fish keep swimming

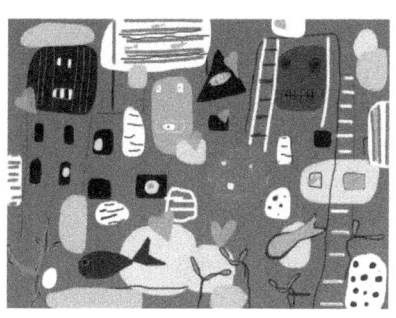

navigating on the asphalt is more
difficult
the buildings are not easy to open

maybe, it would be better to try it
below

mismanosgritanyabasta
tal vez tendré que dejarlas en este apocalipsis

debajo los peces siguen nadando

navegar en el asfalto es más difícil
los edificios no son fáciles de abrir

acaso sería mejor probar debajo

in this urban settlement
we have grown spikes
new heads

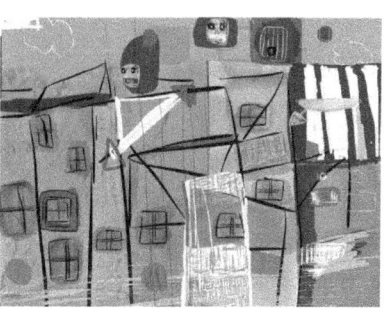

my hairs prick me
hands stretch up from the subsoil
in a terrifying intention to
continue

stunned trapped survivors of this
terrified city

en este asentamiento citadino
nos han crecido púas
nuevas cabezas

mis pelos hincan
se estiran manos del subsuelo

en una voluntad aterradora por seguir

aturdidos atra pados sobrevivientes en esta ciudad despavorida

will we return?

fed up they set off for somewhere
else
I will flee into the cosmic void

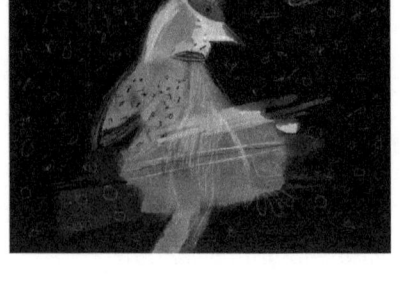

a fugitive I am destined to escape
in a thousand pieces

¿volveremos?

hartos parten a otros lares
yo huiré al vacío cósmico

prófuga he de escapar en mil pedazos

sharksducksstars
where has the sea gone to now so
I can't find it?

others search for their hills

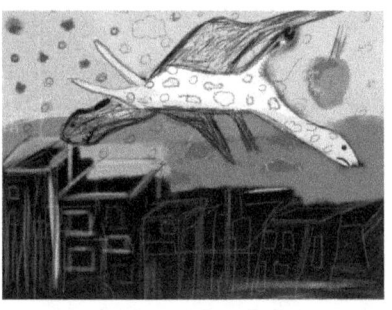

It rains sky blue days that are
nights

the whitewash reproduces swiftly
theresnoroom cellular
chaos-mutation

a tree has been falling

tiburonespatosestrellas
¿dónde está el mar que no lo encuentro?

otros buscan sus cerros

llueve celeste días que son noches

la cal se reproduce raudamente
nohayespacio caos-mutación celular

viene cayendo un árbol

will we remember how to swim
in this poisoned noise?

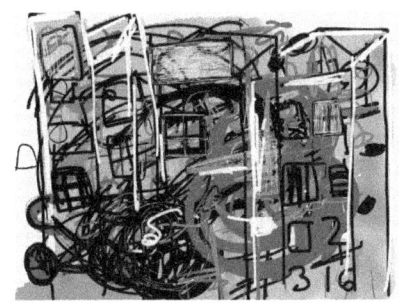

¿recordaremos cómo nadar en este
ruido intoxicado?

may be, it's time to hibernate

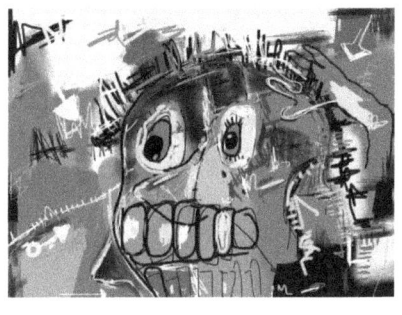

I blur
blend
dilute
drip myself
in a thousand colors

quizá sea momento de hibernar

me desdibujo
difumino
diluyo
chorreo
en mil colores

I still am

todavía soy

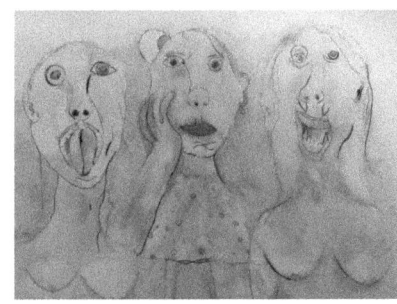

crammed full I frolic
I look inside
There is my house
I can stay
and feed my hatchlings
fight, woman, fight

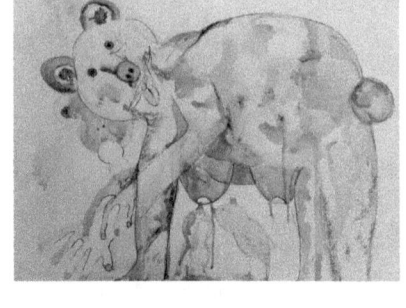

atiborrada retozo
miro dentro
allí está mi casa
puedo quedarme
y dar de comer a mis polluelos
pelea, mujer, pelea

swim or die in stridency

the silence begins to arise
we're alive
we're still swimming

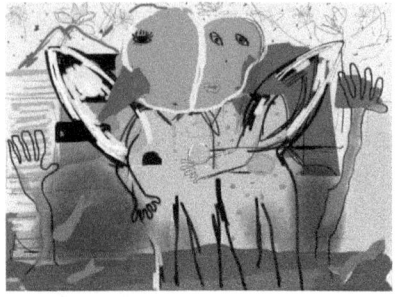

nadar o morir en la estridencia

el silencio empieza a surgir
estamos vivos
seguimos nadando

Subject Index

Author Index